Reflections on Adaptive Behavior

Reflections on Adaptive Behavior

Essays in Honor of J. E. R. Staddon

edited by Nancy K. Innis

The MIT Press
Cambridge, Massachusetts
London, England

For information on quantity discounts, please email special_sales@mitpress.mit.edu.

Set in Stone Serif and Stone Sans on 3B2 by Asco Typesetters, Hong Kong. Printed and bound in the United States of America.

Library of Congress Cataloging-in-Publication Data

Reflections on adaptive behavior : essays in honor of J. E. R. Staddon / edited by Nancy K. Innis.
p. cm.
Includes bibliographical references (p.) and index.
ISBN 978-0-262-09044-5 (hardcover : alk. paper)—ISBN 978-0-262-59026-6 (pbk. : alk. paper)
1. Adaptability (Psychology) 2. Adjustment (Psychology) 3. Behaviorism (Psychology) I. Staddon J. E. R. II. Innis, Nancy K.
BF335.R35 2008
155.19'434—dc22 2007039855

10 9 8 7 6 5 4 3 2 1

Contents

Preface

On May 17, 2003, former graduate students, post-doctoral fellows, and research associates met at Duke University to celebrate the career of Professor John E. R. Staddon. At a day-long symposium, fifteen papers were presented, many of which provided the basis for the chapters in this volume. Papers by José Lino Oliveira Bueno, Jeremie Jozefowiez, Elliot Ludvig, and Ken Steele were also presented.

This volume is a permanent tribute to John Staddon. Eight of the chapters are by former graduate students in Staddon's lab who received their degrees in the 1970s (Innis, Malone, Kello), the 1980s (Reid, Horner), or the 1990s (Machado, Dragoi, Cleaveland). The appendix to chapter 1 lists all Staddon's Ph.D. and MA/MS students and their dissertation or thesis topics. Other chapters are by former post-doctoral fellows (Dale, Wynne, Higa) and research associates (Manabe, Chelaru, Cerutti).

The book opens with a brief biography and an outline of Staddon's research program, which spans nearly 40 years, from the mid 1960s to the present day. The chapters in parts I and II present accounts of research and theory, most of which involve topics, such as choice and timing, which are directly related to Staddon's research program. Part III comprises chapters of a more general nature on behaviorism. In part IV, Staddon's Italian colleague Giulio Bolacchi, whose work until now has only been published in Italian, outlines his theory of interests, a proposal for integrating the social sciences. Bolacchi is Chairman and Program Director of the International Graduate Program in Science of Organization of the Association for the Institution of a Free University in Nuoro. Staddon has participated in this program each year since 1991.

Acknowledgments

I have many people to thank. The Department of Brain and Psychological Sciences at Duke University and the Psychology Department at the University of Western Ontario provided much-appreciated support for this project. Special thanks go to Ute Wittmann Pair at Duke and Daniella Chirila at UWO. All the authors in this volume responded quickly and cheerfully to my requests for help (e.g., reviewing manuscripts and revising papers) as we put the book together. Jennifer Higa, Armando Machado, and Bob Dale, who helped me in innumerable ways, deserve special mention. Most important of all was the contribution of Lucinda Paris—this Festschrift would never have appeared without her support and encouragement.

Nancy K. Innis

Reflections on Adaptive Behavior

1 Theoretical Behaviorist: John E. R. Staddon

Nancy K. Innis

John Staddon—theoretical behaviorist. In the tradition of behavior analysis this appellation might be considered an oxymoron. However, "[e]xperimental analysis *by itself* can never make sense of behavior. Theoretical imagination is also required." (Staddon 1999, pp. 218–219) "*Conjecture,* not just about variables but also about *processes,* is essential." (Staddon 2001a, p. xi) John Staddon's theoretical imagination has set him apart from contemporary animal learning researchers. Who else would characterize his model as a leaky bucket?

Staddon's long career has been devoted to the study of the adaptive function and mechanisms of learning. His epistemological approach, theoretical behaviorism, consists in applying parsimonious black-box models to unravel the principles of learning. In doing this, he has typically taken positions that deviate from the norm. At a time when psychologists were maintaining their distance from behavioral biology, Staddon was promoting optimality theories and urging cooperation between ecologists and psychologists. (See Staddon 1980a.) Now optimality theories in psychology are commonplace. At a time when identifying mechanisms is considered the only legitimate approach to explaining behavior, Staddon is not afraid to invent functional models. At a time when physiological instantiation is the holy grail, Staddon postulates internal states that are purely theoretical.

In his most recent book, *Adaptive Dynamics: The Theoretical Analysis of Behavior* (2001a), Staddon presents theoretical behaviorism in its most recent incarnation and describes research problems to which his models have been applied, including habituation, feeding regulation, choice, spatial search, and timing. Several of the chapters in this present volume, by his former students and colleagues, deal with these topics, revealing his influence on their work. I begin with a brief biography, outlining the development of Staddon's career as both a scientist and a teacher.

Family Background and Education

John Eric Rayner Staddon was born March 19, 1937 at Lavender Cottage in Grayshott, Hampshire, England, the first child of Leonard John (Jack) Staddon and Dulce Norine Rayner Staddon. A sister, Judy, was born four years later. Jack Staddon was a Cockney, born in West Ham, who left home early and joined the army. He was stationed in India and in Rangoon, where he met Dulce Rayner. Dulce was born and grew up in a small village in Burma, although her mother's family was originally from Calcutta. After their marriage, the Staddons settled in England, and were living near Jack's base in Hampshire at the time John was born. Toward the end of 1937 they moved to London, eventually to a house in Cricklewood, an area of northwest London. During most of John's early childhood England was at war, and on more than one occasion, when the bombing became intense, he was sent to live in the country. His father was away much of the time, and from 1942 to 1944 was stationed in India with the Intelligence Corps in Karachi. His mother contributed to the war effort as personal secretary to Sir John Pratt in the Far East Section of the Ministry of Information. John's grandmother, Irene Rayner, to whom he was closely attached, lived with the family and cared for the children.

Growing up in the house in Cricklewood, John was a happy, quiet child who liked to collect "creepy crawlies" and examine them under his microscope—a pastime similar to one that Charles Darwin, one of John's academic heroes, engaged in during his youth. John was also very keen on tropical fish and at one time had six tanks. These interests continued into adulthood; John often has a fish tank at home, and he has a small collection of beautiful old microscopes. As a teenager, he liked to read science fiction, play tennis, and listen to music. Later, when he was at university, he enjoyed riding around the countryside on his Vespa motor scooter.

Early Education

Education was especially important to Dulce Staddon, and the family never scrimped on books. Both she and John's grandmother always read to the children when they were young, and John was reading on his own by the time he was four. After the war, John attended Burgess Hill School in Hampstead where his best friend was Martin Bernal, now famous for his revisionist history *Black Athena*. This was a progressive school suggested by John's uncle, Eric Rayner. At the time Rayner was night editor of the *Daily Telegraph* newspaper, and he later worked for the BBC overseas service. Over the years, to some extent, John followed in his uncle's journalistic footsteps. As an undergraduate he wrote film reviews for the university newspaper, and later he edited Duke University's faculty newsletter for a few years (1991–1994). His interest in writing for a general audience is also evident in two books, *Behaviorism: Mind, Mechanism and Society* (1993a) and *The New Behaviorism: Mind, Mechanism and Society* (2001b).

In 1947, John was 10 years old and would soon face the 11 Plus examinations, which at the time determined the type of secondary school education (grammar, technical, or secondary modern) for which a child in Britain was eligible. Realizing that the Burgess Hill School was not good academically, his mother looked for an alternative. In September 1947, John was enrolled at St. Marylebone Grammar School, a well-established grammar school for boys located near Baker Street, a 3-mile bus ride from his home. When he started at St. Marylebone, John was at something of a disadvantage because he had declined to be exposed to any mathematics at the progressive school. However, within a few months, with the help of a tutor, he had mastered the subject. John completed his elementary and high school education at the St. Marylebone Grammar School.

Undergraduate Years

John enrolled at the University of London in 1955. For his A levels, which qualified him for university, he had specialized in pure and applied mathematics, physics, and chemistry. He started out in engineering. Before long, however, he realized that he could switch to psychology, which was closer to biology, the subject to which he "had been devoted since youth" but had been unable to study at St. Marylebone because the school lacked the necessary facilities (Staddon 1991, p. 1). After two years at university and feeling somewhat jaded, perhaps because he was not making the most of his academic opportunities, John interrupted his studies and joined his parents, who were living in Northern Rhodesia (now Zambia). In Rhodesia he worked for the World Health Organization on a nutrition program. On a trip into the wilderness to collect blood samples, he became very ill, likely with malaria, and would have died had it not been for an observant nurse who recognized his symptoms and obtained the appropriate medication. Returning to England, John completed his undergraduate program and graduated with a B.Sc. in Psychology from University College, London in 1960.

John's record at London was not outstanding, yet graduate school was an obvious choice for someone with an inquiring mind. Through their advertisements on bulletin boards at the University of London, he was attracted to universities in North America. Accepted by all three departments to which he had applied, he chose Hollins College, a small school in Roanoke, Virginia, where he spent a year in the graduate program. His intellectual ability soon became obvious to his professors at Hollins. They encouraged him to apply to Harvard University, and he left Hollins College without completing the master's program.

Graduate School—Harvard University

John Staddon arrived at Harvard in September 1961 and joined a group of dedicated researchers in B. F. Skinner's Pigeon Lab located in the basement of Memorial Hall. His faculty supervisor, Richard Herrnstein, had earned his doctorate under Skinner only 6 years earlier. Most of Herrnstein's students were doing research on choice—this was the year that he introduced the Matching Law, and so John, never the conformer, decided to work on something else. Because of the ubiquity of temporal processes in both classical and operant conditioning, he chose to study temporal discrimination, believing that "understanding the mechanism of timing might provide a key to understanding conditioning in general" (Staddon 1991, p. 1).

Most of the timing experiments John carried out at Harvard involved differential reinforcement of low rate (DRL) schedules of reinforcement. On these schedules, an animal must wait a specified time (DRL value) before making a response in order to receive a reinforcer. In the experiments. His doctoral dissertation, "The effect of 'knowledge of results' on timing behavior in the pigeon," involved experiments in which the DRL value changed cyclically every 5 minutes. A limited hold was added so that the birds were required to respond at times demarcated by both an upper and a lower time limit. The major variable examined was the effect of feedback stimuli, indicating to the bird that it had waited too long before pecking (a brief flash of red light on the key) or not long enough (a flash of green light). The birds showed an ability to track the changing time requirements; however, although knowledge of results improved performance, especially for birds that were not timing well, probe tests showed that it was not the information of too long or too short, but rather the relative frequency of the feedback stimuli, that seemed to control behavior (Staddon 1963). In a reflective comment on his study, Staddon observed:

> The interesting things about this dissertation are of course that (a) the hypothesis to be tested—"knowledge of results"—was cognitive, not at all something that could be inferred from standard conditioning principles; and (b) the results showed it to be wrong. But cognitive ideas about animal behavior, like deleterious recurrent mutations, just keep coming back, only to be refuted almost every time. (J. E. R. Staddon, personal communication, June 2, 2003)

In those days experiments were controlled by electro-mechanical equipment, and wiring the complex DRL program for these studies was "a technical *tour de force*" (Staddon 1991, p. 1). John completed the work for his doctorate by the end of 1963, and received his Ph.D. in experimental psychology from Harvard in 1964. His dissertation research was published in the *Journal of the Experimental Analysis of Behavior* (*JEAB*) in an article dedicated to B. F. Skinner in his 65th year (Staddon 1969a).

The ambition of most young scientists in the 1960s (perhaps even today) was to have a paper published in the prestigious journal *Science*. John Staddon's first academic publication appeared in *Science* in 1964. Following up on the problem of temporal tracking addressed in his doctoral research, he devised a simpler procedure in which pigeons were exposed to a cyclically changing fixed-interval (FI) schedule. Interval durations changed according to a sinusoidal pattern which offered the possibility of applying a linear systems analysis. On this simpler cyclic schedule, pigeons' response rates tracked the changes in inter-reinforcement time, but were out of phase with the schedule cycle; rate was highest when there were fewest reinforcements (Staddon 1964). In most of his subsequent research on timing, Staddon would use variants of a cyclic FI procedure. (See below.)

Living in Cambridge, Massachusetts, John was able to take advantage of opportunities to explore areas of psychology beyond the Pigeon Lab. He was exposed to the field of visual perception when a research assistantship with Jacob Beck provided financial support during his first term at Harvard.

He also carried out neurological research on crayfish in Larry Stark's Electronic Systems Laboratory. An entirely different perspective was obtained when, along with fellow graduate students Jacques Mehler and Charlie Harris, John participated in some of the activities at the Center for Cognitive Studies, recently established by George Miller and Jerry Bruner. In retrospect, however, the most significant experience was a course on artificial intelligence that he attended at the Massachusetts Institute of Technology. The course, developed by Marvin Minsky, was taught that year by John McCarthy. Minsky's notes for the course were later published in the book *Computation: Finite and Infinite Machines* (Minsky 1967). If this course did not directly influence the way Staddon began to formulate his approach to understanding behavior, it certainly was compatible with it. In a brief mimeographed paper dated 1963, the outline for a presentation at Skinner's graduate seminar, John proposed "a simple-minded formalism for talking about behavior." The proposal began as follows:

> An organism both acts upon the environment and is acted upon by it. What is the simplest formalism that will take account of this fact? The following is offered as a possible (by no means original) candidate, in the hope that it constitutes a language in which may be expressed all and only meaningful (testable) statements about behavior. Since it is probably not adequate, its real purpose must be to encompass its own destruction by yielding something more satisfactory.... An organism is considered as a black-box or machine and by convention is described in terms of three constructs: *input* (I), *output* (O), and *internal state* (S).... (Staddon 1963, pp. 1–2)

In this outline we find several of the core elements of the theoretical framework that Staddon has embraced throughout his career. First, look for simple (parsimonious) explanations; second, develop "black-box" models of behavior that include consideration of the internal state of the system; third, recognize that all theories are temporary, eventually to be replaced. John recalls that "Skinner was unimpressed and uninterested" (personal communication, June 2, 2003).

Academic Career

University Appointments

In 1964, John Staddon accepted an appointment in the Psychology Department at the University of Toronto, and he and his first wife, Nada Ballator, whom he had met at Hollins College, moved to Toronto. It was here that their son, Nicholas, was born the following year. A second child, Jessica, was born in Durham, North Carolina in 1969. At Toronto, Staddon for the first time was faced with teaching undergraduate students. In a course on experimental psychology (Psychology 91) he spent considerable time discussing the black-box systems approach that he believed to be the best way to attain an understanding of behavior. The undergraduates were baffled. By early 1965, Staddon had several experiments up and running in the sub-basement of Sidney Smith Hall where the psychology animal laboratories were located. These included studies of timing (involving both DRL and FI schedules), choice, and, before long, the "frustration effect." The following year, he began reexamining Skinner's "superstition" experiment. Staddon's research program, initiated at Toronto and continued at Duke University, will be examined in detail in later sections of this chapter.

Perhaps more than anything else, the interminable winters in Ontario encouraged the Staddons to move back to the South. In 1967, John joined the faculty of the Psychology Department at Duke University in Durham, North Carolina, where he moved quickly through the ranks, becoming a full professor in 1972. In 1983 he was named James B. Duke Professor of Psychology. In addition, he was appointed professor of zoology in 1979 and professor of neurobiology in 1988. From 1985 to 1987, he was chairman of Duke's psychology department. Over the years, he has served on many university-wide committees. In 2002 he was appointed secretary of the Faculty Council.

Editorial Work

Staddon has contributed to psychology as an editor of several journals. In 1979, he joined Chris Bradshaw as US editor of *Behaviour Analysis Letters* (*BAL*), a journal that typically published short accounts of recent research. In 1983, *BAL* amalgamated with *Behavioural Processes* (*BP*). John continued as co-editor of *BP* until 2001, when Clive Wynne took over from him. Wynne (chapter 11), a research collaborator who was at one time a postdoctoral fellow in Staddon's lab, thus provides a continuity of perspective for the journal. In 1991, Staddon joined the editorial board of *Behavior and Philosophy*, taking over as editor of that journal in 1996. Over the years he was frequently on the editorial board of *JEAB*, and he served as associate editor from 1979 to 1982. He has served on the editorial boards of several other journals, including *Behaviorism* and the *Journal of Experimental Psychology: Animal Behavior Processes.*

Leaves and Awards

Throughout his career various awards have permitted Staddon to spend time in psychology departments in several countries; he has visited or held positions in departments in Australia, Brazil, England, Germany, Italy, and Mexico. John chose to spend his first sabbatical leave (1973–74) working with David McFarland, a member of the Animal Behavior Research Group at Oxford University. John had been interested in McFarland's work for some time, believing that "sophisticated feedback analysis [was] possibly a better way to handle the complexities of behavior on reinforcement schedules than the rather crude descriptive principles then current" (Staddon 1991, p. 4). At Oxford he also got to know many of the people who, during the next decade, would become leading figures in behavioral biology as optimality approaches to foraging behavior became popular. One of these individuals was Alasdair Houston, who was an Oxford undergraduate at the time. Houston would later spend a year at Duke in Staddon's lab.

On the invitation of Arturo Bouzas, Staddon spent several weeks at the Laboratorio de Analisis Experimental de la Conducta (Laboratory of the Experimental Analysis of Behavior) in Coyoacan, Mexico in 1981, the year in which he held a Guggenheim Fellowship. In 1985, he received the Alexander von Humboldt Prize, an award that allowed him to spend 1987–88 in Juan Delius's laboratory in Bochum, Germany. This proved to be a very happy year as John recovered from trying times, both personally and as department chair, in the company of Lucinda Paris, his second wife. Follow-up visits to Delius's laboratory, which had moved to the University of Konstanz, were also supported by the Humboldt Foundation.

John's association with the Brazilian psychologist Jose Lino Oliveira Bueno began in 1986, when Bueno invited him to visit the University of São Paulo in Riberão Preto. Other visits to Brazil followed, including one as a Fulbright Distinguished Scholar in 1989. In 1988 Bueno spent a sabbatical year at Duke in Staddon's laboratory. In 1991, Staddon was invited by Giulio Bolacchi (chapter 15) to take part in the Associazione per l'Istituzione della Libera Università Nuorese (Association for the Institution of a

Free University in Nuoro), and every year since then he has spent a week in Sardinia participating in this program. From 1995 to 2000, Staddon held the position of adjunct professor at the University of Western Australia in Perth. He visited that department on two occasions to collaborate with Clive Wynne, who was on the faculty there. They co-edited a book, *Models of Action: Mechanisms for Adaptive Behavior,* which was published in 1998.

Staddon is a fellow of the New York Academy of Sciences, of the American Psychological Society, and of the American Association for the Advancement of Science. He is a member of the Society of Experimental Psychologists and a Trustee of the Cambridge Center for Behavioral Studies.

Theory and Research

Philosophy of Science

Although he received his graduate training at Harvard, the bastion of Skinnerian behaviorism, Staddon did not adopt the atheoretical position to which most behaviorists subscribe. Early on, he pointed out the danger in claiming to reject theory, suggesting that "those who ignore their metaphysical preconceptions are liable to be misled by them" (1969b, p. 484). In a review of Floyd Ratliff's book *Mach Bands,* he praised the virtues of "speculative thought" and "Mach's view of the proper role of theory" (Staddon 1969b, p. 485), which involved "a formula which represents the facts more concisely and plainly than one can with words, without, however, claiming quantitative exactness" (Ratliff 1965, cited in Staddon 1969b, p. 485). Staddon's models are quantitative and they are formal (theoretical). He takes the position that a model need not be isomorphic with physiological processes as long as it can lead to explanation and understanding. The best theories are, of course, parsimonious and capable of accounting for many phenomena. We can see this approach to theory exemplified in many of the models that Staddon has introduced throughout his career, including those presented in *Adaptive Dynamics.* And these will not be the last models from Staddon's pen. It is his belief that theories are ephemeral; they must be constantly under revision. His hope is that "as each model is proposed and, eventually, retired, we may learn a little more about the essential mechanisms of learning—so the next model may be a little bit better, a little bit more securely founded" (Staddon 2001a, p. xi).

Research Program

Temporal Control of Behavior At Toronto, Staddon continued his research on the DRL performance of pigeons, using veteran birds he had brought with him from Harvard. After several publications appeared with the same subject numbers, colleagues began to chide John, asking him why he couldn't afford to get new birds. Indeed, most of his experiments did not require naive subjects, and both rats and pigeons from the Toronto laboratory, including some of the old Harvard birds, went along when Staddon moved to Duke. A survey of his *JEAB* publications of the late 1960s and the early 1970s will reveal the identities of the stalwart pigeons who served in these studies.

Most of Staddon's research on temporal discrimination at Toronto and during his first few years at Duke involved cyclic FI, rather than DRL, schedules. On simple FI schedules, animals typically pause a constant proportion of an inter-food interval before starting to peck the response key. Post-reinforcement pause, a more direct indicator of temporal control, soon replaced response rate as the main datum of interest in the cyclic studies. Changes in pause track changes in the input cycle directly, rather than out of phase as is the case with the response-rate measure. In the first doctoral dissertation supervised by Staddon, Nancy Innis showed that pigeons could successfully track intervals of seven different durations which increased and then decreased across a cycle according to an arithmetic progression (Innis and Staddon 1971). The results of these experiments, and other studies involving schedules with fewer intervals per cycle, identified the conditions under which temporal tracking did or did not occur. However, no progress was made at identifying the mechanism of temporal control. At the time, when computers were not a standard tool in psychology laboratories, data analysis was laborious, simulations were difficult, and so model development was limited.

Working with FI schedules led Staddon to a tangential foray into an area generally associated with runway, rather than Skinner box, research. Just down the hall from his lab at Toronto, John's senior colleague Abe Amsel was studying the "frustration effect." The procedure involved recording the speed at which rats ran down two consecutive runways. There was always food in the goal box at the end of the second runway, whereas the goal box at the end of the first runway contained food on only 50 percent of the trials. Running speed in the second runway was substantially elevated followed non-reward in the first goal box. Amsel attributed this increase to heightened motivation due to frustration on not receiving food; hence the term "frustration effect." Staddon's work with FI schedules led him to suggest a simpler explanation. In an analogy to the double-runway situation, he set up a study in which birds were exposed to pairs of fixed intervals. Reward always was presented for a peck at the end of the second interval; however, it was available after only 50 percent of the first intervals of a pair. Non-rewarded intervals terminated in a time out. Response rate was much higher in intervals that were preceded by non-reward (N) than by those preceded by reward (R). Staddon concluded that this elevation in rate was the result of the absence of inhibitory after-effects of reinforcement, an "omission effect," and that a similar explanation could account for the increase in running speed after non-reward in Amsel's studies (Staddon and Innis 1969).

In subsequent studies at Toronto and at Duke, Staddon further delineated the inhibitory properties of reinforcement and stimuli associated with it. On FI schedules it is, of course, adaptive for the animal to refrain from responding early in intervals when food is never available. Thus, animals attend to and recall cues that allow them to predict food availability. John Kello (chapter 14) carried out omission-effect studies for his doctoral research at Duke in the early 1970s. (See appendix.) In a 1974 article in the *Psychological Review*, Staddon outlined his ideas on the role of memory and attention in timing, emphasizing that inhibitory temporal control by a time marker (e.g. reward) is "a function of the whole preceding temporal context" (p. 376). Like stimulus control in other situations (e.g. matching-to-sample studies), temporal control is determined by the value of the stimulus, retrieval cues, and interference or confusion effects. The omission effect, then, could be the result of confusion as to which stimulus came last (R or N), could be a memory effect, or could be due to overshadowing by attention to the salient stimulus (R).

Interest in timing research took a back seat for over a decade, but in the late 1980s, with the aid of computer models, theoretical progress was at last possible. In part, Staddon was stimulated to return to studies of timing because he saw a number of flaws in the popular scalar expectancy theory (SET) being advanced by John Gibbon, Russell Church, and their associates (Gibbon 1977; Gibbon and Church 1981, 1984). In collaboration with post-doctoral fellows Jennifer Higa and Clive Wynne, research on cyclic schedules was resumed and a series of models of timing advanced. The first experiments were carried out when Staddon was on leave in Bochum. During the previous few years, he had been working on optimality models of choice behavior. (See below.) Now he devised a simple procedure to extend his optimality analysis to temporal discrimination. Wynne, who was also interested in issues of reinforcement maximization having just completed doctoral research on momentary-maximizing explanations of choice at the University of Edinburgh, was happy to collaborate. The procedure, a response-initiated delay (RID) schedule, is as follows: after reinforcement the bird is presented with a red key light; the first peck on the red key changes its color to green and after a fixed time (T) reinforcement occurs, independent of the bird's behavior. The optimal strategy, of course, is for the bird to peck the red key as soon as it comes on. However, birds do not do this; they wait for a period of time (t) before pecking. The duration of this wait time is linearly related to the duration of the inter-food interval ($t + T$). Moreover, Staddon and Wynne found that "the timing process seemed to be both *rapid* and *obligatory*, i.e. the animals were evidently constrained to behave in this way" (Staddon 1991, p. 9). These results suggested that interval timing involved a "one-back" mechanism they called linear waiting (Wynne and Staddon 1988). Support for linear waiting came from experiments carried out with Jennifer Higa (Higa 1996; Higa, Wynne, and Staddon 1991). For example, using a RID schedule in which a single, short "impulse" interval was interpolated into a series of longer intervals, they found that pigeons' wait times were short in the interval following the interpolated interval, but only in that interval.

Over the next few years, Staddon and Higa continued to develop other timing models. The first of these was a model in which post-reinforcement events were seen "to be represented dynamically by a diffusion-like memory process" (Staddon 1991, p. 10). This diffusion-generalization model (which represents time spatially) was developed at the time Staddon was working with Alliston Reid (chapter 3) on a diffusion-generalization model to account for spatial navigation. Tolman's (1948) idea that rats have a cognitive map of their environment, for example of the location of food on a maze, was criticized because he offered no mechanism for reading the map. The model of Reid and Staddon (1997, 1998) provided a mechanism—an associative process based on stimulus generalization (essentially a similarity space). In the diffusion-generalization model of timing (Higa and Staddon 1997), reinforcement augments "activation at a point whose distance from the origin is proportional to time elapsed since the time marker (reinforcer delivery...). Activation diffuses constantly in real time" with rate of responding "represented by the height of the activation surface at each instant of time in the to-be-timed interval" (Staddon, Chelaru, and Higa 2002a, p. 106). In one version of the model, responding was based on a gradient of activation and a threshold. These models had some difficulties; for example, it was not possible to duplicate the performance observed on cyclic-interval schedules or capture all the features of dynamic timing effects.

Scalar expectancy theory assumes, *a priori*, that timing depends on a biological clock. Staddon maintains that "*there may be no separate 'internal clock'* at all;... interval time discrimination is just like any other discrimination," and that animals remember the occurrence of salient time markers and learn "to discriminate between memories of different ages, and thus of different 'strengths'" (2001a, p. 338). Moreover, in most versions of SET time is represented linearly (proportional timing) and the decision whether or not to respond is determined by the ratio of the representations of time in working and reference memory. Staddon's position is that time is encoded in a log-like manner and that there is a constant-difference response rule. There is good evidence for this with interval schedules; for example, a power function relationship between post-reinforcement pause and interval duration has been shown to hold for performance on both simple FI and cyclic FI schedules (Innis and Staddon 1971). Both linear and non-linear models make the same prediction for simple FI schedules. However, SET cannot account for temporal tracking on cyclic schedules.

Power functions are not the only non-linear functions, and Staddon's most recent model is multiple-time-scale (MTS) theory (Staddon and Higa 1999; Staddon, Chelaru, and Higa 2002a). This model combines linear waiting with a short-term memory model originally devised to account for rate-sensitive habituation (Staddon 1993b; Staddon and Higa 1996). In the habituation model the strength of the fading stimulus trace is represented by the output of a set of cascaded leaky integrators (the leaky bucket analogy). The integrator model has also been applied to the dynamics of feeding behavior. Although "behavioral theories stand on their own feet" and are "valid to the extent that they describe behavioral data accurately and economically" (Staddon 2001a, pp. 150–152), it is encouraging to find agreement with physiology. Recently a physiological counterpart of the cascaded integrators idea has been reported for the human visual system (Glanz 1998).

For timing, the integrator model says that "what is learned on periodic schedules is the reinforced and non-reinforced values of the animal's memory trace for the time marker" (Staddon 2001a, p. 341). In line with the approach to research that has guided him throughout his career, Staddon starts by making "qualitative (rather than quantitative) predictions from a theory that uses as few theoretical concepts as possible" (Staddon and Higa 1999, p. 247), looking at its application across a broad range of a situations involving individual subjects rather than group averages. MTS theory can account for a wide range of data from a variety of studies on temporal control. Both Jennifer Higa (chapter 8) and Mircea Chelaru (chapter 9) report related research on timing in this volume.

In the early 1980s, most psychologists, it seemed, were in agreement that scalar expectancy theory could account for interval timing. Then John Staddon began to develop his dynamic models of timing, reactivating many of the issues surrounding temporal control and forcing SET theorists into controversial debate. For example, *JEAB* devoted a large section of an issue to an article by Staddon and Higa (1999) and commentaries on it. Staddon's models are now receiving increased attention and are stimulating research that will finally help us explain how animals time, a process so integral to an understanding of all conditioning processes.

Biological Constraints on Learning Curiosity is the hallmark of a good scientist. Staddon was curious about (perhaps suspicious of) the results reported in a widely cited article by Skinner on "superstitious" behavior in pigeons. Skinner (1948b) reported that pigeons exposed to periodic free presentations of food (a fixed-time (FT) schedule) were observed to display idiosyncratic responses during inter-food intervals. Skinner believed that these responses were the result of the strengthening action of reinforcement and that the experiment provided support for his general-process theory of learning. Staddon took his cue from the ethologists and decided to make detailed observations of what the birds were doing throughout the inter-food interval. Virginia Simmelhag, who was an undergraduate student in one of his courses at Toronto at the time, took on the tedious task of recording the second-by-second behavior of pigeons exposed to such FT schedules. She later completed her master's degree at Toronto on this project. (See appendix.)

The data provided evidence that the behavior occurring just prior to food presentation was not an idiosyncratic response, strengthened by reinforcement, but rather a food-related (pecking) response. Immediately following reinforcement the birds engaged in other, more idiosyncratic behavior. Staddon and Simmelhag (1971) identified two behavioral states associated with these two types of responses, which they labeled interim and terminal. The editor of the *Psychological Review*, where the article reporting these data was submitted, asked Staddon to expand on the brief theoretical account drawing a parallel between operant conditioning and Darwinian selection that they had presented, and he was happy to comply. The published article, which has become a classic, includes an account of many conditioning phenomena within the variation-selection theoretical framework. As well as superstitious behavior, they dealt with classical and instrumental conditioning, the recently reported phenomenon of autoshaping, and a number of schedule-induced behaviors such as polydipsia. The article was received very well and became part of a growing body of findings reporting constraints on learning.

The "superstition" research led Staddon and his students to conduct a number of studies examining schedule-induced behavior, including a doctoral dissertation by Alliston Reid. (See appendix.) In collaboration with Sandra Ayres, a master's student at Duke, Staddon looked at how animals distributed their time among a number of activities during inter-food intervals, when opportunities for several other behaviors were made available. These data allowed him to develop a theoretical account presented in a chapter in *The Handbook of Operant Conditioning*, a book he co-edited with Werner Honig (Honig and Staddon 1977). As well as pointing out that the various behaviors reflect different internal states, Staddon (1977a) emphasized the idea that there was competition among them. A few years later, he developed a model for instinctive drift, the finding that a well-learned operant response to obtain food may begin to deteriorate and be replaced by innate food-related behavior (Breland and Breland 1961). Based on the idea of reciprocal inhibition between competing (incompatible) behaviors, the model is able to predict a change from an operant response to a species-specific behavior (Staddon and Zhang 1991).

Staddon's research on schedule-induced behavior played an important role in advancing the changing conception of both operant and classical conditioning that was emerging during the 1970s, a movement away from the "naive reflexology" that had dominated learning theory during the preceding decades. The results reported by Staddon and Simmelhag (1971) indicated that classical conditioning is "an integral component of the 'variational' mechanisms which allow organisms to generate adaptive behavior in advance of instrumental contingencies" (Staddon 1991, p. 2). Along with other research published at the time (see Shettleworth 1972), this study helped advance the view that there are biological constraints on learning which cannot be ignored. At last psychologists and biologists were talking to one another, and John Staddon was a key figure in bringing about this change.

Optimality and Choice John Staddon was introduced to theoretical accounts of choice behavior when he was a graduate student at Harvard. At the time, Richard Herrnstein was developing his matching law, which describes the fact that in choice situations, such as concurrent reinforcement schedules, animals will match their relative rate of responding to the relative reinforcement rate (Herrnstein 1961). However, Staddon's longtime interest in biology, and the view that animals behave adaptively, led him to develop a theoretical analysis of choice responding based on utility theory. In fact, he first proposed an expected utility model for choice in an article submitted to *JEAB* in December 1967. The reviewers were not persuaded by his theoretical ideas which they considered too speculative and not particularly relevant to the data from the study he was reporting, an experiment involving DRL schedules. They rejected the paper. The data were finally published, sans utility theory, the following year (Staddon 1968). However, stimulated by his interactions with the behavioral ecologists at Oxford during his sabbatical year, John continued to "mull over the relationships between operant conditioning and behavioral ecology" (Staddon 1991, p. 5). Applying optimality theory to the matching law, he suggested that matching could be the result of reinforcement rate maximization and was able to show this for a class of feedback functions (Staddon 1980b). In an effort to make researchers aware of the "intimate relation between the concepts of utility, reinforcement, and Darwinian fitness" (Staddon 1980a, p. xviii), Staddon brought together contributions by economists, psychologists, and behavioral ecologists in an edited volume, *Limits to Action: The Allocation of Individual Behavior*. The result was to facilitate communication between ecologists and psychologists leading to many productive collaborations.

In what he referred to as "a first step on what is likely to be a long and theoretically involved journey" (Staddon 1979a, p. 2), Staddon published his own optimality theory of behavioral allocation, known as the minimum-distance model (Staddon 1979b). This model assumes that animals "optimize not a single variable ... but rather some function of the total repertoire of behavior, subject to limitations of time and the constraints imposed by the schedule" (ibid., p. 50). Attempting to maintain the preferred level of the various activities in this repertoire under schedule constraints, they will act to "minimize the deviation" from the preferred distribution. The minimum-distance model proved successful in explaining a large number of the properties of molar behavior observed on schedules of reinforcement.

John Staddon's contributions to the study of variability and choice has been wide ranging, stimulating research and theory development by both colleagues and competitors. His elegant minimum-distance model has implications, not only for the evolution and ecology of learning, but also for neuroscience. In collaboration with a number of graduate students he has contributed to the real-time analyses of choice behavior in a number of areas; for example, studies of ratio invariance with John Horner (chapter 13), of momentary maximizing with John Hinson, and of history effects on choice with Derick Davis. More recently, in collaboration with his Duke University colleague Dan Cerutti (chapter 6), Staddon has been looking at models of choice that emphasize time to reinforcement as the important factor in determining preference in animals. This emphasis on the ubiquity of temporal processes in learning phenomena has been a consistent element of Staddon's conception of what controls animal behavior throughout his career.

Principles of Learning

John Staddon's books have presented a fresh and reasoned perspective on experimental psychology. In 1983 he published a textbook, *Adaptive Behavior and Learning*, that emphasized theoretical principles of learning rather than experimental techniques or findings. Moreover, unlike most learning theorists who operate on the premise that to be scientific one must only consider mechanistic accounts, he promoted explanations "in terms of outcomes, either evolutionary outcomes (Darwinian fitness) or outcomes in the life of the individual (goal or motives, reinforcers or 'preference structures'—take your pick)" (Staddon 1983, p. x). This willingness to consider functional, along with mechanistic, accounts has consistently been a characteristic of Staddon's approach, rooted, of course, in his longstanding interest in behavioral biology. Then, in 2001, John brought together his most recent theoretical ideas in *Adaptive Dynamics*. This book is "an argument for a simple proposition: that the way to understand the laws and causes of learning in animals and man is through the invention, comparison, testing, and modification or rejection of black-box models" (Staddon 2001a, p. ix). John Staddon has spent his entire career doing just that.

I first met John Staddon when I was "assigned" to carry out my fourth-year honors' thesis research with him at the University of Toronto. The project I had planned to do fell through and John, who had just arrived at Toronto, was looking for a student. No one had approached him initially. According to the neo-Hullians who dominated the animal labs at Toronto at the time, Staddon was a Skinnerian and doing his kind of research was to be avoided at all costs. But I soon became a devoted member of his lab, helping to set things up and enjoying the excitement of discovering how to be a researcher. Our motto in those days came from the nineteenth-century physicist Michael Faraday: "Work. Finish. Publish." John certainly continued to follow that advice.

More than 30 years later, I am grateful for the twist of fate that sent me to Staddon's lab, with its one relay rack and a few "Harvard" pigeons. Little did I know then that the young "Skinnerian," just starting his career, would become the respected scientist we are honoring now. Little did I know that, as well as mine, the lives of many students would be altered as the result of being a part of "Staddon's lab." As my teacher and mentor, John taught me how to think about research, about science—and about life. As a cherished friend, he has always been there for me over the years. Thank you, John, for giving me the opportunity to be a part of it all.

Students and colleagues who have worked in Staddon's lab remember above all the stimulating atmosphere of the weekly lab meetings. As one former student put it, John "was the creative variation that fed the selective minds of the students" (A. Machado, personal communication May 12, 2003). The following chapters reveal the evolution of those minds.

Appendix

Doctoral Dissertations Supervised by J. E. R. Staddon

Innis, Nancy K. Temporal tracking on cyclic-interval schedules of reinforcement (Duke, 1970).

Malone, John C. Contrast effects in maintained generalization gradients (Duke, 1972).

Kello, John E. Observation of the behavior of rats running to reward and nonreward in an alleyway (Duke, 1973).

Davis, J. Michael. Socially-induced flight reactions in pigeons (Duke, 1973).

Starr, Bettie C. Sensory superstition on interval schedules (Duke, 1976).

Reid, Alliston K. Schedule-induced behavior: Amount and order of activities controlled by behavior interaction (Duke, 1981).

Hinson, John M. Momentary maximizing as a basis for choice (Duke, 1981).

Motheral, M. S. Optimal allocation of behavior: Ratio schedules (Duke, 1982).

Kessel, K. Kin selection, dominance and sociality in *Lemur catta* and *Lemur fulvus*: An experimental and observational analysis (Duke, 1982).

Horner, John M. Probabilistic choice in pigeons (Duke, 1986).

Kohn, Arthur. Effect of variable reward amount and delay on repeated choices (Duke, 1989).

Davis, Derick G. S. Probabilistic choice: Empirical studies and mathematical models (Duke, 1991).

Machado, Armando. Behavioral variability and frequency-dependent selection: Laboratory studies with pigeons (*Columba livia*) (Duke, 1993).

Dragoi, Valentin. Dynamics of operant conditioning (Duke, 1997).

Cleaveland, J. Mark. The role of the response in matching-to-sample tasks using pigeons and budgerigars (Duke, 1998).

Talton, Lynn. Timing, reward and the dopamine system (Duke, 2002).

Hopson, John W. Timing without a clock: Learning models as interval timing models (Duke, 2002).

Master's Theses Supervised by J. E. R. Staddon

Innis, Nancy K. Cyclic-interval schedules: The effect of within-session experience with discriminative stimuli (Toronto, 1967).

Simmelhag, Virginia L. The form and distribution of responding in pigeons on response-independent fixed- and variable-interval schedules of reinforcement (Toronto, 1968).

Kello, John. The control of responding on cyclic fixed-interval schedules of reinforcement (Duke, 1969).

Bowen, Charles. When, where, and why of polydipsia (Duke, 1972).

Ayres, Sandra. The effect of periodic food delivery on the behavior of rats (Duke, 1973).

Acknowledgments

I thank Jennifer Higa, John Horner, Armando Machado, and Virginia Grant for helpful comments on earlier versions of this chapter.

I Behavioral Variability and Choice

2 Making Analogies Work: A Selectionist Model of Choice Behavior

Armando Machado, Richard Keen, and Eric Macaux

The growth of knowledge—or the learning process—is not a repetitive or a cumulative process but one of error-elimination. It is Darwinian selection, rather than Lamarckian instruction.

—Karl Popper (1972, p. 144)

This statement of the situation is meant to describe how knowledge really grows. It is not meant metaphorically, though of course it makes use of metaphors.

—Karl Popper (1972, p. 261)

Scientific investigations often rely on analogies. In the seventeenth century, William Harvey conceived of the heart and lungs as water bellows; in the eighteenth century, several physicists conceived of magnetism as a fluid and of a piece of iron as a sponge that could absorb the fluid; in the early twentieth century, Niels Bohr conceived of the atom as a miniature solar system; later in the same century, cognitive psychologists conceived of the human mind as a digital computer. By means of analogy the conceptual structure of a familiar domain—whether water bellows or sponge, solar system or computer—is superimposed onto an hitherto unfamiliar domain, the heart, magnetic iron, atom, or brain. The analogy illuminates the new domain, allowing the scientist to see its elements and their interrelations in a new light. On occasion, significant scientific advances take place.

One of the oldest analogies in the field of learning brings together the evolution of species by means of natural selection, the familiar domain, and operant conditioning or reinforcement learning, the relatively unfamiliar domain. To put it differently, the effects of reinforcement on behavior are conceptualized as analogous to the effects of natural selection on the evolution of species. One version of the analogy runs as follows (see also Campbell 1960; Plotkin 1993; Skinner 1981; Staddon and Simmelhag 1971):

1. In a given environment, a subject's responses vary in terms of their dimensions—effort, duration, latency, force, topography, etc.
2. Some of these response variants may be more fit than others in the sense that they correlate with higher probabilities of reward, shorter delays to reward, greater reward magnitudes, less energy expended, or any other fitness currency.
3. Responses replicate according to their fitness value. On the average, responses with higher fitness replicate more than responses with lower fitness.
4. Learning is conceived as the process whereby the composition of the initial population of responses changes in time, the fittest responses being retained while the less fit are selectively eliminated.

Three concepts are critical in this approach: selection, variation, and memory. Without behavioral variation there is nothing to select, and without memory the products of the selection process cannot be retained.

In this chapter we elaborate the foregoing analogy to try to understand some issues and to make sense of some empirical findings obtained in the study of choice. The chapter is divided into four sections. In the first section, we develop the main theoretical ideas and derive a mathematical model for the simplest choice situation, the concurrent variable ratio variable ratio schedule, also known as the two-arm bandit game. In the second section, we compare the model with a set of findings already reported in the literature. In the third section, we describe the results of a set of new experiments designed to test the model in a more stringent way. In the fourth and final section, we extend the model to choice in concurrent variable interval variable interval schedules and then conclude with some remarks on the model's strengths and limitations.

A Selectionist Model of Choice

In 1938, the learning psychologist E. C. Tolman remarked that everything important in psychology could be "investigated in essence through the continued experimental and theoretical analysis of the determiners of rat behavior at a choice point in a maze" (Tolman 1966, p. 172). Hyperbole aside, Tolman's confession of faith, as he called it, has become reality. For the last 60-odd years, the study of choice in pigeons, rats, and human beings has been a dominant theme of psychological research. Somewhat paradoxically, however, most studies have not addressed Tolman's central concern, the early determiners of choice, but instead have described and analyzed the types of equilibrium (e.g., matching) observed after prolonged exposure to a choice situation. Hence little is known about the factors that influence the *acquisition* of preference in recurrent choice situations and how these factors are interrelated. The analogy between reinforcement learning and evolution by means of natural selection may shed some light on this neglected issue.

Consider the simplest choice situation: A hungry pigeon pecks a Left (L) or a Right (R) key. A peck on the L key delivers a small amount of food with probability r; a peck on the R key delivers the same amount of food but with probability s. This schedule is known as a Concurrent Variable-Ratio Variable-Ratio schedule (Conc. VR VR) with parameters $1/r$ and $1/s$. We let $r > s$ and refer to the L and R keys also as 'rich' and 'lean' keys, respectively. It is commonly found that pigeons, rats, and other animals eventually acquire an exclusive preference for the rich key. That is, if the probability p of choosing the L key equals 0.5 at the beginning of training, then that same probability will equal, or be close to, 1.0 at the end of training (Herrnstein and Loveland 1975). But what determines how fast the preference for the rich or L key is acquired?

To model the learning process, we assume that responses replicate at the end of time epochs of duration ε. This means that if the repertoire of the organism at time t_0 comprises a proportion p_0 of L responses, and therefore a proportion $q_0 = 1 - p_0$ of R responses, then during that epoch the probability of choosing the L key will equal p_0. However, at the end of the epoch, at time $t_0 + \varepsilon$, or t_1, the proportion of L responses in the repertoire will change to p_1 and for the duration of the new epoch the animal will choose the L key with probability p_1; at time $t_1 + \varepsilon$, or t_2, the proportion p_1 of L responses will change to p_2, and the process repeats. In terms of our guiding analogy, the ends of the epochs correspond to the moments organisms reproduce.

What determines the duration of the time epochs, ε? We assume that ε varies inversely with the overall probability of reinforcement, T. Presumably, situations richer in reinforcement engender more arousal (Killeen,

Hanson, and Osborne 1978) or faster internal clocks (Killeen and Fetterman 1988; Gibbon 1995) and therefore shorter intervals between the reproductive moments. The reciprocal of the time epochs ε, that is, $1/\varepsilon$, is the rate at which responses reproduce. We let this rate be a *positive, monotonic increasing function* of T,

$$\frac{1}{\varepsilon} = f(T). \tag{1}$$

As we mentioned before, the population of responses changes at the end of successive epochs. Because a Conc. VR VR schedule involves only two response classes, L and R, the change in the population of responses is fully represented by the change in the proportion of L responses, Δp. To obtain an expression for Δp, we notice that no aspect of the situation other than the schedule parameters is likely to induce variations in fitness between the two classes—the forces required to activate the keys, the distances from the keys to the hopper, the amounts of food delivered by pecking the keys, and the like are all presumed equal; only the reinforcement probabilities associated with the two keys differ. Hence, Δp must depend exclusively on the reinforcement probabilities r and s, which we conceive of as the fitness values of the L and R response classes, respectively.

To derive the expression for Δp, let m responses of class L and n responses of class R be emitted during the first epoch. Naturally, $m/(m+n) = p_0$. Of the m responses on the left key, $(m \times r) =$ will be reinforced; similarly, of the n responses on the right key, $(n \times s)$ will be reinforced. Assume that each reinforced response yields, say, c_1 new responses of the same class. Then the reinforced L responses will yield a total of $(c_1 \times m \times r)$ new L responses and the reinforced R responses will yield a total of $(c_1 \times n \times s)$ new R responses. Table 2.1 summarizes the effects of one cycle of the selection process.

At the end of the first epoch, the new proportion of L responses, p_1, will equal

Table 2.1

Response classes in repertoire	Number at beginning of epoch	Number reinforced during epoch	Number at end of epoch
L	m	$m \times r$	$c_1 \times m \times r$
R	n	$n \times s$	$c_1 \times n \times s$

$$p_1 = \frac{c_1 \times m \times r}{c_1 \times m \times r + c_1 \times n \times s} = \frac{m \times r}{m \times r + n \times s}$$

and the change in p will be

$$\Delta p = p_1 - p_0 = \frac{m \times r}{m \times r + n \times s} - \frac{m}{m+n} = \frac{m \times n(r-s)}{(m+n)(m \times r + n \times s)}.$$

Dividing the numerator and the denominator by $(m+n)$ and noting that $m/(m+n) = p_0$ and $n/(m+n) = q_0$, one gets

$$\Delta p = \frac{\dfrac{m \times n(r-s)}{m+n}}{(m+n)\dfrac{m \times r + n \times s}{m+n}}$$

$$= \frac{m \times n}{(m+n)(m+n)} \frac{r-s}{\dfrac{m}{m+n} \times r + \dfrac{n}{m+n} \times s}$$

$$= p_0 q_0 \frac{r-s}{p_0 \times r + q_0 \times s}.$$

In the last equation, the numerator of the fraction is the difference in reinforcement probabilities, D, and the denominator is the total reinforcement probability, T. Hence, the effect of selection during one epoch may be written more generally as

$$\Delta p = p \times q \times D/T. \qquad (2)$$

This expression has three parts, which may be interpreted in the light of our analogy as follows. Part 1, the term pq, represents the influence of the class proportions on the selective change. The influence is maximal when $p = q = 1/2$ and minimal when $p = 1$ or $p = 0$. Without variability in the response repertoire there can be no selection. Part 2, the denominator of the fraction, corresponds to the mean fitness of the behavioral repertoire, T. The magnitude of the change due to selection decreases as the mean fitness increases. Thus, the closer the organism is to optimal performance, the slower its response population changes. Finally, part 3, the numerator of the fraction, corresponds to the difference in fitness between the classes in the repertoire. Larger differences cause larger changes in the response population such that when $r > s$, $D > 0$ and L responses increase, whereas when $r < s$, $D < 0$ and L responses decrease. The three parts of the preceding equation are also the key components of the general selection model of quantitative evolutionary genetics (e.g., Mettler, Gregg, and Schaffer 1988, chapter 6).

The model composed of equations 1 and 2 may be approximated by a differential equation. To that end, we subdivide each time epoch into small intervals of duration Δt and assume that p changes linearly within each epoch. In this case, $dp/dt = \Delta p/\varepsilon$ and therefore

$$\frac{dp}{dt} = f(T)\left(p \times q \times \frac{D}{T}\right). \tag{3}$$

Equation 3 states that the rate of preference acquisition (dp/dt) depends on the rate at which responses reproduce multiplied by the effects of selection.

The preceding equation makes one incorrect prediction: For constant T, the rate of preference acquisition is directly proportional to the difference in reinforcement probabilities, D—doubling D doubles the rate of change in p, for example. As we illustrate in the next section, the data do not always support this prediction. A more general model that can potentially solve this problem but still preserve the foregoing assumptions is

$$\frac{dp}{dt} = f(T)g(p \times q \times D/T), \tag{4}$$

where g is a *monotonic increasing* function of its argument, positive when $D > 0$ and negative when $D < 0$. For some functions g, dp/dt increases with D but not proportionately. We do not know the exact form of the functions f and g. Here we will explore one of their mathematically simpler possibilities, namely, power functions. That is, we let

$$f(t) = \alpha T^{\beta}$$

and

$$g(p \times q \times D/T) = (p \times q \times D/T)^{\gamma}$$

with α, β, and γ as free parameters. We know that at least function g cannot be the correct one because the direction of selection (i.e., the sign of g) should be determined by the sign of the difference in reinforcement probabilities, D, which is not the case if γ is different from 1. We consider the two power functions only as *numerical* approximations to the correct functions when $D > 0$ and explore their consequences. Moreover, parameter γ is assumed greater than or equal to 1 in Conc. VR VR schedules so that preference grows with D but not necessarily in a proportional way. To summarize, the master equation to be applied to Conc. VR VR schedules is

$$\frac{dp}{dt} = \alpha T^{\beta}(p \times q \times D/T)^{\gamma} \tag{5}$$

with $\alpha, \beta > 0$ and with $\gamma \geq 1$.

Model versus Data

For Conc. VR VR schedules, the model predicts the following results. First, because $D = r - s > 0$, the asymptotic value of p is 1, which means that the animal eventually fixates on the rich alternative (Herrnstein and Loveland 1975). Second, when D remains constant but T increases, the effect of selection decreases, which should slow the growth of p, but reproductive epochs occur at higher rate, which should speed the growth of p. If γ is greater than β, the net effect is slower learning. This prediction agrees with empirical findings (Bailey and Mazur 1990; Mazur and Ratti 1991). For example, Mazur and Ratti (1991) exposed pigeons to a series of four Conc. VR VR schedules in which the difference between the two reinforcement probabilities always equaled 0.06, but T varied systematically. A fifth schedule with parameters $r = 0.19$ and $s = 0.01$ served as a control condition. Figure 2.1 shows the average results obtained with eight pigeons. In general, the data (symbols) suggest that preference for the rich key is acquired more rapidly with lower overall reinforcement probabilities. The curves through the data points show the model's predictions. With a single parameter set, the model fits the data well.

Third, if the absolute values of the schedule parameters change but their ratio (r/s) remains constant, then the model predicts faster acquisition the higher the value of T. For although the quotient D/T remains constant whenever r/s is constant, the time epochs are shorter when the overall reinforcement probability is higher. The results of Mazur's (1992) study support this prediction. In the first part of his study, the ratio r/s was held at 5 while r varied from 0.05 to 0.20; in the second part, the ratio was held at 2 while r varied from 0.04 to 0.16. In either part, a fifth schedule condition with $r = 0.19$ and $s = 0.01$ served as a control.

The top panels in figure 2.2 show the results obtained with eight pigeons. Despite some noise and one inversion (see filled circles on left panel), the data suggest that, for a constant ratio, preference develops more rapidly

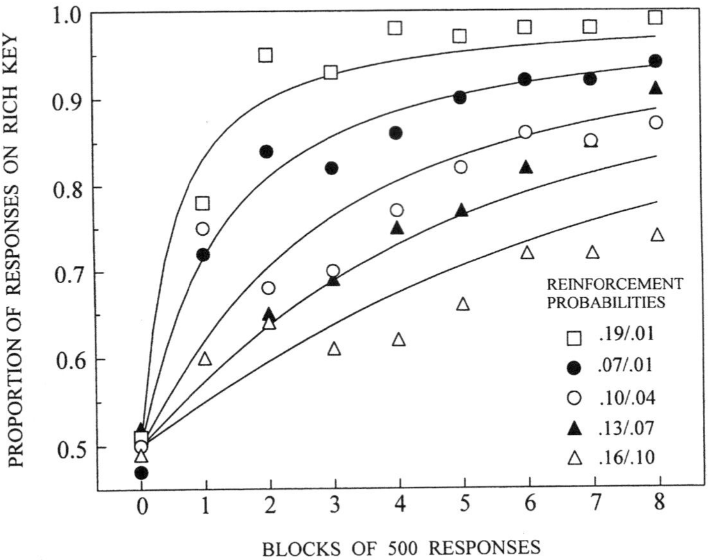

Figure 2.1
The symbols show the acquisition of preference in Conc. VR VR schedules. The numbers are the reinforcement probabilities associated with the two response keys (adapted from Mazur and Ratti 1991). The lines are the model's best fit (see equation 5) with parameters $\alpha = 0.036$, $\beta = 0.59$, and $\gamma = 2.16$.

with higher overall reinforcement probabilities. The curves through the data points are the model's predictions. The model accounted well for the major trends in the data.

The bottom panels in figure 2.2 show preference plotted against the total number of reinforcers. If acquisition depended exclusively on the number of reinforcers, then the four data sets should superimpose. On the left panel, the data clearly did not superimpose, showing in fact the opposite order of that shown in the top left panel. That is, with reinforcers as the time scale, acquisition is faster with lower overall probabilities of reinforcement. The four curves show that the model predicts the observed effect. However, in the bottom right panel the data points superimpose considerably, an effect also reproduced by the model. The difference between the model's predictions in the two cases stems from the differences in the value of parameter β; when β is close to 1, as in the right panel, the curves superpose, but when β is significantly below 1, superposition fails.

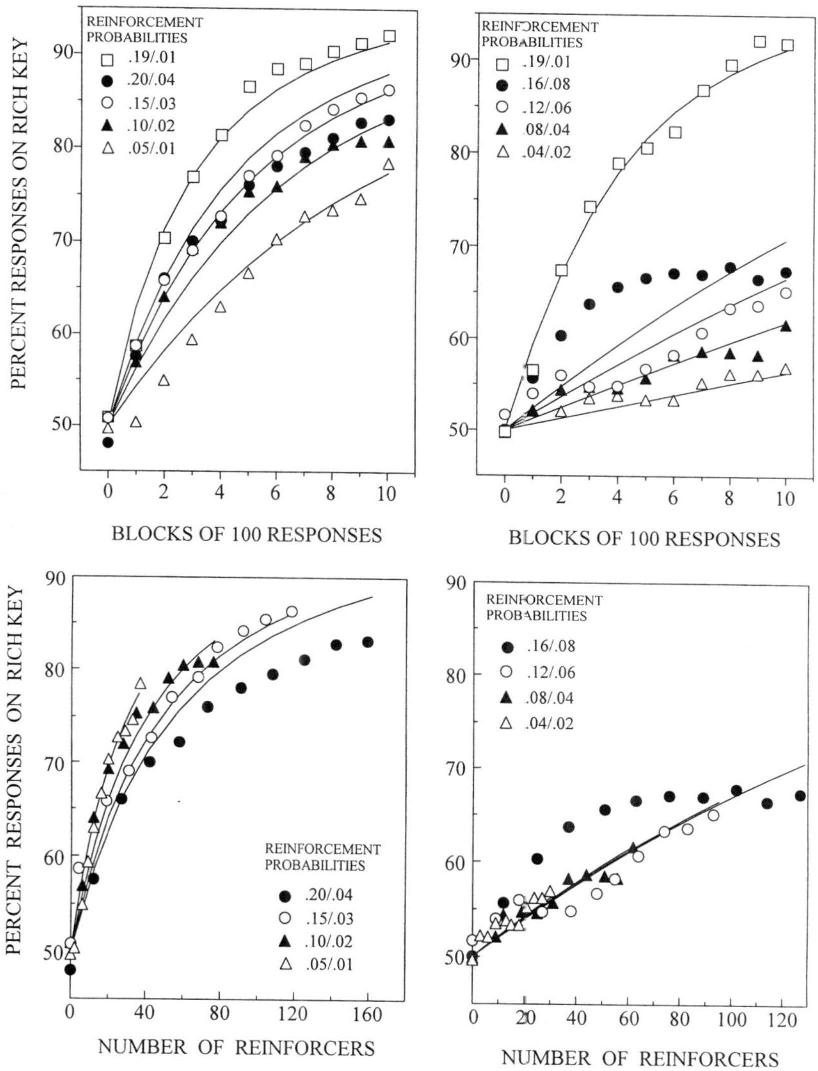

Figure 2.2

Top: The symbols show the acquisition of preference in Conc. VR VR schedules. The numbers are the reinforcement probabilities associated with the two response keys. Bottom: The same data plotted as a function of the total number of reinforcers (adapted from Mazur 1992). The lines are the model's best fit (see equation 5) with parameters $\alpha = 0.026$, $\beta = 0.57$, and $\gamma = 1.89$, for the left panels, and $\alpha = 0.032$, $\beta = 0.95$, and $\gamma = 1.61$, for the right panels.

Further Tests of the Model

A rigorous test of the model's assumptions requires a choice situation in which the experimenter, not the animal, controls the key variables D and T. These variables should then be held constant within a condition and varied independently across conditions. Unfortunately, these requirements cannot be met with the standard Conc. VR VR schedule because the overall probability of reinforcement, T, and hence the ratio D/T, changes with the animal's preference. If the two reinforcement probabilities equal r and s, with $r > s$, then the overall reinforcement probability can range from s (exclusive preference for the lean key) to r (exclusive preference for the rich key).

To circumvent this shortcoming of the standard Conc. VR VR schedule, we designed a choice procedure in which D and T are both independent of the subject's behavior. The top left panel in figure 2.3 illustrates the details. The horizontal axis is an estimate of the animal's current probability of choosing the rich key, p. In the experiments reported below, this estimate equaled the proportion of choices on the rich key during the last 80 trials. The solid lines give the payoff probabilities during the next trial for the rich and lean keys. The distance between the two curves equals D and the dotted line equals T. Regardless of the animal's current preference, D and T remain constant.

The schedule allows the researcher to vary independently the difference between the two payoff probabilities and the total probability. The top right panel of figure 2.3 shows how D may be varied across conditions while T remains constant. For the outer lines, $D = 0.12$; for the inner lines, $D = 0.04$; in both cases, $T = 0.12$. Equation 5 predicts that acquisition will be faster for larger D. The bottom left panel shows how T may be varied while D remains constant. For the two lower lines, $T = 0.05$; for the two upper lines, $T = 0.20$; in both cases, $D = 0.05$. Assuming $\gamma > \beta$, equation 5 predicts that acquisition will be slower for larger T.

We conducted five experiments with the new procedure. The first three employed the usual two key choice situation, with each key associated with a different reinforcement schedule. The last two experiments employed Findley's (1958) procedure with one response key and one changeover key. In two experiments D varied while T remained constant, and in three experiments T varied while D remained constant.

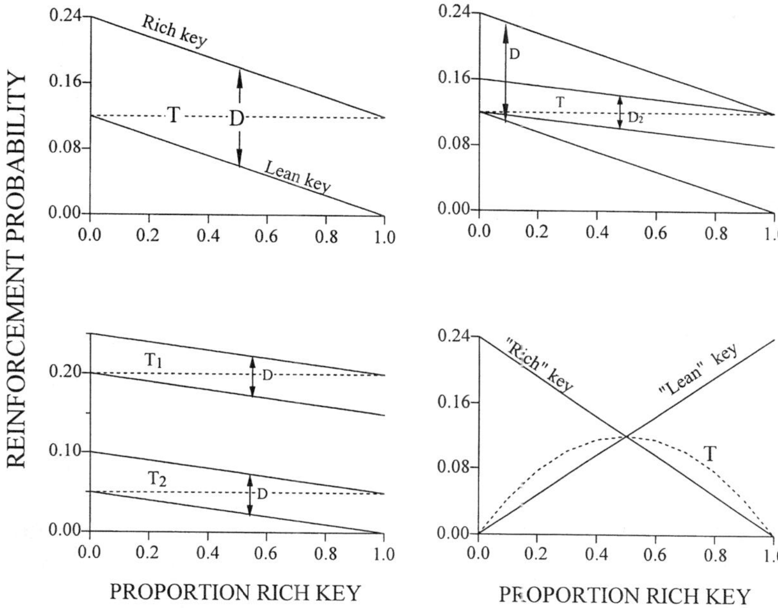

Figure 2.3
Top left: Reinforcement schedule used during the experimental conditions. The horizontal axis is the proportion of choices of the rich key during the last 80 trials. The two lines with negative slope show the probabilities of reinforcement on the next trial given a peck on the rich and lean keys. The difference between the two probabilities is *D*; the dotted line shows the overall probability of reinforcement, *T*. Top right: Two schedules showing how *D* may be manipulated while *T* remains constant. Bottom left: Two schedules showing how *T* may be manipulated while *D* remains constant. Bottom right: Reinforcement schedule used during the transition phases. One key is arbitrarily chosen as the rich key. This schedule is used to bring preference to 0.5 between experimental conditions.

General Method Pigeons (*Columba livia*) were maintained at 80 percent of their free-feeding body weight. They were housed in individual home cages with a 12:12 light-dark cycle. The experiments took place in two identical Med Associates operant chambers equipped with two response keys, a grain hopper, and a house light mounted on the rear wall of the chamber. The keys could be lit with red, green, or white lights. The chamber was enclosed in a sound-attenuating plywood box equipped with a fan that circulated air and helped mask extraneous noises. A 486 Pentium computer using the C++ programming language controlled experimental events and recorded the data.

After the pigeons learned to peck the keys reliably with the reinforcement probability set at 0.1 per peck, the experiment proper began. At the beginning of each trial, the two keys were illuminated with white light. A peck on one key either yielded a reward—access to food for 2.5 seconds—or turned both keys off for a 0.4-second inter-trial interval. Sessions ended after the birds obtained 50 reinforcers.

The experiment was divided into conditions and each condition was preceded by a transition phase. The purpose of the transition phase was to bring choice to indifference. During transition, pecks were reinforced according to the frequency-dependent schedule illustrated in the bottom right panel of figure 2.3. One key was arbitrarily designated as the rich key. The proportion of pecks on the rich key during the last 80 trials determined the reinforcement probabilities for the next trial. As the pigeon responded more on one key, the reinforcement probability on that key decreased while the reinforcement probability on the other key increased. In terms of equations, the probability of reinforcement given a peck on the rich key equaled $c(1 - p)$, $0 \leq c \leq 1$, and the corresponding probability given a peck on the lean key equaled $c \times p$. The two reinforcement probabilities were equal only at indifference, the matching equilibrium of the schedule. The dotted line in the figure shows the overall reinforcement probability, T, which equals $2 \times c \times p \times (1 - p)$. Notice that T is almost constant around the matching equilibrium (i.e., at $p \approx 0.5$, $T \approx c/2$). During each transition phase, c was set so that the overall reinforcement probability at equilibrium equaled the value of T that would be used during the next experimental condition. For example, if T equaled 0.12 during one experimental condition, then c was set at 0.24 during the transition phase that preceded it—as choice proportions returned to indifference during the transition phase, T approached the 0.12 value that would hold during the next experimental condition.

The transition phase lasted for 10 sessions of 50 rewards each and for the first 15 rewards of the eleventh session. The remaining 35 rewards of the eleventh session and all 50 rewards of the next sessions constituted one experimental condition. (The exact number of sessions during each condition varied across experiments; see below.) Although the transition phase always brought preference close to indifference (i.e., $0.45 \leq p \leq 0.55$), the least-preferred key during the last three sessions of the transition phase became the rich key during the following experimental condition.

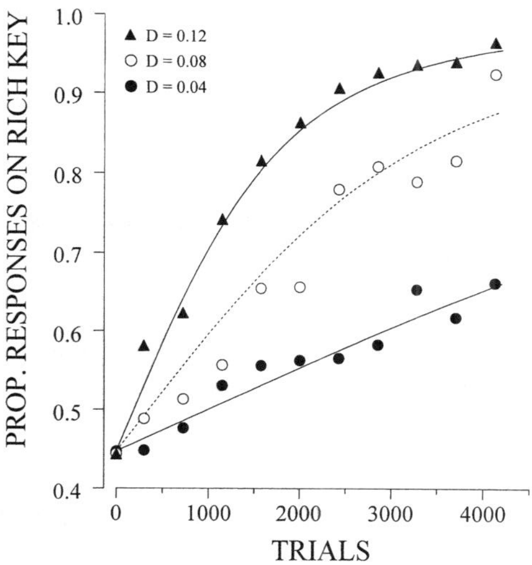

Figure 2.4
The symbols show the median proportion of choices of the rich key during experiment 1. The lines are the model's best fit (equation 5) with parameters $\alpha = 0.018$, $\gamma = 1.5$, and $p_0 = 0.45$.

Experiment 1 The experiment was designed to test the effects of varying the difference in reinforcement probabilities, *D*, while maintaining constant the overall reinforcement probability, *T*. Nineteen pigeons were exposed to *D* values of 0.12, 0.08, and 0.04, while *T* always equaled 0.12. Each pigeon was exposed to the three *D* values in a counterbalanced order, and afterwards it was re-exposed to one of these *D* values.

Figure 2.4 shows the median proportion of choices of the rich key as a function of trials. The data show that acquisition was fastest when *D* equaled 0.12, intermediate when $D = 0.08$, and slowest when $D = 0.04$. In all conditions, the obtained overall reinforcement probability was always close to the schedule value of 0.12.

The curves through the data points represent the model's best fit. Because *T* was constant, the quantity αT^{β} in equation 5 was also constant. Hence, in fitting the model we forced β to equal 1 and estimated only parameters α and γ as well as the initial p_0 value. In other words, the equation used to fit the data was $dp/dt = \alpha(p \times q \times D)^{\gamma}$. A single set of parameters was required to fit the three data sets simultaneously. As the lines through the data points show, the model fit the data well.

The analysis of individual curves revealed three findings: First, there was little between-subjects variability in the $D = 0.12$ condition relative to the $D = 0.04$ and $D = 0.08$ conditions. Second, in both the $D = 0.04$ and $D = 0.08$ conditions some individuals preferred the lean key even after 10 sessions of training. Third, although the model accounted well for the median data, it could not account for the individual data because it could not predict a preference for the lean key.

Experiment 2 The experiment tested the model by examining the effect of varying the total reinforcement probability, T, while holding D constant. Across conditions T equaled 0.05, 0.10, and 0.20; D always equaled 0.05. Sixteen pigeons served as subjects. Each pigeon experienced each condition twice in a counterbalanced order. During the transition phase that preceded each experimental condition (figure 2.3, bottom right panel) the overall reinforcement probability, T, equaled the value that would be used during the following experimental condition.

Because sessions ended when 50 reinforcers had been collected, the number of responses needed to end a session varied across conditions. On the average, it took 1,000, 500, and 250 responses to end a session when T equaled 0.05, 0.10, and 0.20, respectively. Therefore the number of sessions per experimental condition was determined as follows: First, the $T = 0.05$ condition lasted exactly ten sessions. Second, the $T = 0.10$ and $T = 0.20$ conditions lasted a minimum of ten sessions and a maximum of 20 and 40 sessions, respectively. Between the minimum and maximum number of sessions, a condition ended if at least 95 percent of the bird's pecks were on the rich key for three consecutive sessions, or if there were no systematic changes in choice proportion for five consecutive sessions. When one of these criteria was met, and therefore fewer than 20 sessions were conducted with $T = 0.10$, or fewer than 40 sessions with $T = 0.20$, it was assumed that the remaining sessions would have yielded a choice proportion equal to the average choice proportions of the last three completed sessions. This assumption enabled us to compare performance across conditions with substantially different numbers of total trials.

Figure 2.5 shows the median proportion of choices of the rich key. To estimate the probabilities from approximately the same number of trials, the results from the $T = 0.10$ and $T = 0.20$ conditions were combined to match those from the $T = 0.05$ condition. Specifically, each data point for

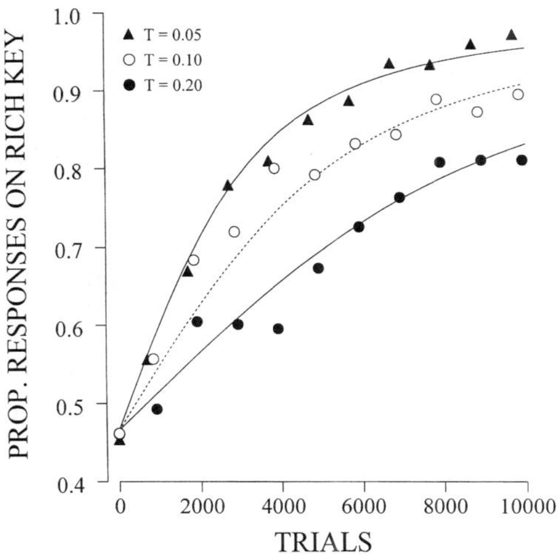

Figure 2.5
The symbols show the median proportion of choices of the rich key during experiment 2. The lines are the model's best fit (equation 5) with parameters $\alpha = 0.001$, $\beta = 0.35$, and $p_0 = 0.48$.

the $T = 0.05$ condition corresponds to one session, each data point for the $T = 0.10$ condition corresponds to two sessions, and each data point for the $T = 0.20$ condition corresponds to four sessions. On the average then each data point is based on approximately 1,000 responses. However, the first data point corresponds to slightly fewer responses because the first session of each experimental condition ended after 35 reinforcers, not 50.

The symbols in figure 2.5 show that the rate of acquisition was fastest when $T = 0.05$, intermediate when $T = 0.10$, and slowest when $T = 0.20$. Even though there is a clear difference by the end of training between the $T = 0.05$ and $T = 0.10$ conditions, performance was similar for the first 4,000 trials. The lines through the data points show the model's best fit. Because D remained constant and only T varied. we forced parameter γ to 1.0 and allowed only α, β and p_0 to vary freely. In other words, the equation used to fit the data was $dp/dt = \alpha T^{\beta} pq$. The model accounted for the major trends in the data.

Because all subjects were exposed to each condition twice, we can compare performance during the first and second exposures to a given condition. In terms of median performance, conditions $T = 0.05$ and $T = 0.10$ replicated nicely, but there was a large difference in the replication of the

$T = 0.20$ condition. During the first exposure, the median for the $T = 0.20$ condition increased and then stabilized around a preference of 65 percent for the rich key. During the second exposure, the median stabilized around 90 percent but the individual data divided clearly into two types of acquisition curves. For 10 of the 16 birds, preference increased rapidly and remained high throughout training. For the remaining 6 birds, preference remained around 65 percent. Further analyses showed that individual differences were highest in the $T = 0.20$ condition and lowest in the $T = 0.05$ condition. This finding is similar to that observed in experiment 1, for the conditions that showed the fastest acquisition also had the least amount of individual differences.

Experiment 3 Experiment 3 was in all respects similar to experiment 2 except that different values of T and D were used. Across conditions T equaled 0.0125, 0.025, and 0.05 whereas D remained constant at 0.0125. A different group of 16 pigeons served as subjects.

Figure 2.6 shows the results. As in experiment 2, each data point represents one, two, or four sessions for conditions $T = 0.0125, 0.025$, and 0.05, respectively. Thus each data point represents approximately 4,000

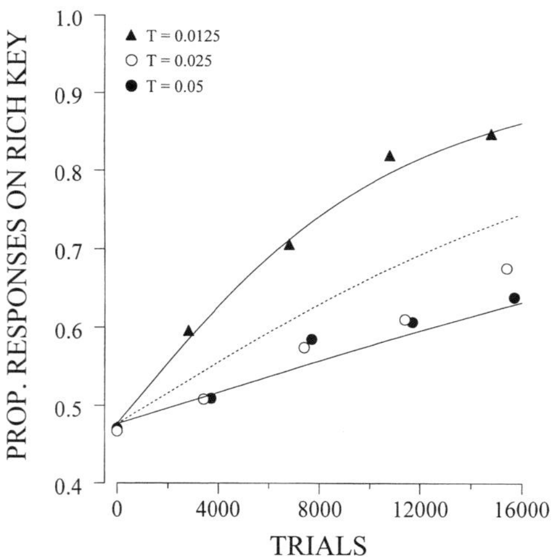

Figure 2.6
The symbols show the median proportion of choices of the rich key during experiment 3. The lines are the model's best fit (equation 5) with parameters $\alpha = 0.059$, $\beta = 1.0$, and $p_0 = 0.48$.

responses (except for the first data point; see experiment 2). It is clear that the smallest T value resulted in the fastest acquisition, but there were no discernable differences between the $T = 0.05$ and $T = 0.025$ conditions.

The lines through the data points show the model's best fit. The model accounted well for the range of the effect of T, that is, for the separation between the lowest and the highest curve. However, because it predicts that when $T = 0.025$ acquisition should be faster than when $T = 0.05$, the intermediate curve deviated systematically from the data.

In terms of individual differences, the $T = 0.0125$ showed the least variance, whereas the $T = 0.025$ and 0.05 conditions showed similar variances. Also, the variance observed in experiment 3 was less than that shown in the first two experiments. In fact, no pigeon ended an experimental condition responding below 40 percent on the rich key. A comparison of the original condition with its replication showed them to be approximately equal.

Experiment 4 The experiment followed the same rationale as experiment 1 except that Findley's (1958) procedure replaced the usual concurrent schedule procedure. The right key was always the response key. Red and green lights projected on that key signaled the reinforcement schedule in effect. The birds could change the operative schedule by pecking once on the left, changeover key, which was illuminated with white light.

Across conditions the difference between reinforcement probabilities varied while the overall reinforcement probability remained constant. Three differences were tested, 0.025, 0.0125, and 0.006; throughout, $T = 0.025$. Sixteen pigeons participated in the experiment.

The symbols in figure 2.7 show the medians from each experimental condition. At every point, preference for the rich key was stronger when the difference between alternatives was large ($D = 0.025$) than when it was small ($D = 0.006$). However, the results from the intermediate, $D = 0.0125$ condition did not differ significantly from the results of the $D = 0.006$ condition. The curves represent the model's best fit—as in experiment 1, we forced β to 1 and let α, γ, and p_0 vary (i.e., the simpler equation $dp/dt = \alpha(p \times q \times D)^{\gamma}$ was used to fit the data). Although the fit was not as good as in experiment 1, note that the range of the predicted effect, the separation between the lowest and the highest curves, matches the range of the data points.

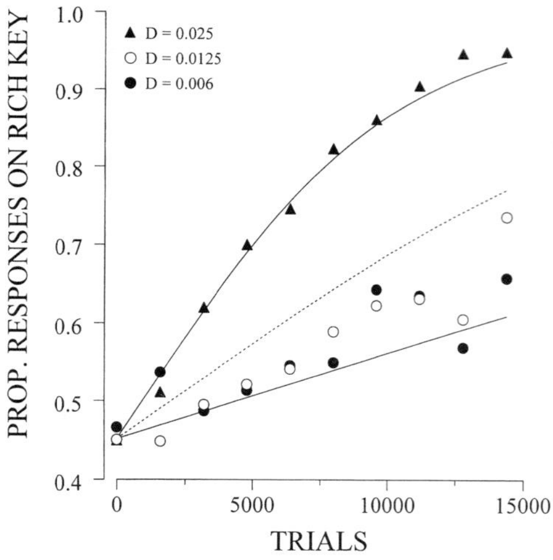

Figure 2.7
The symbols show the median proportion of choices of the rich key during experiment 4. The lines are the model's best fit (equation 5) with parameters $\alpha = 0.009$, $\gamma = 1.1$, and $p_0 = 0.45$.

Experiment 5 This experiment was similar to experiments 2 and 3 except that it used Findley's procedure. Three T values were tested across conditions, 0.05, 0.025, and 0.0125, while D was held constant at 0.0125. The same 16 birds used in experiment 4 served as subjects. Each bird was exposed to each condition twice in counterbalanced order.

Figure 2.8 shows the results. Although the differences among conditions were relatively small, it was the case that higher overall probabilities of reinforcement slowed down the rate at which preference developed. Because D was constant, we forced γ to equal 1 and used the simpler equation $dp/dt = \alpha T^{\beta} pq$ to fit the data. The model accounted for the major trends in the data.

At the individual level, a few birds preferred the lean key or remained indifferent between the two keys, particularly when $T = 0.05$. As in previous experiments, variance among birds was greater the higher the value of T. This result suggests that when the D/T ratio is sufficiently small, the bird's ability to perceive the difference between alternatives may be compromised so much that exclusive preference fails to develop.

When the difference in reinforcement probabilities equals the total reinforcement probability, the Weber-like fraction D/T equals one and the

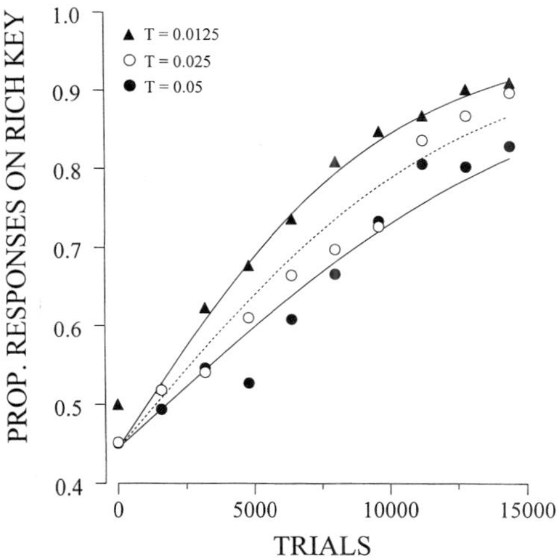

Figure 2.8
The symbols show the median proportion of choices of the rich key during experiment 5. The lines are the model's best fit (equation 5) with parameters $\alpha = 0.003$, $\beta = 0.65$, and $p_0 = 0.45$.

model reduces to $dp/dt = \alpha T^{\beta}(pq)^{\gamma}$. In this equation, the role of T on setting what we have called the "reproductive epochs," or the tempo of learning, becomes evident: a higher reinforcement probability should result in a faster acquisition of preference. The experiments summarized above included five conditions in which $D = T$. Figure 2.9 shows the median data from these conditions and the model's best fits (these are the same curves as in the original figures). The data confirmed the predicted order of acquisition.

General Discussion The five experiments yielded data consistent with those reported by Mazur and collaborators and which we summarized above. To recapitulate:

1. For a constant overall reinforcement probability, acquisition is faster the greater the difference between the two reinforcement probabilities (figures 2.4 and 2.7).

2. For a constant difference between the two reinforcement probabilities, acquisition is faster the lower the overall reinforcement probability (figures 2.5, 2.6, and 2.8).

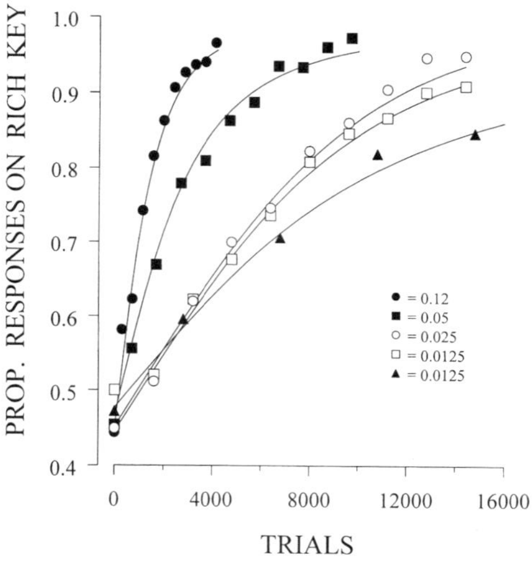

Figure 2.9
The symbols show the data from the condition of each experiment in which $D = T$ and therefore $D/T = 1$. The lines are the model's best fits. The numbers in the legend show the value of T (or D). As predicted, if D/T remains constant, preference is faster the higher the overall reinforcement probability, T.

3. For a constant ratio of reinforcement probabilities, acquisition is faster the higher the overall reinforcement probability (figure 2.9). Because there are only two degrees of freedom among the three quantities—ratio, difference, and total reinforcement probability—this last conclusion could be expressed also by stating that for a constant ratio of reinforcement probabilities, acquisition is faster the greater the difference between the two reinforcement probabilities. Critical, however, is the fact that speed of acquisition does not depend simply on the ratio of reinforcement probabilities.

The selectionist model accounted for these three findings by assuming that acquisition depends on two processes, one that sets the tempo of learning, and another that sets its direction. The former depends on the overall reinforcement probability; the latter on the ratio of the two reinforcement probabilities, or, more specifically, on the Weber-like fraction D/T. These ideas were summarized in the general equation, $dp/dt = f(T)g(pqD/T)$, where f and g are monotonic increasing functions of their arguments. When T is constant, dp/dt depends exclusively on the difference D; because

Table 2.2

Response classes in repertoire	Number at beginning of epoch	Number reinforced during epoch	Number at end of epoch
L	m	$\varepsilon \times \phi_1$	$c_1 \times \varepsilon \times \phi_1$
R	n	$\varepsilon \times \phi_2$	$c_1 \times \varepsilon \times \phi_2$

g is monotonic increasing, the net result is point 1 above. When the ratio D/T is constant, dp/dt depends exclusively on $f(T)$; because this function is positive and monotonically increasing, the net result is point 3 above. Finally, when D is constant, dp/dt depends on both functions, f and g. Increasing overall reinforcement probability, T, increases f but decreases g. For the net effect to yield point 2 above, it is necessary that the relative increment in f (i.e., $\Delta f/f$) should be less than the relative decrement in g ($\Delta_T g/g$). In equation 5, this occurs when $\beta < \gamma$.

Extending the Model

Conc. VI VI Schedules

To extend the model to Conc. VI VI schedules we assume that the L and R keys deliver reinforcers at rates ϕ_1 and ϕ_2, with $\phi_1 > \phi_2$. These rates are the reciprocal of the VI parameters. In addition, we assume that the animal responds at a constant rate (more specifically, according to a Poisson process) and, once it decides to respond, it chooses the L and R alternatives with probabilities p and $q = 1 - p$, respectively (e.g., Gibbon 1995).

In Conc. VI VI schedules, the overall reinforcement rate is approximately constant and equal to $T = \phi_1 + \phi_2$. Hence, according to the model, response reproduction occurs at a rate $f(\phi_1 + \phi_2)$, where f is a positive, monotonic increasing function of its argument.

To determine the effect of selection, we note that during one epoch of duration ε, approximately $(\varepsilon \times \phi_1)$ responses on the L key will be reinforced and $(\varepsilon \times \phi_2)$ responses on the R key will be reinforced.[1] The offspring will be proportional to these numbers. Table 2.2 summarizes the effect of one selection cycle. At the end of the epoch, the new proportion of L responses, p_1, will equal

$$p_1 = \frac{c_1 \times \varepsilon \times \phi_1}{c_1 \times \varepsilon \times \phi_1 + c_1 \times \varepsilon \times \phi_2} = \frac{\phi_1}{\phi_1 + \phi_2}$$

and the change in p will be

$$\Delta p = \frac{\phi_1}{\phi_1 + \phi_2} - p.$$

(For the speed of attaining matching, see Mark and Gallistel 1994.) Expressed as a differential equation, the full, general model is

$$\frac{dp}{dt} = f(\phi_1 + \phi_2) \times g\left(\frac{\phi_1}{\phi_1 + \phi_2} - p\right), \tag{6}$$

where, as before, f and g and are monotonic increasing functions of their arguments.

The preceding equation has the following properties. First, $dp/dt = 0$ when $p = \phi_1/(\phi_1 + \phi_2)$. Hence, at equilibrium the matching law is obtained (Herrnstein 1970). Second, for the same equilibrium value, the model predicts faster learning with higher overall reinforcement rates, which agrees with the empirical evidence (Mazur 1992; Myerson and Miezin 1980). Third, if f and g are the identity functions (i.e., $f(\phi_1 + \phi_2) = \phi_1 + \phi_2$ and $g(\phi_1/(\phi_1 + \phi_2) - p) = \phi_1/(\phi_1 + \phi_2) - p$, then the model reduces to that of Myerson and Miezin (1980). In this case, the rate of preference acquisition will be proportional to the overall reinforcement rate. However, some results described below suggest that f cannot be the identity function. Hence, we let f be the same power function assumed before, that is,

$$\frac{dp}{dt} = \alpha(\phi_1 + \phi_2)^{\beta}\left(\frac{\phi_1}{\phi_1 + \phi_2} - p\right). \tag{7}$$

One of the most common findings obtained with Conc. VI VI schedules is undermatching (Baum 1973). How then can a selectionist model of choice yield undermatching? One way is to assume that responses of one class may on occasion mutate into responses of another class. The causes of mutation may include reinforcers having their effects not only on the last response but on the responses that preceded it, the animal assigning reinforcers incorrectly to responses, or the frequent switching between two alternatives that are very similar on the response and stimulus sides (e.g., pecking two keys, pressing two levers). If mutation occurs at some rate $\mu > 0$, then $\mu \times p$ responses of the L class will change into responses of the R class and $\mu \times q$ responses of the R class will change into responses of the L class (where, as before, $q = 1 - p$). Including mutation in the model and assuming g to be the identity function yields our master equation for Conc. VI VI schedules,

$$\frac{dp}{dt} = \alpha(\phi_1 + \phi_2)^{\beta}\left(\frac{\phi_1}{\phi_1 + \phi_2} - p\right) - \mu p + \mu q,$$

or, equivalently,

$$\frac{dp}{dt} = \alpha(\phi_1 + \phi_2)^{\beta}\left(\frac{\phi_1}{\phi_1 + \phi_2} - p\right) - \mu(2p - 1). \quad (8)$$

Figure 2.10 shows the fit of equation 8 to three data sets reported by Mazur. In the top panel, Mazur (1992) scheduled one reinforcer every 30 seconds, on the average, and then with probability r allocated it to one key, and with the complementary probability allocated it to the other key. The value of r varied across conditions. The symbols in the figure show the average results obtained with six pigeons. To fit the model, we forced β to 1 because the overall reinforcement rate did not change, and allowed α and μ to vary. With two free parameters, the model fit the three data sets well, in particular the severe undermatching displayed by the birds.

In another study, Mazur (1995, experiment 1) repeated the preceding experiment but varied the pigeons' initial preference, p_0. To illustrate, in one condition, 10 percent of all scheduled reinforcers were initially allocated to one key, but after behavior stabilized the allocation probabilities were reversed and that same key yielded 90 percent of the scheduled reinforcers. The middle panel of figure 2.10 shows the results. Consider the triangles. During the last session in which one key delivered 10 percent of the reinforcers, the birds chose that key approximately 22 percent of the time. (See three leftmost triangles in pre-transition phase.) Six minutes into the next session the reinforcement allocation was reversed (see transition phase) and the birds' choice proportion changed from about 17 to 65 percent. By the end of the last post-transition session (see three rightmost triangles), choice proportion had stabilized at about 75 percent.

To fit the model, we forced β to 1 and allowed α and μ to vary. The initial p value was set to the average of the first two data points of the transition phase. As the lines show, the model fit the data well.

In another experiment, Mazur (1995, experiment 2) varied the overall reinforcement rate but maintained constant the allocation probabilities and the pigeon's initial preference. Reinforcers were scheduled once every 30

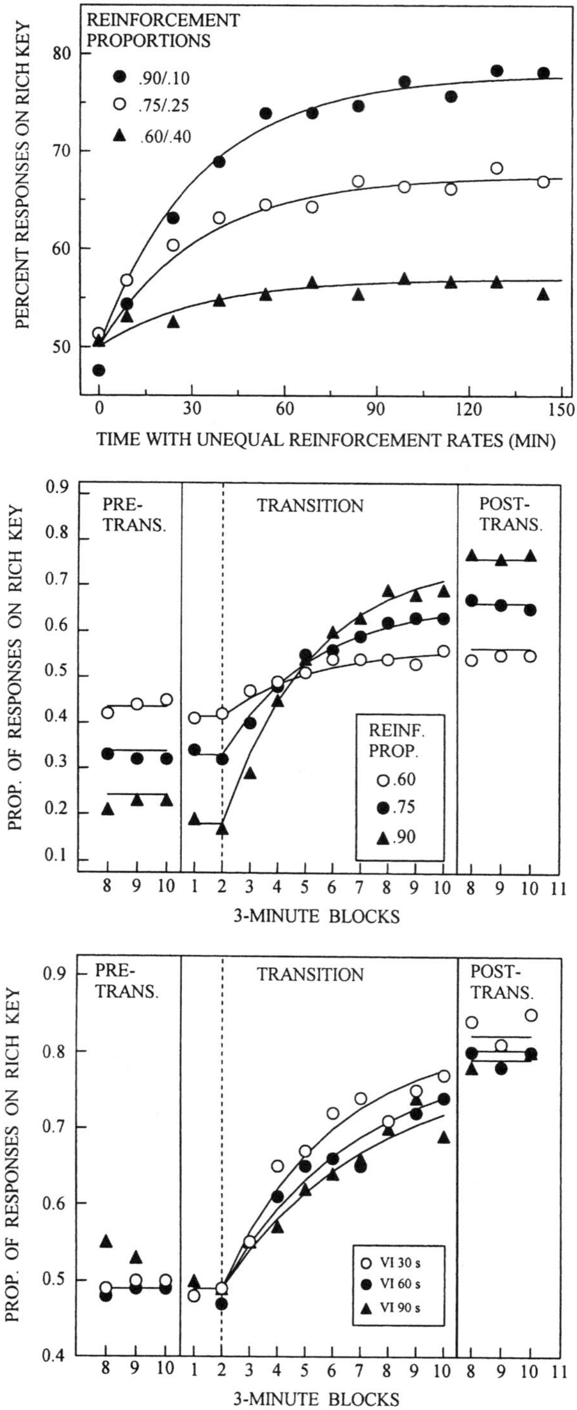
REINFORCEMENT PROPORTIONS
.90/.10
.75/.25
.60/.40
PERCENT RESPONSES ON RICH KEY
TIME WITH UNEQUAL REINFORCEMENT RATES (MIN)
PRE-TRANS.
TRANSITION
POST-TRANS.
REINF. PROP.
.60
.75
.90
PROP. OF RESPONSES ON RICH KEY
3-MINUTE BLOCKS
PRE-TRANS.
TRANSITION
POST-TRANS.
VI 30 s
VI 60 s
VI 90 s
PROP. OF RESPONSES ON RICH KEY
3-MINUTE BLOCKS

seconds, 60 seconds, or 90 seconds on the average. The bottom panel of figure 2.10 shows the results. Although the differences in speed of preference acquisition were not large, certainly not proportional to overall reinforcement rate, it was the case that preference changed faster with higher reinforcement rates. With α, β, and μ as free parameters, the model fit the data well. One interesting feature of both data and model is that the degree of undermatching was smallest when the overall reinforcement rate was highest.

Strengths and Weakness of the Selectionist Model

In its most general form, the model presented above assumed that choice depends on three distinct processes: the reproductive epochs, which set the tempo of learning; the selection cycles, which set the direction of learning; and response mutations which offset to some extent the effects of the selection cycles. The model reproduced the main qualitative trends of the meager data set we have on acquisition of preference in Conc. VR VR and Conc. VI VI schedules. Alternative models of choice—e.g., Bush and Mosteller's (1955) linear operator model, Myerson and Miezin's (1980) kinetic model, Herrnstein and Vaughan's (1980) melioration model, Horner and Staddon's (1987) ratio invariance model, or Mazur's (1992) value model—cannot account for the same pattern of findings.

The model has also inspired the design of an improved procedure to study acquisition, a procedure in which the experimenter, not the animal, controls the two key variables *D* and *T*. Five experiments with the new procedure reproduced the main findings reported before by Mazur and

Figure 2.10
Top: The symbols show the acquisition of preference in Conc. VI VI schedules. Reinforcers were scheduled once every 30 seconds on the average and then assigned to the keys according to the probabilities shown in the legend (adapted from Mazur 1992). Middle: Similar experiment but with different starting preferences. The dotted line shows the moment the probabilities were reversed (adapted from Mazur 1995, experiment 1). Bottom: Acquisition of preference when reinforcers were scheduled every 30, 60, or 90 seconds on the average and then allocated to the rich key with probability 0.9 (adapted from Mazur 1995, experiment 2). The lines are the model's best fits (equation 8) with parameters $\alpha = 0.01$ and $\mu = 0.000076$ (top), $\alpha = 0.033$ and $\mu = 0.0003$ (middle), and $\alpha = 0.0043$, $\beta = 0.40$, and $\mu = 0.00014$ (bottom).

his collaborators concerning acquisition of preference in Conc. VR VR schedules.

But the model also has limitations, chief among which is the exact form of the functions *f* and *g* in equations 4 and 6. To fit specific data, we have assumed that *f* and *g* were power functions of their arguments, but, as already mentioned, these functions cannot be correct. The rate of response reproduction, function *f*, must have an upper bound, and the sign of the difference between the reinforcement probabilities must be preserved in order to set the sign of dp/dt. Additional limitations of the model include its silence concerning the role of extinction in any of the presumed processes. We know, for example, that resistance to extinction depends on the animal's history, for a naive pigeon will stop pecking quickly if the reinforcement probability per peck decreases from, say, 1.0 to 0.01, but will continue pecking if the same probability of 0.01 is reached gradually. As it is, the model cannot account for this common observation. Finally, we note one other limitation of all extant models of choice, their inability to account for the substantial variability within and between animals. Some pigeons, for example, come to prefer the lean key in a Conc. VR VR schedule, and even when a bird systematically prefers the rich key, it may show substantially different acquisition curves when exposed on two separate occasions to the same reinforcement schedules. The sources of this variability remain to be identified and experimentally controlled.

We conclude this study with a speculative note. We believe that the analogy between evolution by means of natural selection and reinforcement learning has the potential to help us understand not only the acquisition of preference, but also other issues related to learning and choice. For example, Machado (1989, 1992) had the analogy in mind when he proposed that operant variability and random-like behavior (e.g., Machado 1989; Page and Neuringer 1985) may be the outcome of frequency-dependent selection or, more specifically, of the differential reinforcement of the least likely responses in the animal's repertoire. To understand his argument, a brief excursion into the familiar domain of evolutionary theory is needed.

A problem that has puzzled evolutionary biologists is what maintains the enormous amount of genetic variability observed both within and between populations of organisms. Simply put, the problem is this: If a new trait is advantageous, in time all members of a population will likely exhibit it; if not, the trait will likely be eliminated. In either case, variability eventually disappears, which is contrary to fact. One way to "solve" the puzzle is to realize that some forms of natural selection instead of reducing genetic variability actually promote and maintain it. These forms of selection, collectively known as frequency-dependent selection, happen when the fitness of a phenotype depends inversely on its frequency in the population. The classic example is Fisher's (1930) theoretical account of the sex ratio,[2] but Clark (1979) also stressed the importance of frequency-dependent selection to explain polymorphisms, behavioral and otherwise, in parasite-host and predator-prey systems. (See also Hori 1993.)

Returning to the unfamiliar domain of operant conditioning, a similar issue has puzzled some psychologists (e.g., Schwartz 1982): How can reinforcement generate or maintain behavioral variability if typically it strengthens the responses that produce it and increases their topographical stereotypy? Machado (1989, 1992) argued that most, if not all, animal studies on operant variability involved a strong form of frequency-dependent selection, for the reinforcement rule always favored the momentarily least likely response alternative. One example of this type of selection is the schedule used during the transition phases of the experiments reported above. (See bottom right panel of figure 2.3.) When reinforcement follows preferentially the responses that are rare or weak, then variability is increased or maintained.

More generally, we believe that the specific quantitative models developed by evolutionary biologists to understand the effects of different forms of natural selection—stabilizing, disruptive, directional, or frequency dependent, for example—are sources of inspiration that remain to be exploited by learning psychologists. The analogy can be used as a heuristic tool to understand *specific* issues in the domain of learning such as how fast preference is acquired, how behavioral variability can be an operant, or how and when molecular response patterns develop in choice situations (Machado and Keen 1999). By pushing the analogy to its limits we will eventually destroy it, for a time will come when our improved models will seize that which is distinctive in the learning domain, in the animal we study, in its current context and in its behavioral history. As the French philosopher Gaston Bachelard (1968, p. 119) once remarked, "intuitions are very useful: they serve to be destroyed.... The diagram of the atom proposed by Bohr a quarter of a century ago [equating it to a miniature solar system] has, in this sense, acted as a good image: there is nothing left of it." The analogy between evolution by means of natural selection and operant conditioning may play a similarly useful role even if in the end it will experience the same fate.

This chapter is dedicated to John Staddon, inspiring mentor and good friend. I [Armando Machado] keep many pleasant memories of my life as a graduate student in John's lab. Some of the most vivid of these memories are about our weekly laboratory meetings—caldrons of new ideas tossed in mostly by our mentor and brought to boiling point by the students. From my regular interactions with John, I came to appreciate his fresh, creative approach to a range of behavioral issues, and I was always amazed by the sheer ingenuity of his quantitative models. Although John and I tended to disagree on Skinner and other philosophical matters, I was always inspired by John's posture as a scientist. Thank you John for being such a wonderful mentor.

Notes

1. This approximation amounts to replacing the VI feedback function by its constant, asymptotic value. A more rigorous model would use the feedback function $r = 1/[\text{VI} + 1/(\lambda p)]$, where r is reinforcement rate, VI is the schedule parameter, λ is the animal's response rate, and p is the probability that it chooses the specific key under consideration. Whenever p is not too close to 0 or 1, r is approximately equal to 1/VI.

2. Fisher argued that the 50%–50% sex ratio is observed because it is the only stable equilibrium. In a population with a majority of females, for example, a genetic mutation that biases the sex of the offspring towards males is favored because males are more likely to reproduce under these conditions. Fisher's argument was recently confirmed by empirical analysis (Conover and Van Voorhees 1990).

3 Variation and Selection in Response Structures

Alliston K. Reid, Rebecca Dixon, and Stephen Gray

Thinking back, I believe I grew up in John Staddon's lab in the late 1970s. Earlier, when I was student in a learning course at Wofford College, my professor required us to select a "hero." Every week we were to present to the class at least one article written by our hero, and I had the luck to begin with Staddon and Simmelhag 1971. It required more than a week, but what a vision of behavioral research it provided! Behavior analysis was combined seamlessly with evolutionary processes, producing a fundamental reorganization of our understanding of traditional reinforcement theory! I took an independent research course with Staddon during summer school at Duke just before my senior year (to "prove myself" to him), and he asked me to write a paper on "Reinforcement as a Feedback Mechanism." This combination of engineering, evolutionary biology, and mathematics centered on the fundamental questions in behavior analysis made me passionate about working with Staddon.

Staddon's lab meetings were unlike any others I have experienced. His view of the experimental analysis of behavior was clear: The aim of behavioral analysis is the explanation of all the behavior of an organism in terms of a limited number of fundamental processes and their rules of interaction. The search for parsimonious mechanism was paramount and carried out with zeal. No mechanism could be incompatible with the haphazard fixes of natural selection. Parsimony was more important than attempts at complete explanations because parsimonious models could be tested, refined, or discarded faster than could complex explanations, thus maximizing the rate of scientific progress.

The research described in this chapter follows the same strategy: a difficult, ostensibly intractable, issue in behavior analysis is broken down into the most parsimonious mechanism(s) that we can identify. Then we see how much of the original problem it can explain without including additional assumptions. The problem of interest in this chapter is the internal structure of learned response sequences. This problem has often seemed intractable because extended training sometimes produces novel behavioral units, in which the response(s) strengthened by reinforcement seem to change into more complex units (see, e.g., Reid, Chadwick, Dunham, and Miller 2001). The obvious difficulty is: How can one model the effects of reinforcement on behavior if the affected behavioral structure changes? To explore and answer this question, we need to look carefully at the circumstances that produce new behavioral units.

What happens to learned response structures when reinforcement contingencies change? We are especially interested in the response structures known as behavioral units, although we are concerned with all structure. For example, the lever-press response in rats becomes a behavioral unit that functions to produce reinforcement in a variety of reinforcement contingencies. With extended training, complex patterns of lever presses or key pecks may become integrated into functional behavioral units (Fetterman and Stubbs 1982; Reed, Schachtman and Hall 1991; Reid et al. 2001; Schneider and Morris 1992; Schwartz 1981, 1982, 1986; Shimp 1982; Stubbs, Fetterman, and Dreyfus 1987; Thompson and Zeiler 1986). Some studies have been specifically designed to demonstrate that the observed response structures act as functional behavioral units. In many other studies researchers have observed high degrees of stability in response structure, even though they did not attempt to prove that behavioral units have developed (Catania 1971; Machado 1993, 1997; Neuringer 1992; Shimp 1982).

The processes responsible for variation and selection in response structures in stable and changing environments have long been elusive. The variability of well-learned sequences of lever presses or key pecks, for example, may be influenced by processes acting at the level of the entire response sequence (which we will call "sequence-level processes") or at the level of the individual operants that make up the sequence ("response-level processes"). The inference of a behavioral unit should require the existence of sequence-level processes. At the least, the term "behavioral unit" implies that the unit (as a whole) will have some degree of response strength (Baum 2002), which is often equated with sequence probability. A sequence-level process such as response strength was clearly implied by Schwartz (1981,

1982, 1986) when he found that complex behavioral units "maintained their integrity" when the reinforcement contingencies were shifted to extinction, or shifted to interval, ratio, multiple, and concurrent schedules that reinforced repetitions of the same behavioral patterns.

Several studies have demonstrated stereotypical behavioral units using a procedure that reinforced pigeons for pecking a two-dimensional stimulus array of lights (Pisacreta 1982; Schwartz 1981, 1982, 1986; Vogel and Annau 1973). Generally, pecks on one key move the light to the right, and pecks on the other key move the light down. Reinforcement is delivered when a particular light (say, at the bottom right location) becomes illuminated. The usual finding is that with extended training, most pigeons produce only a small subset of the large number of possible sequences that would result in reinforcement. These dozen or so sequences are inferred to be complex behavioral units because of the stability of the sequence probabilities from day to day and when shifted to reinforcement schedules that foster repetitions of that behavior pattern.

Does the *stability* of sequence probabilities mean that sequence-level processes are at work? Or, could response-level processes be responsible, sometimes masquerading as sequence-level processes? In the three sections that follow, we ask: What happens to learned response structures when reinforcement contingencies change? What processes produce stability of these response structures, or act to select a new pattern of behavior? We begin by discussing an elegant series of experiments by Allen Neuringer and his colleagues that asked these same questions and demonstrated this stability in response sequences when reinforcement contingencies were shifted to extinction. Then we describe two experiments from our lab that were designed to further identify the processes at work.

Reanalysis of Neuringer, Kornell, and Olufs 2001

In an elegant series of experiments, Neuringer, Kornell, and Olufs (2001) recently made a major contribution to our understanding of variability in response structure. They carried out three experiments, each involving two phases. In the first phase, sequences of three responses across three operanda were reinforced according to some schedule of reinforcement. Thus, 27 response sequences were possible. The second phase was always an extinction condition. They compared the ordering of the sequence probabilities generated under the reinforcement schedules with the ordering observed under extinction. They concluded that "the ordering of sequence probabilities was generally unchanged, the most common sequences during reinforcement continuing to be most frequent during extinction" (p. 79), and that learned response structures maintain their integrity even under extinction. This remarkable finding implies that the processes affecting the production of the response sequences may have acted at the level of the entire sequence, rather than on the individual responses making up the sequences. Yet, this conclusion would imply that each of the 27 sequences had its own independent probability or "sequence strength." It may be reasonable to assume that a few of the most frequent sequences had become complex behavioral units, but we doubted that all 27 sequences could simultaneously act as units. Keeping 27 *simple responses* separate would be a formidable discrimination problem—keeping 27 *sequences* of three responses separate would seem impossible, especially for rats. Some of the sequences were observed rarely, and reinforcement for these infrequent sequences was even less common. Therefore, the basis for their development into complex behavioral units is not clear.

Can these findings be explained parsimoniously without assuming sequence-level processes? Could response-level processes produce all these ordinal sequence probabilities; and if so, could we identify them? Could the ordering of sequence probabilities be explained without assuming that each sequence had response strength? Professor Neuringer graciously provided us with the data from the three experiments so we could carry out additional analyses.

VAR Condition

We began this analysis by searching for order in the response probabilities obtained in their group data. Figure 3.1 is a tree diagram calculated from the obtained sequence probabilities in the VAR condition of experiment 2 (Neuringer et al. 2001). Their experiment compared the sequence probabilities of two groups of rats exposed to two different reinforcement contingencies. The VAR condition reinforced variation in response sequences by providing food only when a variability criterion was met. The YOKE group received the same distribution of reinforcement, but they could obtain food by completing any sequences without regard to the variability criterion. When shifted to extinction, both groups produced nearly the same ordinal

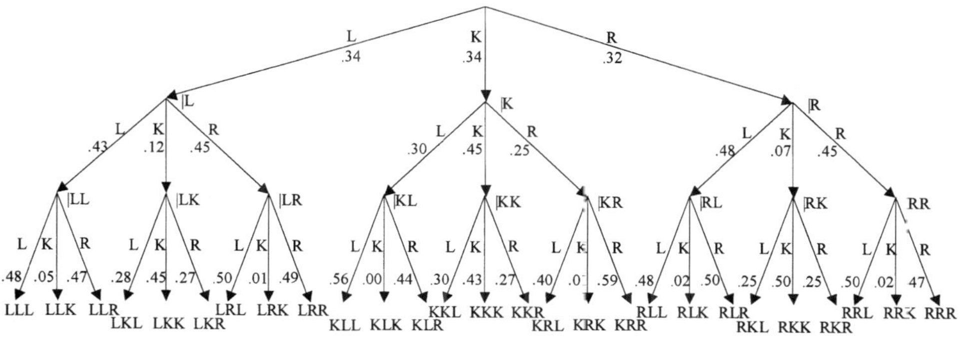

Figure 3.1

This tree diagram represents the sequence hierarchy obtained in the VAR condition of experiment 2 of Neuringer et al. (2001). The top of the tree represents the first response of the sequence, and the bottom represents completed sequences. Each number represents the obtained average conditional probability of a left (L) or right (R) lever press or key (K) response, given that the responses higher in that branch had already occurred.

sequence probabilities as they had under the previous reinforcement schedule. Considering only the VAR condition for now, figure 3.1 shows the obtained probabilities of each of the three responses (Left lever, Right lever, and Key) leading to the 27 sequences at the bottom of the figure.

Close examination of the tree diagram shows that it contained considerable redundancy and symmetry. We made several general observations:

1. Sub-trees were often symmetrical. All probabilities following initial Left and Right presses were remarkably similar (compare the left branch of figure 3.1 with the right branch). At each position in the tree, Left and Right lever presses produced similar probabilities, but Key produced a different probability in most sub-trees. This difference may be related to its location: the key was located on the back wall, whereas the left and right levers were adjacent to the feeder on the front wall.

2. The top tree (representing the selection of the first response in the sequence) had a uniform unconditional probability (~1/3) determined by end-of-trial cues (or cues signaling the beginning of the trial) such as food delivery or timeout. A uniform probability was an optimal solution to the VAR contingency because sequences beginning with L, R, or K would be equally probable, generating high levels of variability.

3. The entire tree diagram seemed to be composed of only three sub-trees, defined by the transition probabilities. By approximating each of the obtained probabilities, we obtained the following three sub-trees:

	Left	Key	Right	Example
Sub-tree A:	1/3	1/3	1/3	Top tree representing first response
Sub-tree B:	1/4	1/2	1/4	Following every choice of K
Sub-tree C:	1/2	$\sim 0^+$	1/2	Following every choice of L or R

Because of this redundancy and symmetry, a model including only these symmetrical sub-trees would be able to reproduce the entire tree to a reasonable approximation.

4. All transition probabilities, with the exception of the first choice, seemed to depend only on the selection of the preceding response. Left presses and Right presses were always followed by sub-tree C. Every Key response was followed by sub-tree B. This observation is similar to a first-order Markov chain. The operanda selected two responses back did not influence the probabilities of the third response in the sequence (i.e., the sub-trees at level three are the same as those at level two). Thus, there was no evidence for a second-order process.

5. Related to the last point, the tree provided no evidence that the rats distinguished between the second and third responses in the sequence because all transition probabilities of both depended only on the most recent response (they were both of the first order).

Clearly, the symmetry and redundancy observed in this condition may not exist under different reinforcement schedules or in apparatus with different operanda. As we examine other studies below, we identify several other response-level processes that are not apparent in the current experiment. The challenge is to find some parsimonious and systematic way of thinking about how all these response-level processes combine to produce the observed variation and selection of response sequences. We have found that a pseudo-Markov model (figure 3.2) is a useful way of thinking about the behavioral effects of a variety of response-level processes on response sequences in discrete trial studies. We identify differences between this pseudo-Markov model and a true Markov chain below. The purpose of this model is to show how a variety of response-level processes can affect a much smaller, fixed set of parameters governing sequence production. The

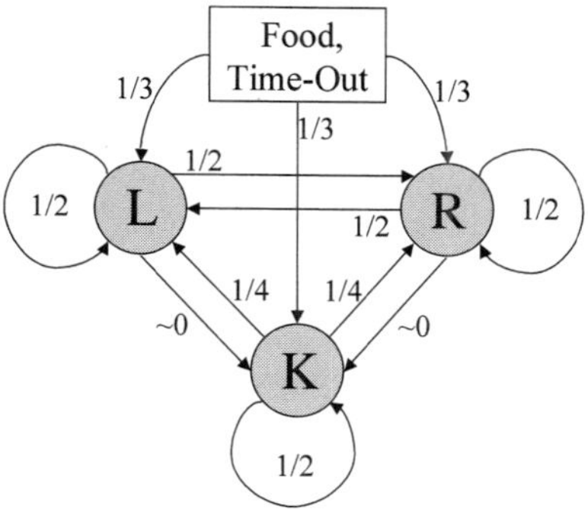

Figure 3.2
This state-transition diagram of a pseudo-Markov model summarizes the conditional transition probabilities between left (L) and right (R) lever presses and the key (K) response. The rectangle represents the stimulus effects of events such as food delivery and time-out that produce unconditional response probabilities. The numbers represent approximations of the values obtained in the VAR condition of experiment 2 of Neuringer et al. (2001).

model also allows us to test how well our simplifying assumptions (such as only three symmetrical sub-trees exist in the tree) characterize the data, because an adequate characterization should accurately reproduce the main findings of the experiments.

Figure 3.2 shows the pseudo-Markov model with the static probabilities listed above for each sub-tree. Sub-tree A is represented by the three identical unconditional probabilities (1/3) leading from the stimuli signaling the beginning of a new trial (Food, Time-out) to each of the three possible responses, L (left), R (right), and K (Key). As in a Markov chain, the probabilities represented by the other arrows are the conditional probabilities of a transition from one response to another, including perseveration on the same operandum. Sub-trees B and C (above) provided the values for these transition probabilities.

Even though this model is simpler than the tree diagram of figure 3.1, one can immediately see that some of the transition probabilities were equal to one another. Only four different probability values are represented in figure 3.2. Because of the symmetry observed in the tree diagram, we could add simplifying assumptions to this implementation of the model for this particular condition. That is, for the VAR condition, let

$p(\mathrm{L}|\mathrm{L}) = p(\mathrm{R}|\mathrm{L}) = p(\mathrm{L}|\mathrm{R}) = P(\mathrm{R}|\mathrm{R}) = 0.47$ (approximately 1/2),

$p(\mathrm{K}|\mathrm{L}) = p(\mathrm{K}|\mathrm{R}) = 0.06$ (approximately 0),

$p(\mathrm{L}|\mathrm{K}) = p(\mathrm{R}|\mathrm{K}) = 0.29$ (approximately 1/4),

and

$p(\mathrm{K}|\mathrm{K}) = 0.42$ (approximately 1/2).

At this point, we have identified the redundancy and symmetry in the tree diagram. We now ask: Can the pseudo-Markov model with only these four parameters reproduce the original ordering of the sequence probabilities observed under the VAR condition that were used to create the tree diagram? Figure 3.3 displays the answer.

The top panel of figure 3.3 compares the original VAR data with the *post hoc* predictions of the model. The model provides a good fit, even though there are small systematic errors. Nevertheless, the order and relative frequency of each sequence are approximately equal to the obtained values. They are as precise replications as we would be likely to obtain from any individual rat.

The usefulness of this conceptual model becomes apparent when we examine the effects of changing the contingency from the VAR condition to extinction. The central point made by Neuringer et al. (2001) was that the sequence hierarchy obtained under reinforcement conditions was approximately maintained under extinction. We would like to know how extinction affects response sequences: Are the effects of extinction equivalent to changing the values of the model's parameters? Or, are additional parameters necessary to account for the slightly altered relative frequencies of the response sequences?

The bottom panel of figure 3.3 shows how well the model fits the extinction data. The model has the same four transition parameters as in the VAR condition above, but we have assumed that extinction has slightly increased the probability of the Key response. Increasing the probability of the Key response naturally decreases other transition probabilities because they must sum to 1.0 for each response. We used the following four parameter values:

$p(\mathrm{L}|\mathrm{L}) = p(\mathrm{R}|\mathrm{L}) = p(\mathrm{L}|\mathrm{R}) = P(\mathrm{R}|\mathrm{R}) = 0.46$ (down from 0.47),

$p(\mathrm{K}|\mathrm{L}) = p(\mathrm{K}|\mathrm{R}) = 0.08$ (up from 0.06),

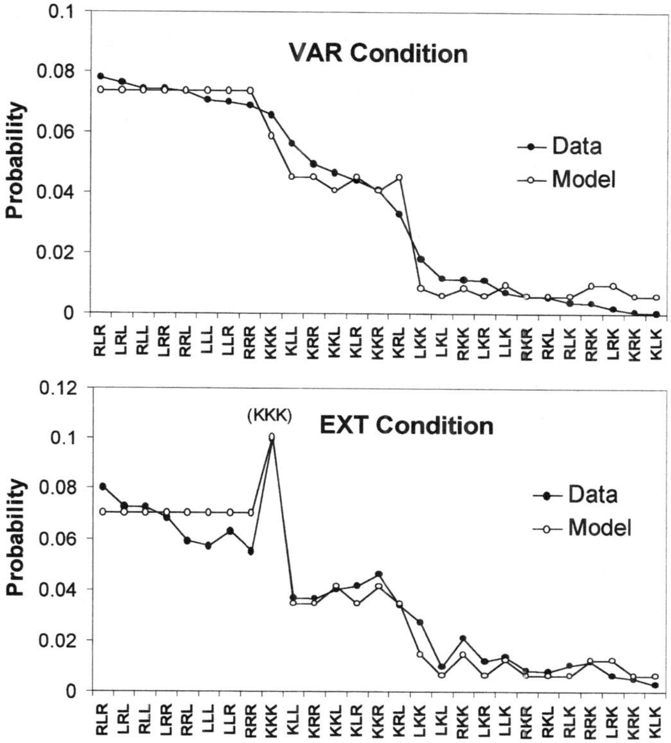

Figure 3.3
A comparison of the *post hoc* predictions of the pseudo-Markov model with the obtained sequence hierarchies from the VAR condition (top panel) and the predicted probabilities in the EXT condition (bottom panel) of experiment 2 of Neuringer et al. (2001).

$p(\mathrm{L}|\mathrm{K}) = p(\mathrm{R}|\mathrm{K}) = 0.225$ (down from 0.29),

$p(\mathrm{K}|\mathrm{K}) = 0.55$ (up from 0.46).

This model, using the same limited number of parameters (which reflect the symmetry observed in the VAR condition), does a good job of reproducing the sequence hierarchy and relative frequencies obtained under extinction—even though the model was not generated from the Extinction data. The model even reproduces the greatly elevated frequency of the sequence KKK observed in the data.

The model appears to be a useful way of thinking about how all these response-level processes combine to produce the observed variation and selection of response sequences. The model points out that the difference between the VAR and Extinction curves in Neuringer et al. 2001 can be explained by assuming that extinction slightly increases the probability of the Key response (a response-level process). This conclusion is consistent with the authors' observation that extinction tends to increase low probability activities: Pressing the key had the lowest probability of the three responses. We conclude that the ordinal sequence probabilities obtained in the VAR and Extinction conditions can be explained by response-level processes, without the conjecture of sequence-level processes.

YOKE Condition

Each rat in the VAR condition of Neuringer et al. (2001) was paired with a yoked partner that received the same distribution of reinforcement but without a variability criterion. The Yoke animals were permitted to vary their sequences but they were not required to do so. The questions of interest were (a) whether this more permissive reinforcement contingency would maintain the ordering of sequence probabilities when shifted to extinction as those observed in the VAR condition; and (b) whether similar increases in variability would occur during extinction.

Figure 3.4 is a tree diagram calculated from the obtained sequence probabilities in the YOKE condition. Close examination of the diagram shows that it also contains redundancy and symmetry, but less than that observed in the VAR condition. We make three general observations:

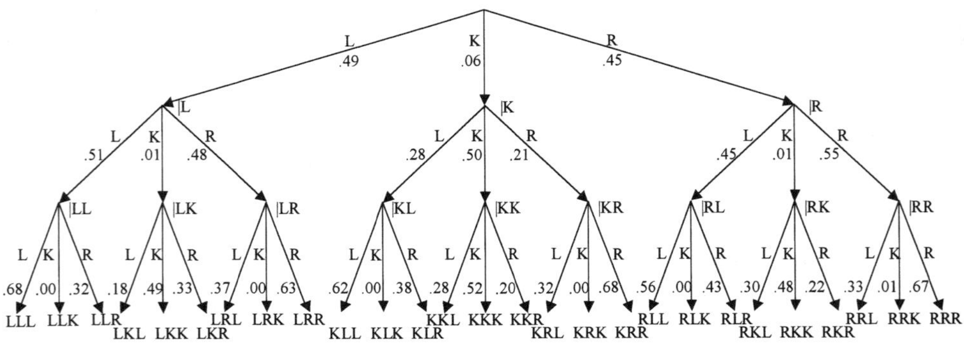

Figure 3.4
This tree diagram represents the sequence hierarchy obtained in the YOKE condition of experiment 2 of Neuringer et al. (2001).

1. There appeared to be at most four sub-trees because most sub-trees contained approximately the same transition probabilities. By approximating each of the obtained probabilities, we obtained the following four sub-trees:

	Left	Key	Right	Example
Sub-tree A:	1/2	$\sim 0^+$	1/2	Top tree representing first response
Sub-tree B:	2/3	$\sim 0^+$	1/3	Following L in third position
Sub-tree C:	1/3	$\sim 0^+$	2/3	Following R in third position
Sub-tree D:	1/4	1/2	1/4	Following every choice of K

Sub-trees B, C, and D appeared to reflect a simple tendency to persist on the same operandum last selected but otherwise avoid the Key.

2. The bias toward perseveration was stronger in the third response position than in the second position. This observation is important because it implies that a simple first-order process would not be sufficient: we needed to consider either a second-order process or non-stationary transition probabilities that would depend on the current position within the sequence.

3. The probabilities of each response in the third response position did not depend upon the particular sequence of the two previous responses, but only on the last response. Therefore, there was no longer any reason to consider a second-order process (for this data set). A simpler approach was to assume that the probability of repeating a response depended upon the number (1 or 2) of responses already produced. This implied that transition probabilities were not stationary: prob(persist) = f(position in the sequence). Since this data set provided only two points in the response sequence involving non-stationary probabilities (the second and third positions), it was not possible to determine the underlying function. Therefore, we did not attempt to derive the function; instead, we simply represented the two positions by their obtained transition probabilities (sub-trees B and C) and acknowledge that the second and third response positions differed in the tendency to repeat the last response.

The observations above provided all the details necessary to see if the pseudo-Markov model would be a useful method of combining each of the response-level processes that appeared responsible for the ordering of response sequences in the YOKE condition. The redundancy in the tree diagram allowed us to represent all response probabilities as four sub-trees. Thus, this condition required one more sub-tree than did the VAR

Table 3.1
Parameter values for the YOKE condition in Neuringer, Kornell, and Olufs 2001.

Sub-tree	Description	Response	YOKE	Extinction
A	Unconditional probabilities for first response	Left Key Right	0.49 0.06 0.45	0.4 0.24 0.36
B	Probability of second response given initial response of L or R (Probabilities of L and R were reversed following L or R.)	Left Key Right	0.5295 0.001 0.4695	0.5295 0.001 0.4695
C	Probability of third response given an initial response of L or R (Probabilities of L and R were reversed following L or R.)	Left Key Right	0.6395 0.001 0.3595	0.5995 0.001 0.3995
D	Probability of second or third response given a previous response of K	Left Key Right	0.25 0.5 0.25	0.25 0.5 0.25

condition, because the probability of persisting on a lever was greater in the third response position than in the second position. Sub-trees B and C represent these different levels of persistence. Table 3.1 provides the parameter values for both the YOKE condition and for the subsequent Extinction phase.

The top panel of figure 3.5 compares the model's *post hoc* predictions with the relative frequencies obtained in the YOKE condition. The good fit by the model implies that our identification of the response-level processes and their influence on response probabilities at each position in the sequence were adequate to reproduce the observed sequence hierarchy.

The bottom panel of figure 3.5 compares the model's predictions with the data obtained when the YOKE group was switched to extinction. Again, the model fits the data well, even though our simplifying assumptions were generated from the YOKE data, rather than the Extinction data. The model helps us recognize that the difference between the YOKE and Extinction curves in Neuringer et al. 2001 can be explained by assuming (a) that extinction slightly increases the low probability of the Key response in the first response position (sub-tree A) and (b) that the increasing tendency to persevere on the left or right levers in the second and third response positions of the YOKE condition (the difference between sub-trees B and C) was not as strong during extinction.

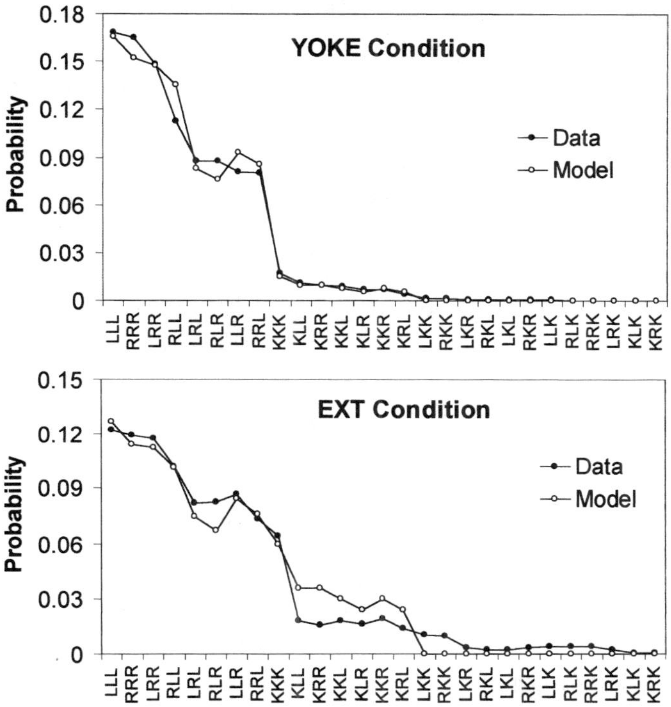

Figure 3.5

A comparison of the *post hoc* predictions of the pseudo-Markov model with the obtained sequence hierarchies from the YOKE condition (top panel) and the EXT condition (bottom panel) of experiment 2 of Neuringer et al. (2001).

We conclude that the ordinal sequence probabilities obtained in the YOKE and Extinction conditions can be explained by response-level processes, without the conjecture of sequence-level processes.

Summary

Our reanalysis of Neuringer et al. 2001 has been helpful in two main ways toward understanding of the processes responsible for variation and selection of response structures. It has demonstrated that the processes responsible for variation and selection of the response sequences observed in each condition (measured by the ordinal sequence probabilities) can be attributed to identifiable response-level processes, without the necessity to postulate sequence-level processes. Response-level processes masqueraded as sequence-level processes. The authors identified some of these response-level processes and some are new: the tendency to avoid the key, the tendency to repeat the same response just emitted, the tendency to treat left and right lever presses the same (the symmetry in the sub-trees), and the tendency to produce more low-frequency responses during extinction.

The second benefit of this analysis is the creation of a conceptual, "pseudo-Markov" model that allows many response-level processes to act on a smaller, fixed set of parameters. Even though this model resembles a Markov chain, it is designed specifically for response sequences in discrete-trials procedures, which violate requirements of formal Markov chains. For example, stationary Markov chains are of fixed order. Yet in a discrete-trials procedure, the first response in a sequence must always be of order zero, since no response has occurred since food was delivered. The second response can be at most of the first order, since only one response has occurred that could have an influence. The third response could at most be of the second order, and so on. Unlike true Markov chains, our pseudo-Markov model allows reinforcement to "reset" the model's state through unconditional probabilities. Transition probabilities do not all have to be the same order, and some may be stationary while others are non-stationary. The model is based on the branching process used to create the descriptive tree diagrams of figures 3.1 and 3.4. The model provides a framework with the flexibility to allow many response-level processes to act in concert on a smaller, fixed set of parameters. It is most useful when we can show that a process affects a particular parameter, such as a particular transition probability or stimulus effect. We have identified some of these response-level processes above, but the list is far from complete.

This model provides a conceptual framework for us to examine additional response-level processes in the next two sections, which describe two experiments designed to further identify the processes responsible for the variation and selection of response structures.

Experiment 1: Effects of Reinforcing a New Target Sequence

Our central question concerned what happens to response structures when reinforcement contingencies change. So far, we have examined only shifts to extinction. When the reinforcement contingencies change in other ways, other processes might affect the variation and selection of response structures. In this experiment, we implemented Reid's (1994) modification of the repeated acquisition procedure (Thompson 1973). We trained eight rats to complete a particular three-response sequence on two levers for several weeks until the accuracy of each trial was stable. Then we exposed them to the "split-session" condition, which imposed two different sequence contingencies in each session. Subjects earned the first 30 reinforcers by producing the training sequence, just as in training sessions. Then the target sequence was changed without warning to another three-response sequence, selected at random, for the remainder of the session. Sessions lasted until either 150 pellets were delivered or 90 minutes had elapsed. During each session, every lever press caused all three panel lights to blink off for 0.3 second. Reinforcement followed the correct completion of the target sequence. A 5-second timeout, with panel lights off, followed incorrect sequences of three responses. No feedback was provided within a trial to indicate correct or incorrect responses. This daily procedure was repeated until all subjects were exposed to every new target sequence twice. Thus, each phase lasted for 16 daily sessions. This procedure was repeated for all subjects in subsequent phases in a balanced Latin square design, with each phase involving a different training sequence.

The design of this experiment provided three situations in which we could look for response-level processes within the same sessions of the split-session condition: in training trials preceding the switch to a new target sequence, such as the last 10 trials before the switch, in extinction trials (trials after the switch but before the subject had been reinforced for successfully completing the new target sequence, and in trials in which subjects had been reinforced for producing the new target sequence—a combination of extinction and reinforcement effects.

This experiment asked two questions: Is there a relationship between the type of training sequence and the errors produced during training? Are the response positions in the sequence equally sensitive to the change in contingency? By utilizing only two levers instead of the three operanda used by Neuringer et al. (2001), we were also able to test Catania's (1971) hypothesis that response strengths of repeated instances of the same operant class should summate. That is, when subjects are trained to complete a (say) Left-Left-Right sequence, the response strength for pressing the left lever should not depend only on its position in the sequence. Instead, the response strength of the first left press should (approximately) sum with the response strength of the second left press because they are two instances of the same operant class. This summation should result in a subsequent probability of selecting Left that is not determined exclusively by its position in the sequence. When incorrect sequences are produced, a disproportionately large number should share the same dominant response as the training sequence.

We began our analysis by asking the question: Were each of the response positions in the sequence equally sensitive to the change in contingency? This question may be answered by examining the persistence of responding (resistance to change) in each position as a function of the response required in the new target sequence. The top panel of figure 3.6 shows how the persistence of responding in each position depended upon whether the same or a different response was required in that position in the new target sequence. The vertical line represents the trial in which the thirtieth pellet was delivered. Points to the left of this line represent responding before the shift to the new target sequence, and points to the right represent the persistence in responding after the shift. Filled symbols represent trials in sessions in which the new target sequences required the *same* response in the first, second, or third position as that required by the training sequence. No change in behavior was required for each of these response positions, and persistence declined only slightly. Open symbols represent trials in sessions in which the new target sequences required a *different* response in the first, second, or third position than that required by the training sequence. Subjects showed less persistence (equivalently, less resistance to change) in the third response position (closest to food) than in any other response position. This effect can be observed by the more rapid decrease in the curve with open circles than in the other curves.

At first glance, the persistence curves of figure 3.6 seem to indicate a graded degree of persistence as a function of position in the sequence (first > second > third). However, the sensitivity of each response position should be represented by the difference in height between the "Same" curves and the "Different" curves (i.e., "First Same" minus "First Different"; "Second Same" minus "Second Different", etc). The bottom panel of figure 3.6 presents this sensitivity measure for the first 70 trials after the transition to a new target sequence. The third response position (closest to food) was clearly more sensitive to changes in the contingency than were the other response positions, which did not differ from one another. Contrary to in-

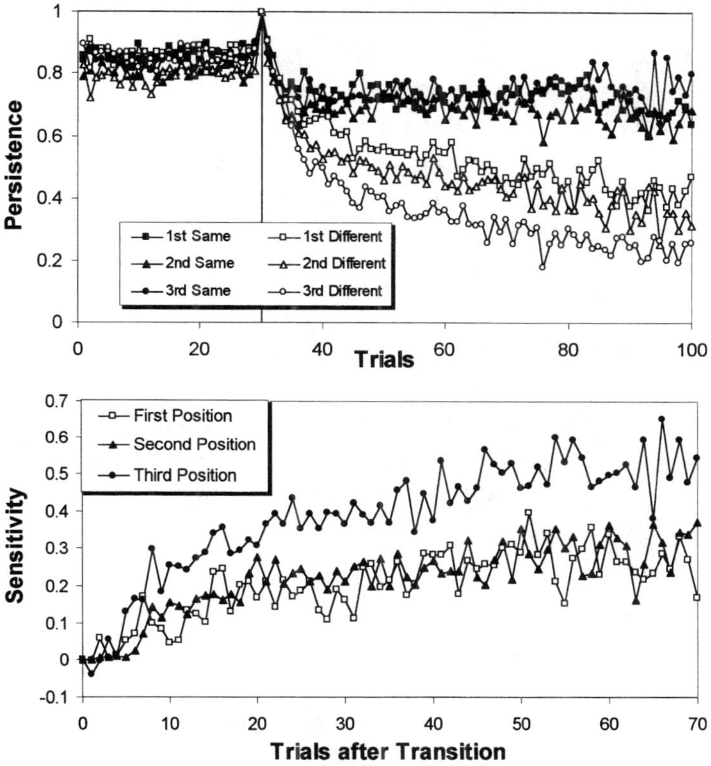

Figure 3.6
The top panel shows how the persistence of responding in each position of a three-response sequence depended upon whether the *same* or a *different* response was required at that position in the new target sequence. Filled symbols represent trials in sessions in which the new target sequence required the *same* response in the first, second, or third position as that required by the training sequence. Open symbols represent trials in sessions in which the new target sequence required a *different* response in the first, second, or third position than that required by the training sequence. The bottom panel shows the sensitivity of each response position to the change in contingency.

tuition, the response position closest to reinforcement was the least resistant to change.

Differential sensitivity to the change in contingency of response position in the sequence may be a powerful response-level process (or, more likely, a combination of different extinction and reinforcement processes). In an experiment similar to the current one, Reid (1994) demonstrated that the response position closest to reinforcement was the first to change. That is, when rats were switched to a new target sequence requiring a different response in only the first or the last position of the sequence, the last response position showed less persistence and greatest sensitivity to the change in the contingency (faster learning of the new sequence). The current results replicate and extend Reid's findings. The new target sequences in Reid (1994) always differed from the training sequence by only one response (in the first or last position). However, in the current study, new target sequences differed by one, two, or all three responses. The current results extend Reid's (1994) findings by clearly demonstrating differential sensitivity of response position even when the new target sequence is extensively different from the training sequence.

The most common response-level process postulated in response sequences is that reinforcement differentially strengthens responses closer in time to reinforcement than those less contiguous—a relation often described as the delay-of-reinforcement gradient. Accordingly, the persistence of responding at each position in the sequence (resistance to change) should differ when subjects are shifted to extinction. Researchers have disagreed on the effects of extinction because shifts to extinction involve both the previous strengthening effects of reinforcement and the weakening effects of non-reinforcement. For example, Fantino and Logan (1979) provided a clear prediction of one effect: "In a complex chain . . . if the delivery of the food pellet were discontinued, the whole chain should be extinguished. The lever-press, the last response in the sequence, should be the last response to extinguish." (p. 171) The authors went on to propose a general principle: "In general, responses at the end of the chain are most readily acquired and are most resistant to extinction." (p. 173) Even though the data depicted in figure 3.6 directly contradict this prediction, Nevin, Mandell, and Yarenski (1981) did observe greater resistance to change in the terminal links of chain schedules than in the initial links when subjects were provided with extra food in the home cage or within the session. Nevertheless, other researchers such as Williams (1999) and Williams, Ploog, and Bell (1995) have observed a backward progression of extinction in chain schedules. This implies that the last response in the sequence (or chain schedule) is the first to change in extinction, and the first response is the last to change.

The current experiment allows us to measure the effects of extinction on each response position within the sequence for each subject separately. For each session, we counted the number of trials after the transition to a new target sequence until that subject made changes in the first, second, or third response positions. Because changes may be influenced by stochastic factors, we decided not to restrict our count to the first change in that response position. Instead, we maintained separate counters for the first, third, sixth, and tenth change in each response position. In order to isolate extinction effects from the effects of reinforcing new sequences, reinforced trials were not included.

This analysis is shown in figure 3.7. These data are compatible with a backward progression of extinction. When exposed to extinction, the first

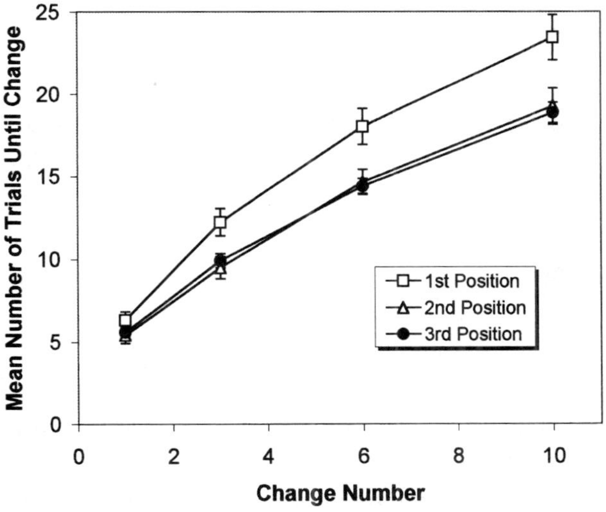

Figure 3.7
The mean number of trials after the transition to a new target sequence until subjects made changes in the first, second, or third response positions of the training sequence. Separate counters were maintained for the the first, the third, the sixth, and the tenth change in each response position. Reinforced trials were not included in these counts.

response position required more trials before the response changed (i.e., before the subject switched from the response learned during training to the other lever) than that required for changes in the second and third positions (which did not differ from each other). These data are compatible with the assumption that backward progressions of extinction are produced by systematic decrements in response strength at each position, but an alternative explanation is possible. Our extinction trials produced end-of-trial cues, namely time-out, which could act as a discriminative stimulus to set the occasion for the first response in the sequence. These cues would be present for the first response in the sequence, but not for the second or third response positions. The elevated persistence observed in the first position in figure 3.7 may have been due to the additional effects of the discriminative stimulus, rather than due to the decremental effects of extinction on response strength at each position within the sequence (Williams et al. 1995). Unfortunately, the design of this experiment does not allow us to rule out either potential explanation, but experiment 2 (below) explicitly examines the effects of end-of-trial cues in discrete-trials procedures.

Error Analysis

Even though subjects were exposed to the Training condition until stability criteria were met, errors in the production of the sequences occurred. Were response-level processes responsible for this variability? Was there a relationship between the type of training sequence and the errors produced? The answer is "Yes" to both questions. We examined the errors made in several ways. We began by creating tree diagrams (figures 3.1 and 3.4) to identify redundancy and symmetry, as we had observed in the data of Neuringer et al. (2001). But we found that we could not simplify the trees —the trees were not composed of a small number of redundant sub-trees, and the probabilities of left and right presses in each sub-tree were usually not symmetrical.

Catania (1971) helps explain the lack of redundancy and symmetry in our tree diagrams by identifying a response-level process in operation in his sequences. Our subjects were trained to complete a three-response sequence on two different levers. Therefore, every sequence had to contain at least two presses of the same lever. Catania (1971) demonstrated that the response strengths of discriminated operants occurring in different positions of a sequence contribute independently to subsequent responding. Thus, when a sequence contains more than one instance of the same operant class (e.g., two left lever presses), the response strengths of the two instances of this operant (left press) approximately summate. Therefore, when subjects are trained to complete a Left-Left-Right sequence, the subsequent probability for pressing the left lever would not depend exclusively on its original position in the sequence. Instead, the response strength of the first left press is approximately added to the response strength of the second left press, resulting in a subsequent probability of selecting left that is not determined exclusively by its previous position in the sequence. If Catania's (1971) hypothesis is correct, then errors in sequence production should strongly favor sequences that share the same dominant response as the training sequence.

To test Catania's (1971) hypothesis, we compared the number of incorrect sequences occurring during training (in the ten trials in all split sessions before the shift to a new target sequence) that shared the same dominant response to those that favored the other (different) lever. Because we were interested in errors, we disregarded all correct sequences. Thus, three possible sequences remained that shared the same dominant response, and four possible sequences contained repetitions on the other lever. The left side of figure 3.8 shows the proportion of trials generated during training that shared the Same or Different dominant response as the training sequence. We have simplified description of the sequences in order to eliminate redundancy. Thus, "AAA" represents all LLL and RRR sequences; "ABA" represents all LRL and RLR sequences; "ABB" represents all LRR and RLL sequences; and "AAB" represents all LLR and RRL sequences. The "AAA" sequences are not shown because errors rarely occurred during these training sequences. The left side of figure 3.8 shows that the proportion of incorrect sequences that shared the *Same* dominant response as the training sequence was substantially greater than the proportion favoring the *Different* response. This powerful effect was observed even though there were fewer "Same" sequences to "choose" from than "Different" sequences (three versus four). Thus, Catania's (1971) hypothesis is strongly supported.

This response-level process explains why the tree diagrams were not symmetrical. The probabilities of left and right presses in sub-trees were not equal because their probabilities were not independent in each position in

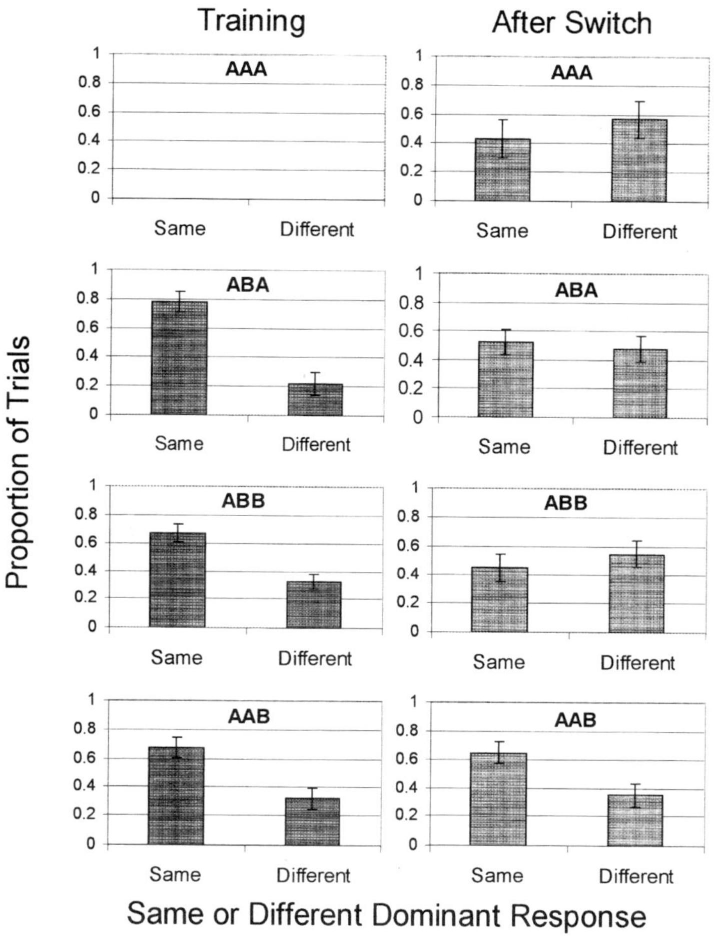

Figure 3.8

The proportion of trials containing incorrect sequences sharing the *same* or *different* dominant response as the training sequence occurring in split sessions before (left panels) or after (right panels) the switch to a new target sequence.

the sequence. Requiring subjects to repeat the same operant within a sequence complicates the tree and makes the relation between response strength and position in the sequence more difficult to ascertain.

The right side of figure 3.8 shows the same analysis, but in the ten extinction trials following the switch to a new target sequence (in the same sessions as in the left side of the figure). Sequence AAB continued to produce incorrect sequences sharing the same dominant response as the training sequence, but this effect did not occur in the other three types of sequences. This difference may be due to slower learning after training on AAB. Reid (1994) demonstrated that when rats were trained to complete AAB then shifted to a new target sequence, learning occurred slower than with other training sequences. (See also McElroy and Neuringer 1990; Neuringer 1991.)

Was the accuracy of responding equal at each position in a sequence? To answer this question, we again examined the ten trials in all split sessions before the shift to a new target sequence. The graphs on the left side of figure 3.9 show that accuracy did depend upon the position in the sequence, but it also depended strongly on the type of training sequence. Errors during training were rare in all positions for sequence AAA. Accuracy increased systematically as the sequence progressed in sequence ABB, but accuracy decreased systematically in sequence AAB.

The right side of figure 3.9 shows the proportion correct across the three response positions occurring in the first ten extinction trials following the switch to a new target sequence. Proportion correct in this situation was based on the requirements of the training sequence, even though the sequence was no longer reinforced. The pronounced decrease in accuracy across sequence AAB observed in training was also observed in the extinction trials following the switch. The overall pattern of accuracy with each sequence type generally replicated that observed during the training trials, but with slightly more variability during extinction.

ABB versus AAB

We have just seen two ways in which the sequences ABB and AAB have been surprisingly different. Figure 3.8 showed that Catania's (1971) hypothesis about response strength (above) played an important role in sequence generation following the shift to new target sequences for AAB, but not for ABB. And figure 3.9 showed that the accuracy at each position

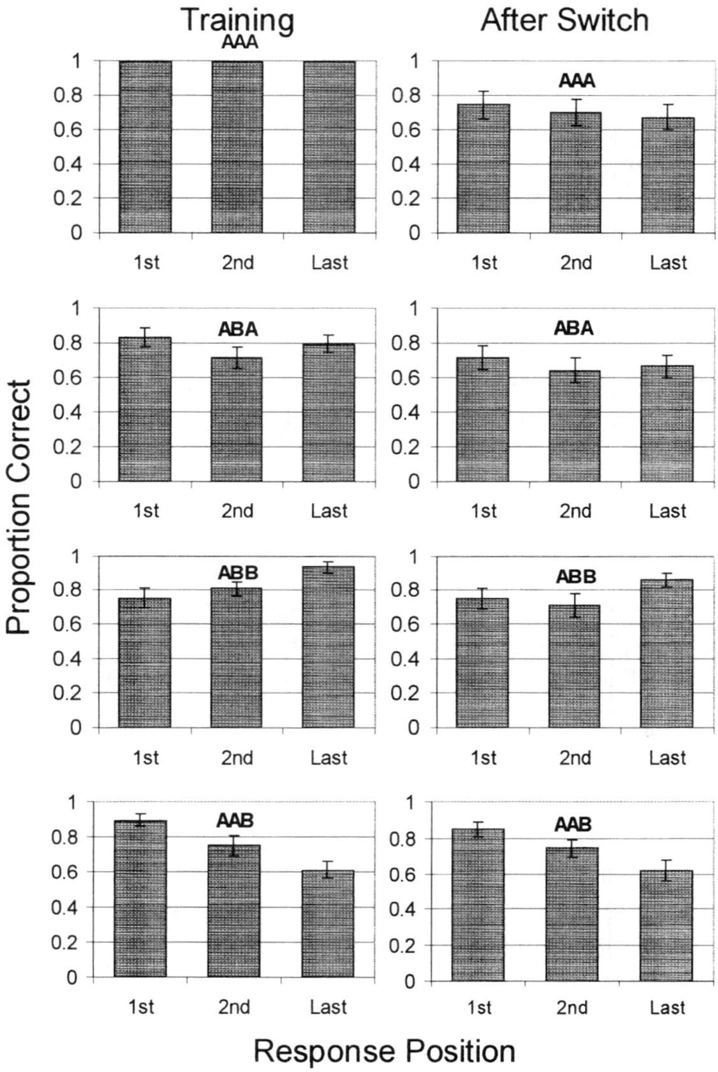

Figure 3.9
The proportion of correct responses in the first, second, or third response position in the sequence before (left panels) or after (right panels) the switch to a new target sequence, based on the requirements of the training sequence.

Table 3.2
Comparison of the types of incorrect sequences occurring when trained to complete AAB or ABB. These training sequences were correlated with statistically significant ($p < 0.05$) increases or decreases in the frequency of particular sequences. AAB and ABB often had opposite effects on the production of incorrect sequences.

Training sequence	Incorrect sequence	Effect	Mean no. of trials	$x^2(6)$
AAB	AAA	↑	41	140.9
ABB		↓	9	19.5
AAB	ABA	↑	39	59.5
ABB		↓	1	94.3
AAB	BAB	↓	8	42.1
ABB		↑	29	102.5
AAB	BBB	↓	7	38.4
ABB		↑	42	209
AAB	BBA	↓	6	63
ABB		↓	5	51.9

was an increasing function of position in the sequence for ABB, but a decreasing function for AAB. Reid (1994) had earlier demonstrated that rats learn new target sequences faster when previously trained on ABB than when training on AAB. Why would these sequences have such different effects when they seem so similar? The sequences have more in common than not: they share the same first and last responses and both require a single changeover from one lever to the other—they differ only in the position of this changeover within the sequence.

In addition to the differences above, we also found that the errors that occurred after extended training on the two sequences differed considerably and reliably. Errors were not random—they depended strongly on the training sequence. We counted the number of incorrect sequences of each type occurring in the last 20 training trials in all split sessions for each training sequence. Table 3.2 identifies those incorrect sequences that were highly probable and those that were improbable. Training on ABB and AAB often had opposite effects on the types of incorrect sequences produced during training. Training on AAB produced significantly more sequences of AAA, ABA, BAB, and BBB; training on ABB produced significantly fewer of those same sequences. Yet opposing effects were not always observed. The two training sequences showed two similarities: The probabilities of producing sequence BBA were significantly lower than average with both training sequences, and when trained to complete AAB, subjects frequently produced ABB (and vice versa). (See also McElroy and Neuringer 1990; Neuringer 1991.)

Summary

Experiment 1 identified several response-level processes that influence the variation and stability of response sequences:

- The degree of persistence of responding in each position in the sequence depended upon whether the same or a different response was required in the new target sequence.
- When exposed to extinction, the first response position required more trials before the particular response changed than that required for changes in the second and third positions.
- The proportion of incorrect sequences that shared the *Same* dominant response as the training sequence was substantially greater than the proportion favoring the *Different* response (Catania's hypothesis).
- The accuracy of responding at each position in a sequence depended upon the position in the sequence, but it also depended strongly on the type of training sequence.
- Even though the sequences ABB and AAB appear to be more similar than different, they produced surprisingly different effects. Some of these effects may be explained *post hoc* by the response-level processes identified above (particularly Catania's hypothesis), but the experiment did not specifically test these explanations.

Experiment 2: Effects of Degrading End-of-Trial Cues on Sequence Variability

The list above of response-level processes is clearly incomplete. In the discussion above, we alluded to a process that may help explain some of the unanswered questions about the source of incorrect sequences observed above. In discrete-trials procedures, each trial terminates with end-of-trial cues such as food delivery or timeout. When subjects are shifted to extinction conditions or required to complete a new target sequence, these end-of-trial cues may be degraded—trials no longer terminate with food delivery (Williams et al. 1995). Therefore, position in the sequence may not have as much stimulus control over responding—the subject may not begin the sequence correctly or may "get lost" in the sequence. Experiment 2 tested this hypothesis by systematically manipulating the cues terminating sequences in a discrete-trials procedure. We asked: How does degrading end-of-trial cues influence which sequence is generated next? How does this effect depend upon characteristics of the training sequence? To answer these questions, we exposed six naive rats to six phases with two conditions in each phase: baseline training and probe sessions. In the baseline training condition, each subject learned to complete a single three-response sequence on two levers until responding stabilized and accuracy exceeded 80 percent for five consecutive days (requiring 14–52 days). Experiment 1 had indicated that two of the eight possible three-response sequences, LLL and RRR, might produce too little variation to be informative in this study. Therefore, we restricted the training sequences to the six remaining sequences. The six subjects were trained to complete each of the six sequences in separate phases presented in a balanced Latin square design. Sessions ended after 100 pellets were delivered or 150 trials were completed. Each lever press pulsed the three panel lights off for 0.3 second, and no feedback was provided within a trial about the accuracy of responding. Correctly executed sequences resulted in the presentation of a tone for 0.3 second and the delivery of a food pellet. Incorrect sequences resulted in 10-second timeout with the panel lights off, and the tone was not presented. Thus, the tone was an end-of-trial cue that was always paired with correctly executed sequences and food delivery.

Following baseline training, subjects were exposed to daily probe sessions for 7–16 days per phase. The contingencies were generally the same during probe sessions as during baseline training. However, every twelfth correctly executed sequence served as an unreinforced probe trial that degraded the end-of-trial cues in either of two ways: (a) the brief tone was presented but no reinforcement was delivered ("tone probes"), or (b) neither the tone nor reinforcement were presented ("no-tone probes"). The brief tone was presented randomly on half of these unreinforced probe trials. We were interested in the sequence that the subject produced following reinforced trials and these two types of probe trials. Our question was "How do end-of-trial cues influence the next sequence generated?"

Degrading the end-of-trial cues in probe trials produced systematic reductions in the accuracy of the subsequent trial in all subjects. The baseline accuracy of trials with normal end-of-trial cues in probe sessions averaged 81.5 percent across subjects. Probe trials ending with the brief tone but without food delivery reduced accuracy on the subsequent trial to 64.6 percent. Probe trials with neither the tone nor food delivery reduced accuracy to 52.0 percent. Much of the reduction in accuracy was due to a failure to begin the next sequence with the correct response in the first position. When an incorrect sequence was produced following tone probes, 61.9 percent had an error in the first position of the sequence. This value increased to 73.3 percent following no-tone probes. Some of these errors in the first position were produced by inappropriately repeating the last response of the probe trial (tone probes: 62.2 percent; no-tone probes: 70.1 percent).

Figure 3.10 shows how errors in sequence production depended upon the training sequence. It shows how the incorrect sequences were distributed over the seven remaining possible sequences for the three conditions in the probe sessions (trials ending normally with tone and food, tone probes, and no-tone probes). Each training sequence produced a distinctive pattern of errors in all three conditions. Thus, errors were not generated at random—rather, they depended on characteristics of the training sequences. When end-of-trial cues were degraded, each training sequence produced a similar distribution of errors across sequence types as that observed when end-of-trial cues were intact. We infer from this observation that the processes responsible for generating incorrect sequences were qualitatively the same in all three conditions. Degrading end-of-trial cues did increase the number of incorrect sequences (in ways identified above), but other processes appear to be responsible for the overall pattern of errors observed for each type of training sequence.

In experiment 1, we found that Catania's (1971) hypothesis about the summation of response strengths was a powerful response-level process influencing the production of sequences. We could determine whether this process was important in this experiment. Did those sequences requiring two responses on the same lever produce errors that also had two responses on the same lever? Figure 3.11 shows this relation for each subject and each sequence type (i.e., ABB, AAB, ABA) for both types of probe trials. Catania's (1971) hypothesis was supported in 33 of 36 situations.

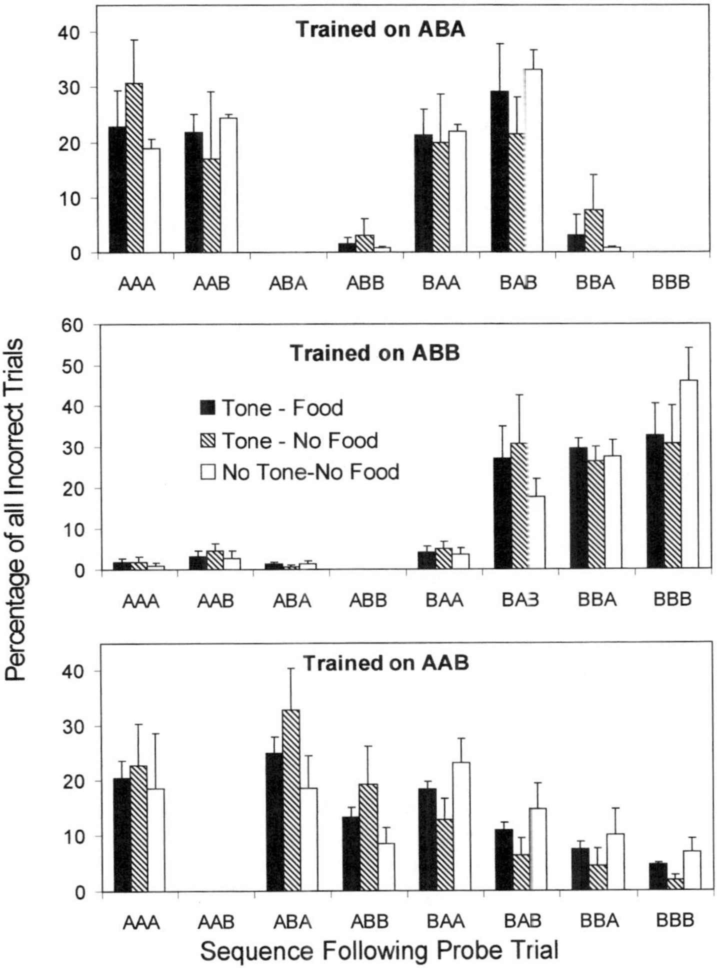

Figure 3.10
The training sequences produced different distributions of incorrect sequences as end-of-trial cues were manipulated in three conditions.

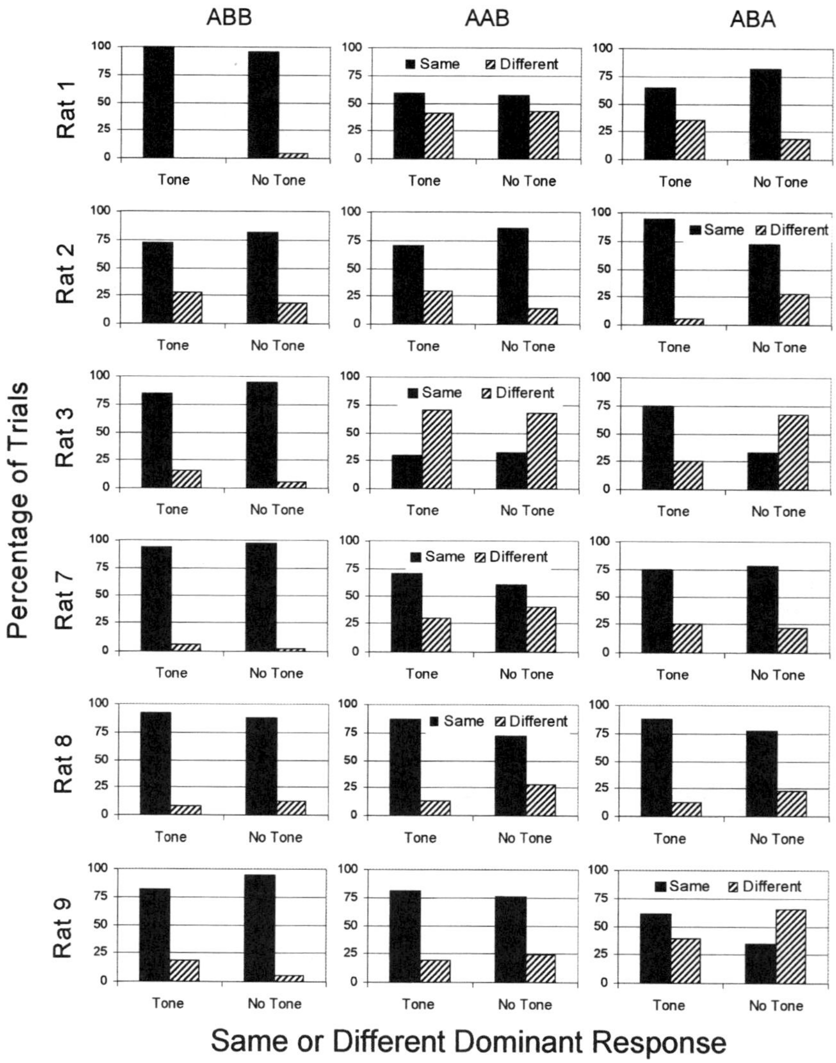

Figure 3.11

The percentage of trials containing incorrect sequences sharing the *same* or *different* dominant response as the training sequence following two types of probe trials for each subject and each type of training sequence. Training sequences requiring two responses on the same lever produced sequence errors that also had more responses on that lever than on the different lever.

Sequence ABB showed the strongest effect: for all subjects nearly all of the incorrect sequences following both types of probe trials contained two or more "B" responses. The same, but reduced, effect was observed for five of six subjects following sequence AAB (Rat 3 was the exception). Following sequence ABA, all subjects showed the effect in probe trials ending with the tone, and four of the six rats showed the effect following no-tone probes. With this ABA sequence, all subjects (particularly Rats 3 and 9) also showed a strong tendency to continue alternating on the levers (producing the sequence BAB; see figure 3.10), especially when the end-of-trial cues were most degraded. We conclude that the summation of response strengths was a powerful response-level process influencing the subsequent generation of sequences in both situations of degraded end-of-trial cues.

Summary

Each training sequence produced a distinctive, highly predictable pattern of errors. The patterns of errors observed in this experiment were the same as those observed in experiment 1. Errors were not generated at random. The errors did depend upon characteristics of the training sequence. The relation between the training sequence and the incorrect sequences produced was not based on simple sequence-level processes such as generalization across sequences or some similarity/dissimilarity metric. That is, they were not simply a function of the number of changeovers required or the position of a changeover in the sequence. Degrading the end-of-trial cues had two main effects: It produced approximately the same types of incorrect sequences as those observed when the cues were intact. This observation implies that normally occurring errors may be caused by failure to correctly identify the end of a trial (or failure to properly begin the next trial)—a problem of stimulus control. These errors depended upon the training sequence in two simple ways: They shared the most frequent response of the training sequence, and many had errors in the first position produced by inappropriately repeating the last response of the preceding probe trial. Both of these factors are response-level processes, rather than sequence-level processes. Thus, response-level processes were responsible for the variation and selection of response sequences when end-of-trial cues were intact and when they were degraded.

Conclusions

We have now examined three situations in which the processes responsible for variation and selection of response structures in stable and in changing environments were response-level processes rather than sequence-level processes. In each case, sequence-level processes appeared at first glance to be implicated, but we discovered that response-level processes were ultimately responsible. For example, Neuringer et al. (2001) demonstrated that the hierarchy of individual sequence probabilities established during reinforcement conditions was generally maintained during extinction. This observation is consistent with the hypothesis that each sequence had become a behavioral unit, with its own strength independent of the strengths of the constituent responses. However, we have shown that identifiable response-level processes were sufficient to explain the stability of the sequence hierarchy, so an assumption that each sequence had its own response strength was unnecessary.

Sequence-level stability may be produced by response-level processes. Sequence-level processes may not necessarily be involved. Therefore, the observation of stability in sequence probability (e.g. Neuringer et al. 2001; Pisacreta 1982; Schwartz 1981, 1982, 1986; Vogel and Annau 1973) should not be a sufficient criterion to conclude that each sequence has become a behavioral unit with its own strength. Stability across situations (Zeiler 1986) is not sufficient to demonstrate that a sequence has strength because response-level processes acting on arbitrary responses may be responsible for the stability. The classification of a sequence as a behavioral unit should imply the involvement of sequence-level processes. Even though response probability may be a suitable measure of response strength for simple operants, sequence probability is *not* a sufficient measure of strength of complex response sequences. Any sequence will have some probability even though it may not have strength independent of its constituent responses.

Complex behavioral units involving sequence-level processes do exist. They have been demonstrated in a variety of reinforcement contingencies and species. For example, Fetterman and Stubbs (1982) and Schneider and Morris (1992) (see also Shimp, Fremouw, Ingebritsen, and Long 1994; Stubbs et al. 1987) reinforced sequences of two responses in a reinforcement schedule in which matching of response sequences was pitted against matching of individual key pecks. With extended training, matching was obtained with response sequences rather than with individual key pecks. Sequence matching was a clear example of a sequence-level process. Reid et al. (2001) (see also Reed et al. 1991) demonstrated the development of complex behavioral units by showing how inter-response times (IRTs) between lever presses became organized around sequence boundaries when the boundaries were demarcated or not. This temporal organization of behavior reflects sequence-level processes.

It is easy to imagine situations in which the formation of complex behavioral units would be highly adaptive. For example, in a stable environment that reinforces a consistent pattern of behavior, the formation of complex units may be an effective way of maximizing reinforcement rate. If the reinforcement schedule is changed in such a way as to reinforce multiple instances of the same behavioral pattern (such as a ratio schedule), it may not be surprising that the pattern maintains its integrity (Pisacreta 1982; Schwartz 1982, 1986), whether sequence-level or response-level processes are ultimately responsible. It has not been clear, however, what happens to the unit when the reinforcement schedule changes in such a way that this behavioral pattern no longer produces the highest reinforcement rate. This chapter has examined situations of this type: shifts to extinction, to a new target sequence, and situations in which end-of-trial cues were degraded. Even though organisms may form complex behavioral units, it appears that animals adapt to these changing contingencies through a combination of response-level processes, rather than through processes that maintain the strength of the complex behavioral unit.

The processes acting on the individual response are more easily observed in sequences composed of unique operant responses, rather than sequences requiring the repetition of responses in the same operant class. This is because reinforcement may act on each response independently, so repetitions of responses may produce (approximate) summation of their subsequent response probability (Catania 1971; Catania et al. 1988). This was a powerful effect observed in experiments 1 and 2 (e.g., figures 3.8 and 3.11). The simplicity of the symmetrical, redundant tree diagrams of Neuringer et al. (2001) existed because they used a different operandum for each response in the sequence. In future studies, researchers may want to provide separate operanda for each response to ensure the independence of responses.

The pseudo-Markov model described above is not proposed as a well-developed behavioral model. Rather, it is a useful conceptual framework to see how a variety of response-level processes can act *in combination* to influence the stability and variability of response structures by their effects on a fixed, limited set of parameters. For example, we found that changes in particular conditional transition probabilities were sufficient to reproduce the main findings of Neuringer et al. (2001). The results of experiment 2 were due to changes in the effectiveness of end-of-trial cues (or equivalently, beginning-of-sequence cues), which are represented in the model as the unconditional response probabilities resulting from the discriminative stimuli beginning a sequence. The pseudo-Markov model provides a useful conceptual framework for understanding the combination of processes producing variability and selection of response sequences. Importantly, it helps us understand that the study of reinforcement's effects on behavioral patterns may not be intractable after all. The model may allow us to identify the point (within an experiment and within individual subjects) in which response-level processes can no longer account for behavioral patterns, and sequence-level processes will demonstrate that new behavioral units have developed.

We began by asking: How can one model the effects of reinforcement on behavior if the affected behavioral structure changes? The formation of complex behavioral units from simpler reinforced operants may be an infrequent occurrence, occurring substantially less often than we had assumed. Over the last century, chaining theory had encouraged us to view learned response sequences as highly ordered and inflexible, so the "problem" of the behavioral unit was viewed with trepidation. Yet the research literature contains relatively few clear demonstrations of the formation of new complex units. (For a review, see Reid et al. 2001.) We now know that chaining theory was wrong in the way it implied that sequence order would be inflexible. Terrace and his colleagues (Straub and Terrace 1981; Swartz, Chen, and Terrace 1991; Terrace 1984) have repeatedly demonstrated the adaptive way in which pigeons and monkeys can skip to later positions in the series when "links" of the chain have been removed. Thus, our attention on the *stability* of response structures may have been excessive—the ability to *vary* behavioral patterns (even well practiced patterns) appears to be a more common and more adaptive characteristic of learned serial behavior.

Acknowledgments

Special thanks to David Allen at Eastern Oregon University for our wonderful conversations about Markov chains and the modeling of data from discrete-trials procedures.

Experiment 1 was part of Rebecca Dixon's senior thesis at Eastern Oregon University. Portions of these data were presented at the Annual Meeting of the Association for Behavior Analysis in 1998. Experiment 2 was part of Stephen Gray's senior thesis at Wofford College. Portions of these data were presented at the Annual Meeting of the Association for Behavior Analysis in 1999.

4 Control of Response Variability: Call and Pecking Location in Budgerigars (*Melopsittacus undulatus*)

Kazuchika Manabe

Variability is necessary to the evolution of species. One kind of variability is polymorphism. The functional basis of polymorphism is frequency dependent selection in which an infrequent type within a species has a survival advantage over a more frequent type. (For an example involving fish, see Hori 1993.) Variability in behavior is also necessary for shaping novel responses in operant conditioning (Mazur 1998). One procedure to reinforce novelty is frequency-dependent reinforcement (Staddon 1983). In this procedure, only a response that is different from a previous response is reinforced (e.g., Machado 1989; Morris 1989; Neuringer 1991; Page and Neuringer 1985). Various response topographies have been shown to be sensitive to frequency-dependent reinforcement. For example, key-peck, lever-press, and chain-pull response sequences can be differentially reinforced in rats (Morgan and Neuringer 1990), beaching, flipping, tail-walking, and tail-slapping in dolphins (Pryor, Haag, and O'Reilly 1969), and block-building in children (Goetz and Baer 1973).

Frequency-dependent reinforcement can be used to produce novel vocal response in small birds too. The first half of this chapter introduces several methods for differentially reinforcing various calls in budgerigars. The last half shows that pecking location of budgerigars can also be brought under the control of frequency-dependent reinforcement.

Control of Call Variability

Vocal plasticity in birds depends on whether vocal learning within a species is open-ended or closed-ended. Open-ended learners, such as canaries and starlings, can modify their vocalizations throughout adulthood. (See Chaiken, Bohner, and Marler 1983; Nottebohm 1984; Nottebohm and

Nottebohm 1978; Waser and Marler 1977.) On the other hand, closed-ended learners, such as white-crowned sparrows and zebra finches, learn their song during a sensitive period shortly after birth and show little or no change throughout adulthood (Nordeen and Nordeen 1992; Price 1979). Vocal learning in the open-ended learners can be affected by social factors (Baptista and Petrinovich 1986; King and West 1989; Marler 1990, 1991; West and King 1996). For example, black-capped chickadees converge their different calls into a common call if they are placed together in a flock (Mammen and Nowicki 1981; Nowicki 1989). The same convergence was found in budgerigars (Farabaugh, Linzenbold and Dooling 1994). An African gray parrot's complex vocal behavior has been shaped by social reinforcement involving human trainers (Pepperberg 1993). In addition to social factors, operant reinforcement can be effective in modifying vocal behavior. (For a review, see Adret 1993.) The following section presents methods of training vocal behavior in birds including the frequency-dependent reinforcement technique developed by Manabe, Staddon, and Cleaveland (1997) and Manabe and Dooling (1997).

Training Call Variability

In these experiments the training of variability in vocal behavior involved two different methods: one-template training or selective reinforcement of a particular call-type (Manabe and Dooling 1997) and differentiation of calls or reinforcement of call variation (Manabe et al. 1997). In the first method, only calls that were within a defined range of similarity with regard to a specific template call were reinforced. With this training, call variability decreased. In the second method, calls that were outside a defined similarity range with regard to the previous *N* reinforced calls were reinforced. Training with the second method increased variability in the obtained call types. These procedures are described below.

The subjects in these experiments were adult male budgerigars (*Melopsittacus undulatus*). The birds were obtained from a local pet supplier and maintained in aviaries either at Duke University or at the University of Maryland. Each bird was caged separately. The birds had free access to water and grit in their home cages. During these experiments, the birds were maintained at 90 percent of their free-feeding weights.

Birds were trained in a small experimental chamber (typically 14 centimeters wide, 12 centimeters high, and 17 centimeters deep) constructed of wire mesh and mounted in an acoustic chamber. An electret condenser microphone was used to record and monitor vocal behavior. A food hopper containing millet was mounted on the floor.

The output of the microphone was sent to a digital signal processing (DSP) board. Call recognition was based on serial power spectra calculated using the fast-Fourier-transform (FFT) or zero-crossing method. (For details, see Manabe 1997; Manabe and Dooling 1997; Manabe et al. 1997.)

After the birds were habituated to the experimental chamber and reliably ate from the feeder when it was raised, manual shaping of vocalizations began. Typical sounds from the large aviary were played in the test chamber to initiate calling. Whenever the birds called back to the aviary tape, the experimenter raised the feeder. When birds began to emit calls reliably in the absence of playback calls, the calls were reinforced automatically.

Selective Reinforcement of Calls

After several sessions in which all incoming signals were classified as contact calls and were reinforced, a typical call was selected as a "template" call. This was done using multidimensional scaling (MDS: SYSTAT for Windows Version 5.0, Wilkinson 1988). First, a matrix of similarity values from all the calls in a session was constructed and scaled using MDS. Similarity was quantified between any two calls in terms of the relative overlap of 20 successive power spectra (for details, see Manabe 1997; Manabe and Dooling 1997; Manabe et al. 1997). In the resultant two-dimensional plot, the center call in the largest call-cluster was selected as the template.

In the next phase, calls were reinforced only when the call was similar enough to the template call. In this phase, four light-emitting diodes signaled the onset of a trial, and trials were separated by a 2-second inter-trial interval. Vocalizations occurring during inter-trial intervals were not reinforced and prolonged the onset of the next trial by 1 second. For a call produced during a trial, similarity was calculated in real time as described above with the similarity criterion initially set at a very low value so that even calls that were minimally similar to the template were reinforced. As the bird's performance improved (i.e., more calls met the criterion), the criterion was gradually increased.

MDS plots of calls and the template for one bird (Kanae) are shown in figure 4.1. The top panel plots the last 37 calls obtained in the first template training session. The bottom panel shows the last 37 calls obtained in the

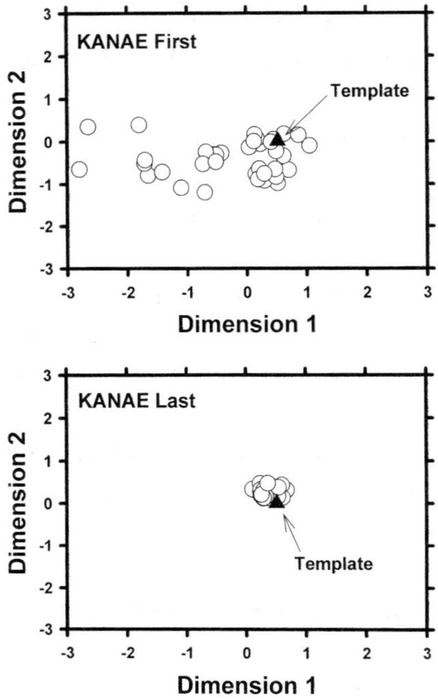

Figure 4.1
Two-dimensional MDS plots for calls of subject Kanae in the first session (top) and the last session (bottom) of template training. Closed triangles indicate the template call. Open circles indicate calls produced by the budgerigar. The calls analyzed were the last thirty seven calls in each session and the template call. Those calls in the first and the last sessions were calculated at the same time. On the MDS plot, similar calls are plotted closely. Adapted from Manabe and Dooling 1997.

last training session. Open circles indicate calls produced by the bird and the closed triangle the template call, respectively. Calls in the last session are distributed close to the template call, whereas calls in the first session are distributed over a broader area. These data show that template training decreased the variability of calls.

Differentiation of Calls, or Reinforcement of Call Variation

To differentiate calls, a frequency-dependent, or *N*-back, reinforcement procedure was used. Here, *N* refers to the number of preceding, reinforced calls that a current call had to be different from in order to produce food reward. So, in a one-back condition, a call was reinforced only when it was different from the last reinforced call. In the beginning, calls were reinforced even if the current call was only a little different from the previously reinforced call. When most calls met the criterion, the difference criterion was gradually increased. At the end of the condition, calls were reinforced only if the current call was quite different from the previously reinforced call. In a two-back condition, birds were required to make a vocalization that was different from the two previously reinforced vocalizations. So, birds needed to make at least three different vocalizations to get food in the two-back condition.

In a reinforcement-based *N*-back procedure, such as described above, the minimum number of call types required for a bird to consistently receive reinforcement is $N + 1$. As N increased, the number of call types that birds produced did in fact increase. Figure 4.2 shows MDS plots of calls produced by a budgerigar trained in a one-back and then in a two-back condition. Each symbol indicates each call that the bird made, and the plots were based on a quantitative measure of similarity between calls. (See Manabe and Dooling 1997; Manabe et al. 1997.) The upper panel shows calls obtained from the last session of the one-back condition. The middle panel shows calls obtained from the first session of the two back condition, and the bottom panel shows calls obtained from the last session of the two-back condition. In the one-back condition, the bird produced two distinct clusters of calls, indicative of two general call types. When the condition was shifted from one-back to two-back, one of the two clusters (distributed on the right area on MDS plot) came to be more broadly distributed in the first session of the two-back condition. This suggests an increased variability among calls formerly belonging to a single call cluster. In the last session of the two-back condition, three distinct clusters of calls are now evident. One unchanged from the one-back condition and two others created by the break-up and divergence of the second, original call cluster.

Pecking Location: A Replication of Call Experiments

In the call experiments, variability of calls was successfully controlled by both differential reinforcement of a specific call and a frequency-dependent reinforcement procedure. The present section shows that variability of pecking location can also be controlled by reinforcement contingencies (Manabe and Kawashima 2001, 2002).

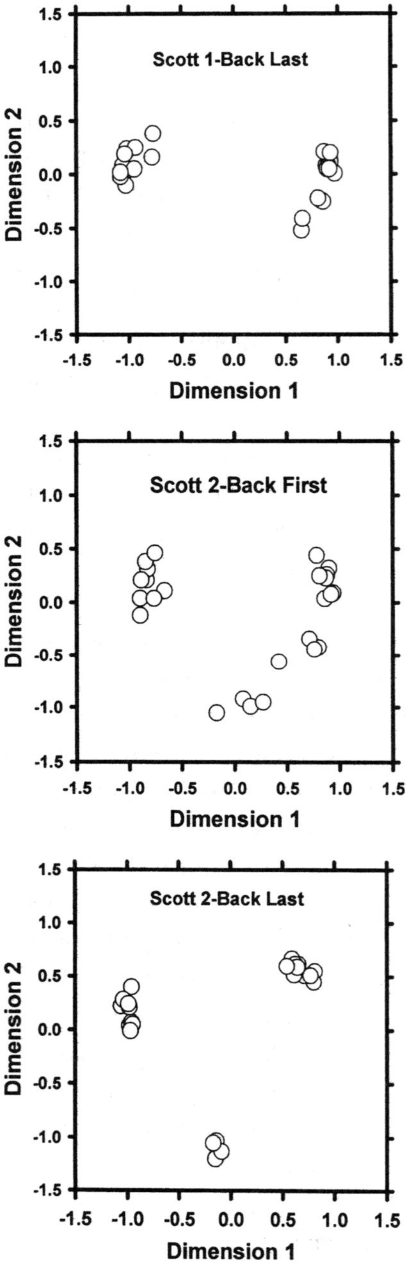

Figure 4.2
Two-dimensional MDS plots for calls of subject Scott in the last session of one-back (top), the first session of two-back (middle), and the last session of two-back (bottom) conditions. Open circles indicate calls produced by the budgerigar. Adapted from Manabe, Staddon, and Cleaveland 1997.

Subjects and apparatus were almost the same as in the call experiments, except that a touch screen was used instead of a microphone. (For a description of the touch screen system, see Morrison and Brown 1990.) A liquid-crystal monitor with touch screen was placed against the front panel of the chamber that had a 12-by-12-centimeter opening. The budgerigars could peck the surface of screen through the square opening. When the screen was white, the birds were required to peck the screen surface to get food.

After shaping the pecking response to the screen surface, budgerigars were trained in two different *N*-back procedures. In the first procedure, a peck was reinforced when it was made to locations that were more than a pre-defined distance from the previous pecked *N* locations (response-based *N*-back). This response-based contingency was formally the same as those previously reported in the literature (e.g., Machado 1989; Morris 1989; Neuringer 1991; Page and Neuringer 1985). In the second *N*-back procedure, a peck was reinforced when it was made to locations that were greater than a pre-defined distance from the previous, *reinforced N* locations (reinforcement-based *N*-back). The reinforcement-based *N*-back procedure was the same as the *N*-back contingency described earlier for the call experiments.

In both *N*-back procedures, subjects could get food by increasing the number of locations pecked as *N* increased. For example, pecking to the left area (L) and pecking to the right area (R) could be reinforced in both one-back conditions. However, for $N > 1$ the reinforcement-based *N*-back was a more stringent criterion. In the two-back condition, subjects had to peck three different areas in the reinforcement-based *N*-back procedure in order to obtain food reward. In the response-based *N*-back procedure, response patterns, such as a peck to a different location after a repetition of the same location (e.g., LLR) would produce reinforcement, as well as pecking in three different areas. The distance criterion for reinforcement was gradually increased within a given *N*-back training bout. After the mean distance among pecking locations was stabile, *N* was increased.

Figure 4.3 shows the last session in the response-based one-back condition (the top panel), the first session in response-based two-back condition (the second panel from top), the twentieth session in response-based two-back condition (the third panel from top) and the last session in response-based two-back condition (bottom panel). Each symbol indicates a single

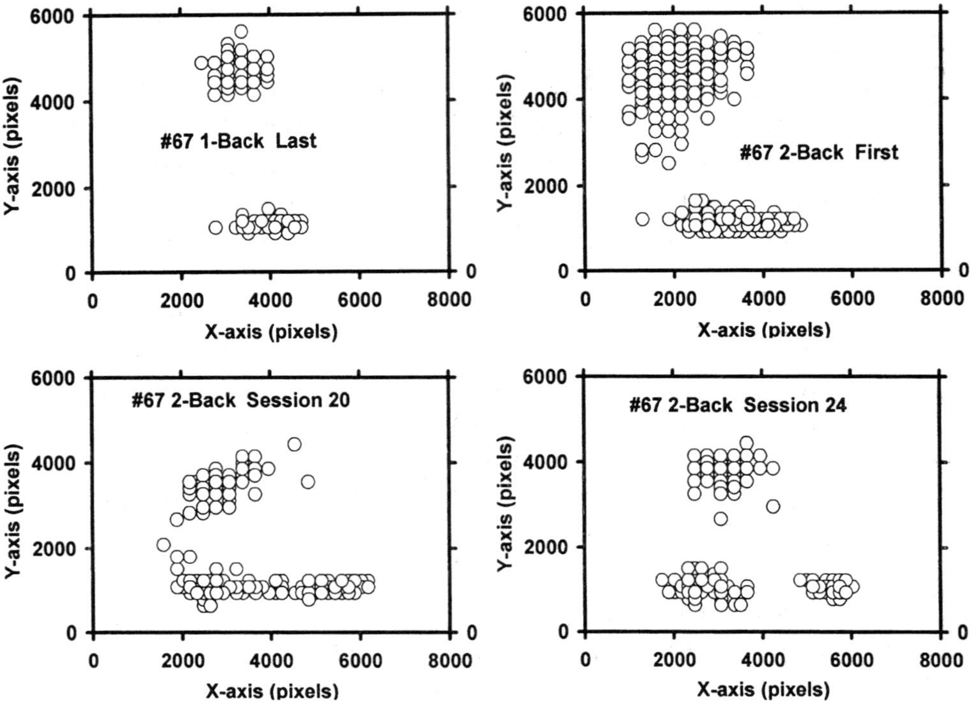

Figure 4.3
Pecking location on the screen in the last session of one-back (top), the first session of two-back (second), the twentieth session of two-back (third), and the last session of two-back conditions (bottom) in the response-based condition. Open circles indicate locations pecked by the budgerigar. The values of pixel on both axes are matched to the number of dot on the computer screen. Adapted from Manabe and Kawashima 2002.

peck, and the location in the plot gives the pecking location. At the end of the one-back condition, the bird pecked two different areas, top and bottom on the screen. When the condition was shifted from one-back to two-back, pecking location came to be more broadly distributed. In the last session of the two-back condition, the subject was pecking a top area and two different areas that clustered at either end of the region at the bottom of the screen. A similar result was found in the *N*-back call experiment.

In the three-back condition, only three different areas were pecked in the response-based condition. (See upper panel in figure 4.4.) On the other

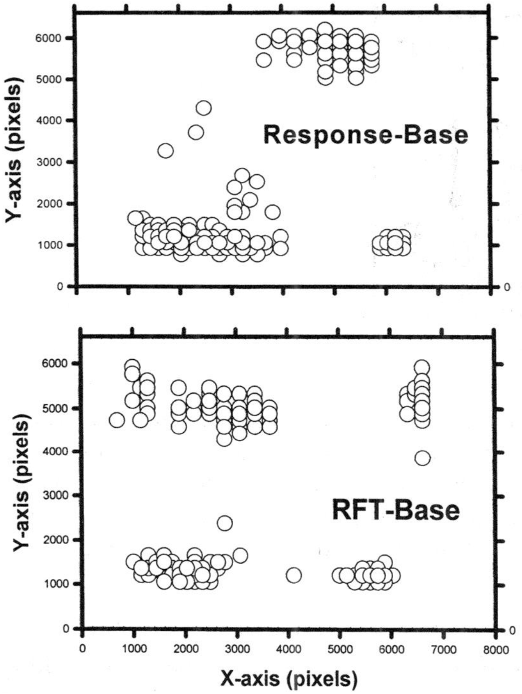

Figure 4.4
Pecking location on the screen in the last session of the response-based three-back condition (top) and the last session of the reinforcement-based three-back condition (bottom) for the same budgerigar. Open circles indicate locations pecked by the budgerigar. Adapted from Manabe and Kawashima 2003.

hand, birds came to peck four different areas in the reinforcement-based three-back condition. (See lower panel in figure 4.4.)

Figure 4.5 concerns the response-based three-back condition for one subject. It shows the bird's pecking location and the conditional probability of switching to a different peck location or staying in the same peck location given a peck at each pecked location. These probabilities are indicated by the numbers on the plots and by the relative thickness of the lines. A, B, and C denote different clusters that the subject pecked. The probability of a peck to the B location after a peck to the C location was 0.97, and after a peck to the A location it was 0.82. These probabilities indicate that the subject almost always pecked the B location after pecks to the A and C locations. The probability of a peck to the A location after a peck to the B

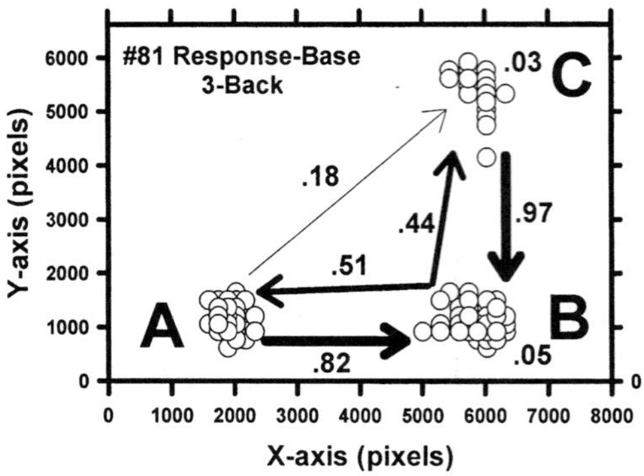

Figure 4.5
Pecking location on the screen in the last session of the response-based three-back condition. Open circles indicate locations pecked by a budgerigar. Numbers in the plot denote the conditional peck probability. Bold lines indicate higher probability, thin lines lower probability, respectively. A, B, and C denote different clusters that subjects pecked. See text for details. Adapted from Manabe and Kawashima 2002.

location was 0.51, while pecks to the C location after pecks to B was 0.44. About half of pecks after a peck to the B location were made to A and C locations. The probability of a peck to the C location after a peck to the A location was only 0.18. There were no pecks to the A location after a peck to C. The probability of a repeat peck to B was 0.05 and that to C was 0.03. There were no repeat pecks to the A location. These data indicate that the subject developed a relatively fixed response pattern—a pattern of alternating B pecks randomly intermixed with A and C pecks. Other birds showed similar fixed response patterns. Such response patterns could get food in the response-based three-back condition. In a three-back condition with a BABC response pattern, the last peck to the C location was reinforced. With the BCBA response pattern, the last peck to the A location was reinforced.

Figure 4.6 shows pecking location in ascending order from continuous reinforcement (CRF) to a four-back condition and returning in order back to CRF in a reinforcement-based condition (Manabe and Kawashima, in preparation). Subjects produced at least $N+1$ pecking locations in the reinforcement-based N-back procedure. The number of pecking areas increased from one to many in the ascending order. In the descending order, the number of packing locations decreased except for the transition from the two-back to the one-back condition. The number of pecking areas was three in both the two-back and one-back conditions. A hysteresis effect was found.

General Discussion

In the vocalization studies, one-template training increased the similarity between calls and the template call and decreased variability (figure 4.1). On the other hand, reinforcement-based *N*-back training increased call variability (figure 4.2). As with other response topographies, budgerigars' calls are sensitive to selective reinforcement and frequency-dependent reinforcement by food. These results indicate that food reinforcement, like social reinforcement in a budgerigar flock, is effective for modifying calls. A similar process was found in both call and pecking location topographies. This result suggests that the reinforcement contingency works for both responses in the same manner.

In the response-based three-back procedure, subjects adopted fixed patterns of pecking instead of increasing the number of pecking locations to get food (figure 4.5). On the other hand, in the response-based two-back procedure, subjects increased the number of pecking locations. (See bottom of figure 4.3.)

In the response-based condition, at least two dimensions of a response, namely pecking location and response pattern, can be used to get food. According to a functional definition, both adopting a response pattern and increasing the number of pecking locations are the same operant that leads to the same consequence (Skinner 1972). However, the question of why the same response-based procedure with different *N* did not affect different response dimensions in the same way remains to be answered.

In a study with humans, Christopher and Neuringer (2002) simultaneously reinforced varying three dimensions of drawing of a rectangle—area, shape, and location. When variability of one dimension was reinforced, variability of the other dimensions also increased. In the present response-based two- and three-back procedures, however, subjects were sensitive to only one of two dimensions at the same time. One possible explanation for this difference may be the following: In the study by Christopher and Neuringer (2002), varying the response in three dimensions was simultaneously reinforced. Subjects already had a response repertory in three dimensions. On the other hand, in the present response-based *N*-back procedure,

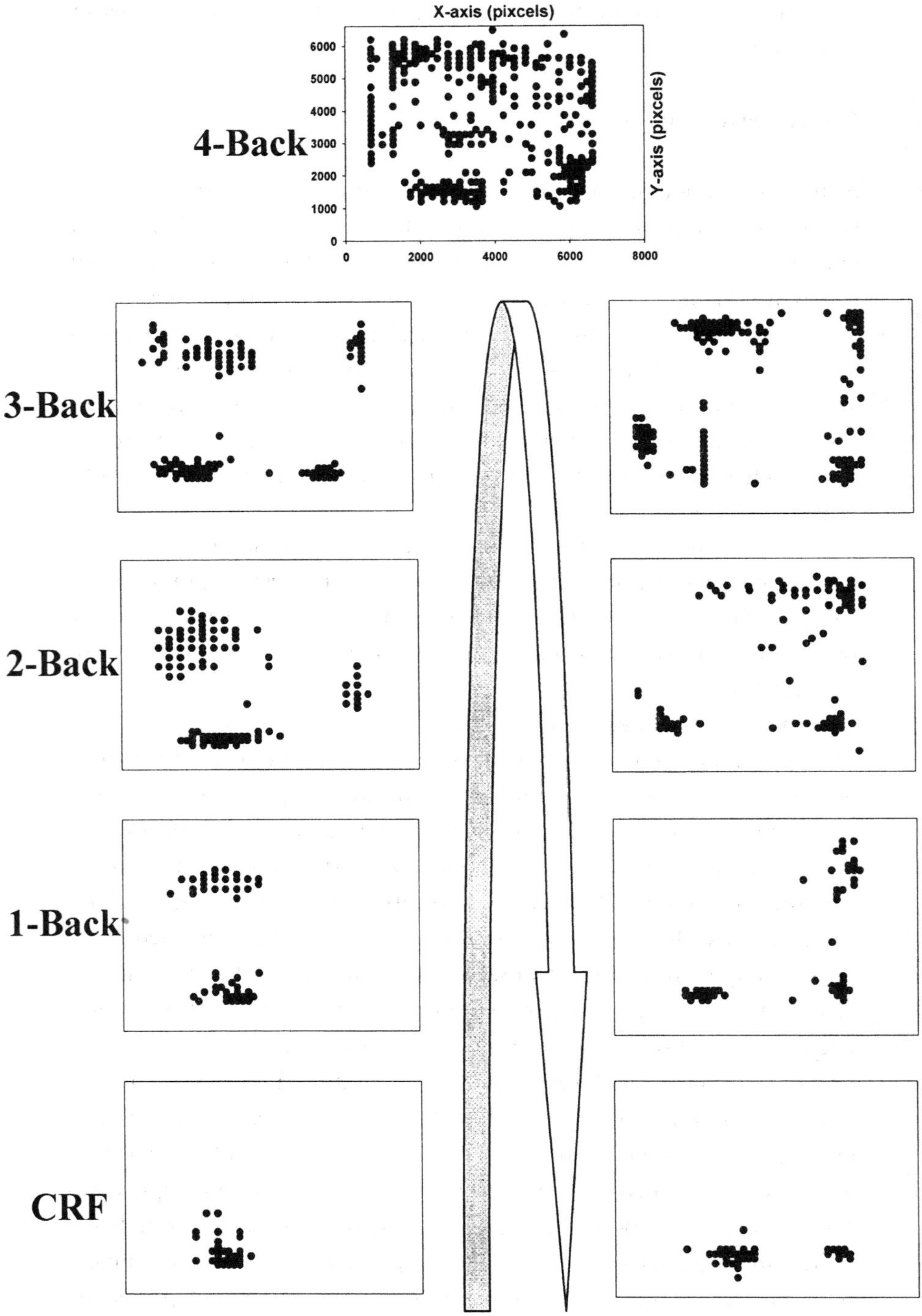
X-axis (pixcels)
Y-axis (pixcels)
6000
5000
4000
3000
2000
1000
0
0
2000
4000
6000
8000
4-Back
3-Back
2-Back
1-Back
CRF

subjects had not been reinforced for varying a response in both dimensions at the same time. Such a history of reinforcement may be a factor causing the difference.

In addition to reinforcement history, the level of variability may be a factors. Grunow and Neuringer (2002) suggested that the success of conditioning depends on the levels of variability of the response. The number of opportunities to be reinforced should be positively related to the rate of novel responses under the present schedule. If variability in the dimension of response location is higher than that of response pattern, responses to novel locations will be more frequently reinforced. If variability in the dimension of response location is lower than that for response pattern, on the contrary, a certain response pattern will be more likely to be reinforced. As a result, only one response dimension may come under control of the present contingency. There may be two methods to examine this possibility. The first is to change the levels of the variability of two response dimensions. The other is to make a difference in the reinforcement rate between the two response dimensions. One of the methods for the latter is the reinforcement-based *N*-back procedure. In this procedure, only response pattern is ineffective for getting food. In the present experiment, subjects came to increase the number of pecking locations in all the reinforcement-based *N*-back conditions. These results may support the above hypothesis that the level of variability of responding is a critical factor for the response to emerge. However, how subjects come to use only one of two response dimensions is still an open question.

The response pattern or increasing the number of pecking locations observed in the present *N*-back procedure may be shaped by a combination of factors, such as extinction caused by a repetition of pecking to the same location and reinforcement for pecking to a different location. Extinction usually increases the level of variability of responding. (See Morgan and

Figure 4.6
Pecking location on the screen for continuous reinforcement (CRF), one-back, two-back, three-back, and four-back conditions from bottom to top. The line in the middle indicates the training order. The training was conducted from CRF, one-back, two-back, three-back, and four-back conditions in an ascending order (left side) and four-back, three-back, two-back, one-back, and CRF conditions in a descending order (right side). Dots represent locations pecked by a budgerigar. Adapted from Manabe and Kawashima, in preparation.

Lee 1996 and Neuringer, Kornell, and Olufs 2001.) On the other hand, reinforcement decreases the level of response variability (e.g., Antonitis 1951; Margulies 1961). To examine the effects of reinforcement contingency on pecking location and on response pattern, the dynamic process in the present frequency-dependent reinforcement procedure should be examined. One way may be a yoked experiment in which yoked subjects receive food reinforcement whenever the experimental subjects peck, regardless of pecking location or response pattern (e.g. Neuringer 1990). The mechanism controlling response variability should be explored further.

John Staddon proposed a competition theory for behavioral contrast in the late 1970s (e.g. Hinson and Staddon 1978). The theory asserted that an increase in response rate in the unchanged component of multiple schedules is due to a reallocation of facultative activities from the rich to the lean component. I was interested in his theory, and tried to confirm it using pigeons. Co-workers and I observed the activities of pigeons in behavioral contrast situations in a Skinner box. Unfortunately, we could not confirm Staddon's theory in the experiment. (See Manabe, Kuwata, Kurashige, Chino, and Ogawa 1992.) In addition, my post-reinforcement pause data did not match those reported by Staddon (Manabe 1990). I met and talked with Dr. Staddon when he visited Japan in 1992. Fortunately, he gave me a chance to visit to his lab as a post-doc. Although I already had a position at a university in Tokyo at the time, I decided to work with Dr. Staddon and to learn as much as I could from him. As a post-doc at Duke University, I had difficulty communicating in English. However, Dr. Staddon kindly supported me and gave me a chance to continue experiments with budgerigars, research I had initiated in Japan. When I discussed experimental design and data with him, I was very happy, for I could see that Dr. Staddon was a pure scientist. I am proud that I was able to work with him. The experiments discussed in this chapter originated in Staddon's lab at Duke University in 1993–94.

5 Rules of Thumb for Choice Behavior in Pigeons

J. M. Cleaveland

In this chapter I present evidence in support of what I term the *active-time model* of concurrent variable-interval (VI VI) choice in pigeons. First, though, a bit of background. I had never actually met my soon-to-be graduate advisor before arriving at Duke. The only evidence I had of this mysterious person consisted of a pile of papers bearing the name "J. E. R. Staddon." Ratio invariance. Hill climbing. Adjunctive behaviors. Waiting time. Value transfer. Who was this man?! Coming as I was from a laboratory that was as branded ("Matching Law") as clearly as a corporation, I simply could not infer a consistent pattern. However, during my tenure as a graduate student in "the Staddon Lab," I came to appreciate that there was a method to John's madness—a method that was simultaneously reverent of scientific possibilities and irreverent toward dogmatism. Remain flexible, use what works, simplify, and strive for quantitative rigor. The work that I will describe below is my own humble attempt to follow these prescripts.

Currencies and Rules of Thumb

Behavioral ecologists often speak of "currencies" in reference to animal behavior. The term is easy enough to define, but conceptually tricky. Simply stated, a currency is a substitute for phylogenetic fitness at the proximal time scale. The reasoning is as follows: Since natural selection tends to bias a population in the direction of more fit phenotypes. And since behavior is an element of a phenotype that has been so selected, it follows that the occurrence of a given behavior will tend to maximize some variable that is correlated with fitness. A currency, then, is the variable that an animal's behavior is hypothesized to maximize (or minimize) within a given context.

Stated more loosely, a currency is the "goal" or "purpose" of a given behavior within a given environment.

Although evolutionary theorists approach proximal behaviors through a logical derivation, optimality models and their derived currencies have proven empirically predictive. So, for example, one can account for the time that a parent starling spends foraging in a food patch by hypothesizing that the starling is maximizing net rate of food delivery to its nestlings (Kacelnik 1984). The same currency (i.e., net rate of food acquisition) also correctly predicts whether a pied wagtail will permit another bird to temporarily share its territory (Davies and Houston 1981). Some other currencies found to be experimentally useful are efficiency (e.g. in honeybees: Schmid-Hempel, Kacelnik, and Houston 1985), and survival (gray squirrels: Lima, Valone, and Caraco 1985; juncos: Caraco, Martindale, and Whitham 1980).

From a psychological perspective, however, the concept of currencies uncomfortably straddles two categories: that of a controlling stimulus and that of a reinforcer. Within psychology a reinforcer is defined as a stimulus that affects the future probability of a contingent behavior. So, for example, a psychologist would say that at the beginning of the summer a female crab spider finds the sound of a bumble bee reinforcing, but that it finds that sound less reinforcing at the end of the season when the female spider's behavior typically turns from foraging to building a nest (Morse and Stephens 1996). A behavioral ecologist, though, might say that the change in the spider's behavior was evidence that the currency, or phylogenetic goal, underpinning the spider's behavior had changed.

Currencies and reinforcers, then, are conceptually similar. However, is it correct to state that a currency *controls* behavior in the same manner that a reinforcer *controls* behavior? A currency is, after all, an inferred variable while a reinforcer is a real thing that can be measured out and exposed to a bird or spider. If fact, behavioral ecologists recognize this point when they distinguish between currencies and "rules of thumb." Whereas one might say that the currency of a foraging bird is net energy rate, the rule of thumb used by the bird refers to the actual mechanism or decision rule that generates this result. So, for example, a bird might consistently switch out of a food patch after catching x grams of food items. If in the bird's natural environment food weight correlates with food energy, then this variable might serve as the rule of thumb that controls behavior and simultaneously maximizes the currency of net energy rate. But of course food weight need not correlate with food energy, so one might imagine a clever laboratory environment in which the bird optimizes net weight per unit time (i.e., its rule of thumb) while not optimizing its net energy per unit time (i.e., its currency). (For further discussion of rules of thumb, see Stephens and Krebs 1986, pp. 172–182.) Such a finding would speak to the animal's rule of thumb but it would in no way invalidate the issue of whether or not the animal's behavior was directed toward optimizing a currency (e.g., net energy rate).

The distinction between currencies, rules of thumb, and reinforcers is a subtle one, but one that bears repeating. Currencies are molar variables. Rules of thumb are more molecular variables, and reinforcers can be both momentary and molar in nature. That is, behavioral control operates simultaneously across different time scales. This does not necessarily imply that the operative mechanisms are the same at each time scale (contra Skinner 1981; see Cleaveland 2002), but it does suggest that behavior can be suboptimal at one time scale and simultaneously optimal at another.

From Currencies to Concurrent VI VI Behavior

As just noted, behavioral ecologists hypothesize currencies in an attempt to understand the molar variables that control behavior. In general these variables are arrived at initially through logical derivations via optimality assumptions and inferences made by the experimenter. In contrast, in operant psychology the most well-known descriptor of molar choice behavior has been derived empirically and is termed the matching law (Herrnstein 1961). The matching law is elegant and simple. It states that animals tend to arrange their choices in proportion to the relative amount of reinforcement each alternative delivers. This finding has been documented with reinforcers that differ in magnitude (Neuringer 1967), with spatial responses (Baum and Rachlin 1969), and with temporal responses (Cantania 1963). Formally, the matching law is given by the following equation (Baum 1974):

$$\frac{B1}{B2} = b\left(\frac{R1}{R2}\right)^{a}, \tag{1}$$

where *B*1 and *B*2 stand for the frequencies of two behaviors, *R*1 and *R*2 stand for the contingent reinforcement frequency associated with *B*1 and *B*2, *b* represents any bias that the animal might have for one of the two reinforcers, and *a* represents the sensitivity of the individual to the ratio of reinforcement frequencies. In this generalized form, the matching law describes a wide range of molar choice behavior. (See Williams 1988.)

Given the widespread success of both the matching law and behavioral currencies in describing molar patterns of choice behavior in animals, a natural question is whether and/or how the two are related. There is, in fact, some evidence that matching and currency assumptions describe two sides of the same coin. Houston (1986) showed that the generalized matching law (equation 1) correctly fits the time allocation of pied wagtails feeding within a flock and feeding within a territory. He further suggested that survival, not overall feeding rate, was the currency being maximized. One can also show mathematically that in concurrent VI VI schedules, matching produces the choice distribution that maximizes the overall rate of reinforcement. (See Williams 1988.) And yet, within operant psychology there remains a debate about whether currency assumptions or matching is the more fundamental and necessary principle(s) for explaining choice behavior in animals (e.g., Heyman and Luce 1979; Herrnstein 1990).

This debate is, of course, rather silly because it merely confirms what to a behavioral ecologist is obvious. Given the phylogenetic constraints that define an organism, the proximal environmental range over which a given rule of thumb optimizes a given currency will be limited. It is this latter point that is often overlooked by proponents of "matching theory." (See Staddon 1992.) The task of the psychologist and the behavioral ecologist is ultimately the same: to elucidate the mechanisms that produce behavior and the local environments under which those mechanisms are operative. Psychology is not helped by ignoring the fact that ontogeny has a phylogeny (Cleaveland, Jäger, Rössner, and Delius 2003).

Three Rules of Thumb for Concurrent VI VI Behavior

In the remainder of the chapter I will consider three rules of thumb that might underlie the choice behavior of pigeons experiencing concurrent VI VI schedules of reward. They are melioration, momentary maximizing, and the active-time model. As the preceding discussion illustrates, one should be cautious in asserting that a single rule of thumb accounts for all (in this case) food-related behavior patterns. I will certainly not make that claim. However, I will suggest that under four specific laboratory conditions, pigeons' choice behavior can best be explained by the active-time model. Let me define my rules of thumb.

Melioration

Melioration hypothesizes that the choice behavior of pigeons under concurrent VI VI schedules of reinforcement is controlled by differences in local rates of reinforcement (Herrnstein and Vaughn 1980; Vaughan 1981). Melioration is derived directly from the matching law by noting that both behavioral frequencies (B_i) among a set of alternatives and time allocation (T_i) to these alternatives tend to match contingent reinforcement frequencies (R_i). That is, for two alternatives, it follows from equation 1 that matching holds when

$$\frac{B_1}{B_2} = \frac{T_1}{T_2} = \frac{R_1}{R_2} \tag{2}$$

and

$$\frac{R_1}{T_1} = \frac{R_2}{T_2} \tag{3}$$

—in other words, when the rate of reinforcement per time spent at alternative 1 equals the rate of reinforcement per time spent at alternative 2. By simply always choosing the alternative with the higher local rate of reinforcement, an organism will tend to produce matching at the molar level.

Momentary Maximization

Momentary maximization (Shimp 1966, 1969) hypothesizes that a pigeon's choice behavior under concurrent VI VI schedules is controlled by a comparison between reinforcement probabilities at each of the available alternatives at the moment of choice. An animal following a momentary maximizing strategy would select the choice with the highest momentary probability of reinforcement. Under constant probability VI schedules (e.g., those produced by Fleshler and Hoffman (1962)) the probability of reinforcement is given not by the time since the last reinforcer, but by the time since the most recent response to each alternative. Reinforcers in such VI schedules are programmed according to

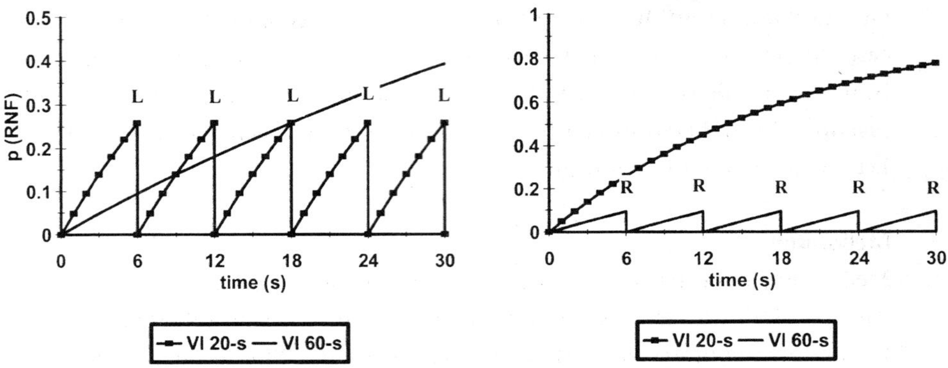

Figure 5.1
This figure uses equation 4 and shows how the probabilities of reinforcement change at two concurrent choice alternatives: a VI 20-second schedule and a VI 60-second schedule. For simplicity the plots assume a response every 6 seconds to only one of the choice alternatives (i.e., perseveration). So, for example, the left plot assumes that the subject selects the VI 20-second schedule (L) every 6 seconds and never responds to the VI 60-second schedule. This figure illustrates the important point that immediately following a choice, the probability of reinforcement at that alternative drops to 0.

$$P_i = 1 - e^{-(t_i/\lambda_i)}, \qquad (4)$$

where P_i, the probability of reinforcement at choice$_i$, depends on the time, t_i, since last choosing choice$_i$, and on the average reinforcement rate, λ_i, assigned to choice$_i$. In order to apply equation 4 to concurrent choice experiments, one simply iterates equation 4 for each choice. Figure 5.1 shows how the probabilities of reinforcement change when an animal responds solely at either of two alternatives in a concurrent VI 20-second VI 60-second schedule. The figure assumes that the subject responds at a fixed rate of one response every 6 seconds as in, say, a discrete-trial procedure. Figure 5.1 shows that as a subject continues to respond at one alternative, which I will term the *active schedule*, the probability of reinforcement grows for the non-selected, or *background schedule*. An animal following a momentary maximizing strategy should switch from the active schedule to the background schedule as soon as the latter has a higher probability of reinforcement. So, for example, in figure 5.1 the animal should switch out of the VI 20-second schedule after three responses.

Active Time

The active-time model is a constrained version of momentary maximizing suggested in Cleaveland 1999. Rather than assume that pigeons keep track of and constantly compare multiple inter-response times, the active-time model lessens the "cognitive load" on the pigeon and asserts that only the time since the most recent choice, i.e., the active schedule inter-response time (IRT), controls choice during concurrent VI VI schedules. Shimp (1981) has shown that the most immediate IRT in concurrent VI VI schedules can control delayed matching-to-sample choices for up to 8 seconds. But the main evidence for the active-time hypothesis is given by changes in switching probabilities as a function of active and background IRTs (Cleaveland 1999).

During concurrent VI VI schedules the alternate schedule always has the higher probability of reinforcement immediately after a choice (figure 5.1). This is true regardless of whether the just-emitted choice was to the rich or lean schedule because, given equation 4, responding resets the IRT of the selected choice, thus resetting the reinforcement probability at the just-chosen alternative to zero. As the active IRT then begins to increase, two results are predicted. First, if the active schedule is the richer of the two schedules, the higher rate of gain associated with its reinforcement probability will eventually provide it with the higher probability of reinforcement. Conversely, if the active schedule is the poorer of the two schedules, then the other choice will always have a higher probability of reinforcement regardless of the length of the active IRT. In summary, then, the active-time hypothesis predicts that after a choice to the rich schedule, switch probabilities will be high and then decline as the active IRT increases. After a choice to the poor schedule, switch probabilities should be high and remain high as the active IRT increases. These are precisely the results reported in Cleaveland 1999, as shown in figure 5.2.

Simulations and Data Sets

Let us now consider how the three rules of thumb outlined above fit the choice behavior of pigeons during concurrent VI VI schedules of reinforcement. I will use four concurrent VI VI data sets for this purpose: matching, molecular choice structure (Hinson and Staddon 1983a,b; Shimp 1969), run-length data (Cleaveland 1999; Heyman 1979; Nevin 1969, 1979), and

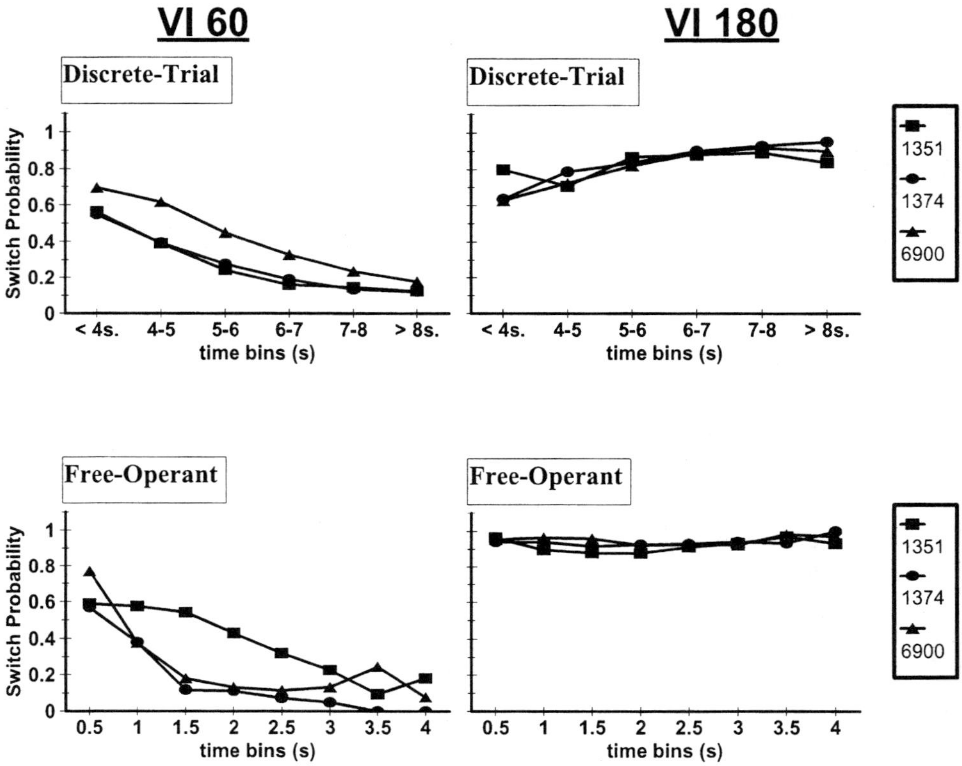

Figure 5.2
In the terminology of this chapter, the time immediately after a choice is termed *active time*. These plots show the likelihood that a pigeon switched from one concurrent VI schedule (the active schedule) to the other given increases in active time. The two upper plots were derived from a discrete-trial experiment with inter-trial intervals equal to, on average, 6 seconds. Conversely, the two lower plots were derived from a free-operant experiment. Adapted from Cleaveland 1999.

a paradoxical result obtained from multiple concurrent VI VI schedules (Belke 1992; Gibbon 1995).

My consideration of these data sets will, of course, be selective, and where necessary I will rely upon simple simulations of the three rules of thumb in order to judge whether they can produce behavior in line with a particular data set. As with the data sets, the simulations are not meant to be exhaustive, but rather to provide extremely basic tests of the three rules of thumb being considered. The assumptions used in order to simulate me-

Table 5.1
Some basic simulation results for three rules of thumb. 'Window' refers to the "memory window" over which local reinforcer rates are calculated. 'Proportion' is proportion of rich schedule choices. *M* value is explained in the text.

Melioration				Momentary maximizing		Active time	
Schedule	Window	Proportion	*M* value	Proportion	*M* value	Proportion	*M* value
20–60	10	0.72	0.34	0.68	0.99	0.63	0.77
	15	0.78	0.24				
	20	0.84	0.17				
30–60	10	0.66	0.33	0.61	0.99	0.63	0.73
	15	0.73	0.23				
	20	0.79	0.16				
40–80	10	0.63	0.34	0.61	0.99	0.63	0.73
	15	0.69	0.26				
	20	0.72	0.21				
60–180	10	0.60	0.43	0.68	0.99	0.63	0.79
	15	0.65	0.35				
	20	0.68	0.28				

lioration, momentary maximizing, and the active-time model are described in the appendix.

Data Set 1: Matching and Molar Maximizing

As was noted earlier, the matching law reliably fits the choice behavior of pigeons under concurrent VI VI schedules of reward. Further, one can derive the matching law from an optimality analysis of concurrent VI VI schedules in which the assumed currency is overall rate of reinforcement obtained. (See Williams 1988.) Therefore, any rule of thumb for pigeons under concurrent VI VI schedules must yield matching at the molar level.

Since melioration is directly derived from the matching law, it follows that this behavioral mechanism should produce molar matching. Table 5.1 shows that simulations of melioration across three concurrent schedules do indeed produce choice ratios that approximate the scheduled reinforcement ratios. However, table 5.1 also shows that the degree to which melioration produces matching depends to a large extent on the temporal/

response span over which local rates of reinforcement are calculated. Keeping VI values constant, larger time windows will produce more and more extreme preference for the richer schedule ("overmatching") while shorter time windows produce indifference ("undermatching"). This effect of "window size" can be intuitively understood by considering two extreme cases: a window for a single response and a window equal to the duration of an entire experimental session. With a window of 1, local "rates" of reward are almost always 0, and choice behavior would presumably be random (this would depend upon the specific implementation of melioration). This would produce indifference between the two choices. Conversely, with a time window equal to the duration of the session, the rich schedule would very quickly have a local rate of reinforcement that was always greater than the poorer schedule, which would lead to exclusive preference for the alternative associated with the rich VI.

As with melioration, momentary maximizing can be derived from the matching law. Equation 2 shows that when matching holds, reinforcement per unit of behavior at alternative 1 equals the reinforcement per unit of behavior at alternative 2. This is equivalent to stating that when matching holds, the probability of reinforcement at alternative 1 equals the probability of reinforcement at alternative 2. Therefore, by always choosing the alternative with the momentarily higher probability of reinforcement, an organism should tend to oscillate around matching at the molar level. In fact, table 5.1 shows that for the simulations considered here, momentary maximizing produced choice distributions that were consistently below matching (i.e., undermatching). This is due to the fact that pigeons, and the simulation used here, do not respond at an infinite rate. Undermatching is, however, actually a more robust finding than matching, at least for pigeons behaving under concurrent VI VI schedules of reward (Baum 1979; Williams 1988).

Finally, it is not intuitively obvious whether an active-time model should yield matching behavior or not. Much would depend, of course, on the exact function relating active IRTs to switch probabilities. However, as table 5.1 shows, for the simulations considered here (see appendix) an active-time mechanism consistently produced choice proportions that matched reinforcement proportions. Interestingly, despite the similarities between momentary maximizing and the active-time model, the latter consistently produced "better" matching.

In summary, then, all three rules of thumb—melioration, momentary maximizing, and active time—can be shown to generate choice distributions under concurrent VI VI schedules that are consistent with the matching law.

Data Set 2: Molecular Structure of Choice

Whereas matching is derived from thousands of responses, molecular analyses of choice look for regularities in responding after a handful of responses. Such analyses of the behavior of pigeons under concurrent VI VI schedules have indeed found regularities in subjects' responding (Shimp 1969; Silberberg, Hamilton, Ziriax, and Casey 1978). The most frequent pattern of responding that is found with pigeons and concurrent VI VI schedules is the pattern given by the ratio of the schedule values—a response pattern that when iterated yields the matching law. VIs of equal value will produce more alternations than any other choice pattern. VIs with a 2:1 ratio (i.e., one VI schedule has an average programmed rate that is twice the alternative) tend to produce choice sequences dominated by two pecks at the rich schedule followed by a single peck at the poor schedule.

The molecular response structures predicted by momentary maximizing may be graphically represented if we define an indifference line at which the probabilities of reinforcement for the two choices are equal (Staddon, Hinson, and Kram 1981). Setting P_1 equal to P_2 and simplifying yields

$$t_1 = t_2\left(\frac{\lambda_2}{\lambda_1}\right), \tag{5}$$

where t_i is the time since the last response to choice 1 or choice 2, and λ_i is the programmed reinforcement rate for choices 1 or 2. Note that the slope of the indifference line in the resultant *clock space* (a plot with time on both axes, in this case inter-response times) is given by the ratio of the programmed schedule values, λ_2/λ_1. If t_1 is greater than t_2, multiplied by this ratio, then the probability of reward for choice 1 will be greater than the probability of reward for choice 2.

Graphically, in a clock space, the choice represented by the nearest axis, without crossing the indifference line, has the higher probability of reinforcement. Thus, in figure 5.3 the *y*-axis schedule (i.e., VI 60-second) will have the higher reinforcement probability at all points to the left of the

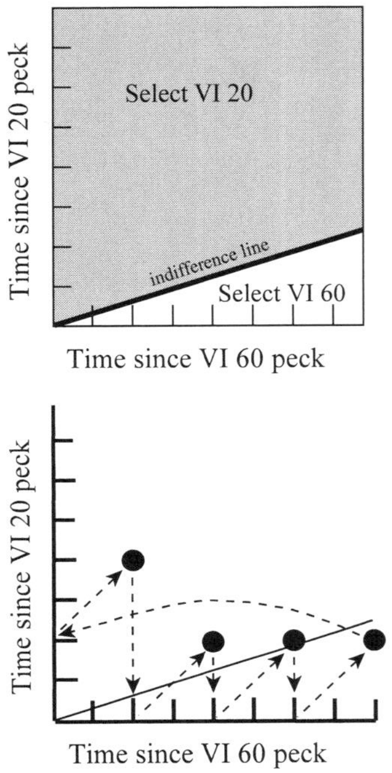

Figure 5.3
An illustration of how equation 5 permits one to create clock spaces that graphically represent the relation between reinforcement probabilities and inter-response times. All points to the left of the indifference line indicate IRT combinations whose derived reinforcement probability differences favor the VI 60-second schedule. Conversely, all points below the indifference line represent IRT combinations whose derived reinforcement probability differences favor the VI 180-second schedule. The bottom plot shows how an animal responding at a fixed rate (one response every two time units) will generate a regular sequence of choices if it consistently picks the alternative with the higher probability of reinforcement.

indifference line, while the *x*-axis (i.e., VI 180-second) schedule will have the higher reinforcement probability at all points below the indifference line.

Momentary maximizing, as illustrated in figure 5.3, predicts that if an animal responds at a constant rate, then a single response sequence will emerge that is equal to λ_2/λ_1. These were in fact the most frequent response sequences reported by Shimp (1969) and Silberberg et al. (1978). However, an animal need not respond at a constant rate, and in such circumstances momentary maximizing does not predict a regular molecular response pattern. In order to determine whether pigeons that do not respond at a regular rate are nonetheless adhering to a momentary maximizing rule of thumb, Hinson and Staddon (1983a) developed a statistic, M, that captures the degree to which a pigeon's choice behavior tracks momentary reinforcement probabilities. M is in essence the accumulated proportion of reinforcement probability differences obtained at each choice. The statistic is given by

$$M = \frac{\sum \text{Correct}}{\sum \text{Correct} + \sum \text{Incorrect}}, \tag{6}$$

where "correct" $= |P_i - P_j|$ if choice$_i$ when $P_i > P_j$ or choice$_j$ when $P_j > P_i$ while "Incorrect" $= |P_i - P_j|$ if choice$_i$ when $P_j > P_i$ or choice$_j$ when $P_i > P_j$. If a subject's behavior tracks momentary reinforcement probabilities, M will approach 1.0. Behavior that is indifferent to momentary reinforcement probabilities would produce M values of 0.5, while sub-optimal behavior would produce M values less than 0.5.

Naturally, table 5.1 shows that simulated choices made via a momentary maximizing rule of thumb yield M values essentially equal to 1.0 (differences from 1.0 are due to the fact that only one IRT clock stops during reinforcement "time"). In fact the momentary maximizing simulations are too good. Hinson and Staddon (1983a,b) found that pigeons in free-operant concurrent VI VI situations tended to produce M values between 0.7 and 0.9 late in training. These findings were replicated by Cleaveland (1999). Cleaveland also found that pigeons in discrete-trial procedures (procedures that force a relatively constant response rate) tended to produce M values of approximately 0.50. This latter finding is clearly at odds with a momentary maximizing rule of thumb.

Simulations of an active-time model, however, yield M values more in the range of those produced by actual birds. Table 5.1 shows that across the simulated schedule values, an active-time rule of thumb produces M values between 0.7 and 0.8. Furthermore, Cleaveland (1999) showed that differences in M values produced by birds experiencing free-operant versus discrete-trial procedures could be accounted for via an active-time model.

Finally, in the simulations considered here, melioration clearly does not produce molecular choice patterns consistent with the data of real birds. Even when the simulated choice distributions produced matching at the molar level, melioration yielded M values between 0.3 and 0.4. When the simulated choice preferences overmatched, M values were between 0.2 and 0.3.

Data Set 3: Run Length and Choice

The response sequencing observed by pigeons in concurrent VI VI schedules is one type of molecular choice data. Another involves the probability of switching given a number of pecks at a single choice. This latter variable is often referred to as run length or perseveration. It has been well documented that switching probabilities are independent of run length in pigeons that are experiencing concurrent VI VI schedules (Cleaveland 1999; Heyman 1979; Nevin 1969, 1979; Silberberg et al. 1978). That is, the probability of switching out of one schedule in a concurrent VI VI experiment appears to be independent of the number of pecks made to that schedule. Figure 5.4 illustrates this result with real birds experiencing a concurrent VI 60-second VI 180-second schedule. It plots the probability of a switch given the amount of time a bird has spent responding to a single alternative. In both discrete-trial and free-operant procedures the plots are flat. For instance in the free-operant case, birds were just as likely to switch out a rich schedule after responding to it for 1 second as they were after responding to it for 6 seconds.

Figure 5.5 presents simulated data using melioration, momentary maximizing, and an active-time model. The data were generated from a simulated concurrent VI 60-second VI 180-second schedule (the other schedules simulated for this chapter produced similar results). Figure 5.5 plots the probability of a switch from the rich schedule to the poorer schedule given increasing run lengths at the rich schedule. As can be seen, only the active-time model and melioration generate simulated switch probabilities that remain flat as run length increases.

Momentary maximizing does not predict the run-length data of real birds for the following reason. As figure 5.1 illustrates, when a bird responds at one schedule the reinforcement probability of the background schedule grows. In other words, perseveration on one schedule is equivalent to increases in the background IRT. Momentary maximizing predicts that as the background IRT increases, the animal should eventually switch to that schedule. Allowing for errors by the animal in mapping IRTs to reinforcer probabilities, one would not expect an immediate switch. However, momentary maximizing certainly predicts a positive correlation between

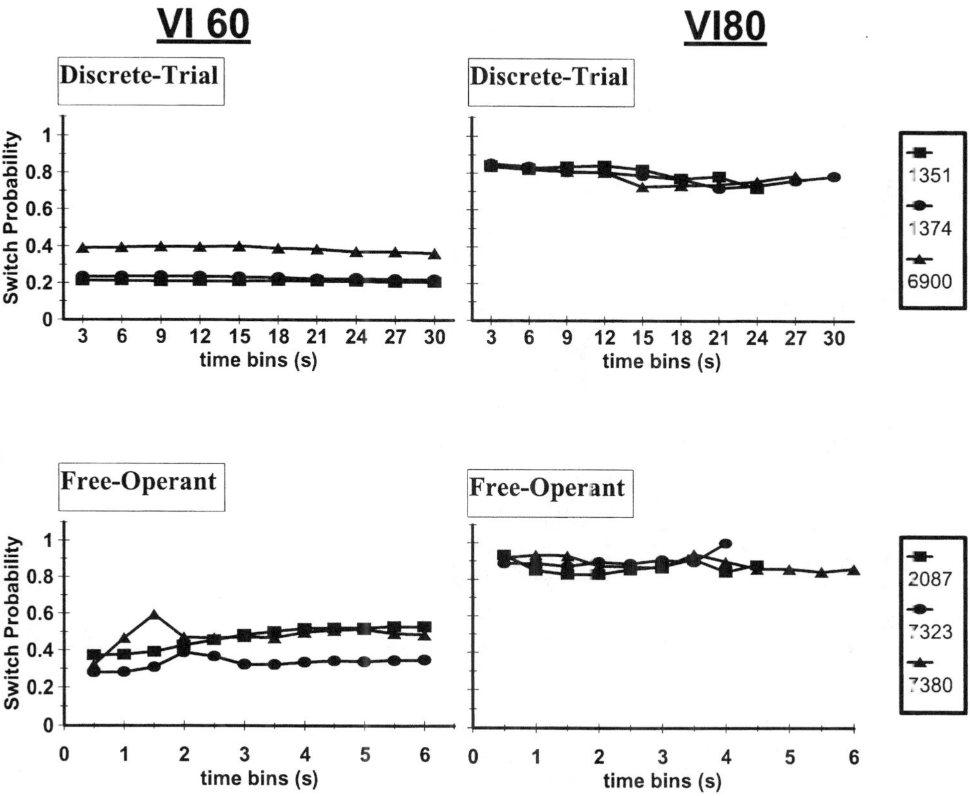

Figure 5.4

Switch probabilities are independent of run lengths. The figure illustrates this point with data for three birds from concurrent VI 60-second VI 180-second schedules. The two upper plots are derived from a discrete-trial experiment, and the two lower plots were derived from a free-operant experiment. The *x* axis gives the amount of time (i.e., run length) that a subject had responded exclusively to one of the two schedules. Adapted from Cleaveland 1999.

background IRTs and switch probabilities, and the simulation of momentary maximizing used here did produce such a correlation. To my knowledge no experimental support for the momentary maximizing, run-length prediction has been obtained (although see Heyman and Tanz 1995).

As was noted earlier, the choice distributions predicted by melioration are heavily dependent upon the window size over which local rates of reinforcement are calculated. The simulated run lengths used to create figure 5.5 came from a simulation that used a window size of 15 pecks. Smaller

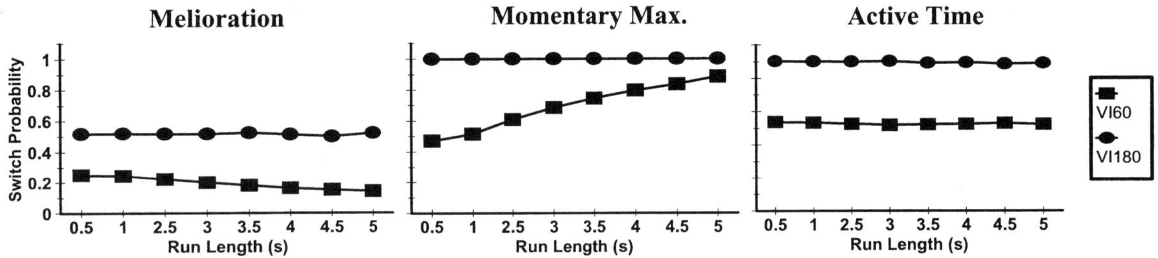

Figure 5.5

This figure shows data from a simulated concurrent VI 60-second VI 80-second schedule and a choice rule given by either melioration, momentary maximizing, or an active-time model. The graphs plot changes in switch probability given increasing run lengths at either schedule. In agreement with the behavior of real birds (figure 5.4) switch probabilities remained flat when a melioration or active-time choice rule was employed. In contrast, using a momentary maximizing choice rule produced an increase in switch probabilities as run length increased on the VI 60-second schedule.

window sizes, assuming no change in VI schedules, tended to move the function associated with the VI 60 schedule (shown in figure 5.5) up toward an asymptote of 0.5. This is intuitively obvious: with a window size of 1, switch probabilities depend only on overall switching probabilities, which were set at 0.5 in the simulations. Conversely, large window sizes lowered the function associated with the VI 60 toward 0. This too is intuitively obvious: with very large window sizes, switching probabilities depend only on the programmed rates of reinforcement at each alternative. Melioration, in this case, would have the animal show exclusive preference for the richer schedule.

In contrast with momentary maximizing, the active-time hypothesis by definition asserts that pigeons are insensitive to background IRTs. In fact the active-time model makes the rather strong claim that the flat switch probabilities shown by pigeons under concurrent VI VI schedules are a sampling artifact. What matters is not the run length but the IRT following the last peck of the run. VI schedules tend to produce steady rates of responding. Thus, the average IRT after the last peck of all run lengths of $N = 3$ will tend to be the same as the average IRT after the last peck of all run lengths of $N = 20$. Since the active-time model asserts that it is this final IRT value that determines the probability of a switch, switch probabilities for run lengths of $N = 3$ will be the same as those for run lengths of $N = 20$, or indeed for run lengths of any size. Despite different run lengths, one is sampling, on average, the same active-time IRT.

Data Set 4: The Result of Belke (1992)

The final data set that I will consider concerns a paradoxical result reported by Belke (1992) and replicated by Gibbon (1995). Belke's study used multiple concurrent VI VI schedules. In this experimental paradigm, pigeons are repeatedly exposed to bouts of concurrent VI VI schedules. For example, a bird might experience bouts of a concurrent VI 20 VI 40 intermixed with bouts of a concurrent VI 40 VI 80 with each bout lasting 60 seconds. In the Belke study, four stimuli were associated uniquely with each of four VI schedules. Only two stimuli were ever presented together. The concurrent VIs experienced by his birds were identical to those just mentioned: VI 20 VI 40 and VI 40 VI 80. The matching law fit the molar choice proportions that were generated by Belke's subjects. However, Belke also introduced several unreinforced probe "bouts" in which the two stimuli associated with the VI 40 schedules were paired. Choice distributions during the probe trials revealed that Belke's birds preferred the stimulus associated with the VI 40 that had been trained in the concurrent VI 40 VI 80 schedule. The preference of the pigeons for this VI 40 stimulus over the other was 4:1.

Belke's result is paradoxical for several reasons. First, it clearly violates the matching law, as the absolute rates of reward associated with the two "different" VI 40 schedules are by definition the same. Yet the birds distributed their probe choices as if one VI 40 schedule was richer than the other. Secondly, melioration just as obviously fails to fit the Belke data. Belke reported that after training and prior to probe trials local reinforcement rates favored the VI 40 stimulus trained with the VI 20 schedule rather than the VI 40 stimulus paired with the VI 80 schedule. Melioration, then, predicts a choice distribution during probe bouts that is in the opposite direction of what the birds actually produced. Finally, momentary maximizing cannot account for the Belke data as it assumes that birds learn a single function for each VI stimulus that relates the time since the last choice of that schedule (IRTs) to changes in the probability of reinforcement on that schedule. Given equivalent VI schedules birds should learn equivalent rein-

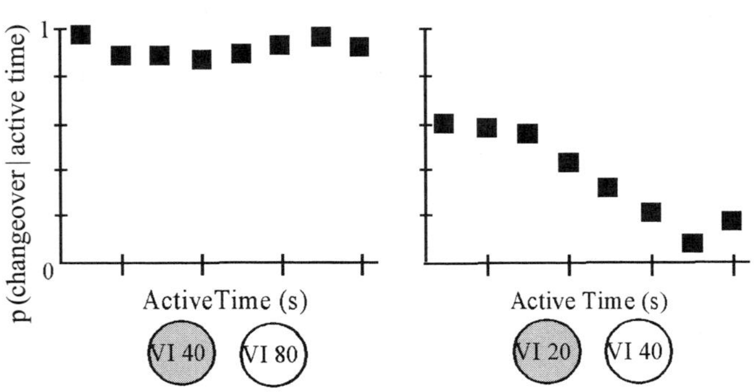

Figure 5.6
This diagram illustrates the experiment of Belke (1992) and the switch functions predicted by an active-time rule of thumb. As described in the text, these switch functions would tend to yield a preference for the VI 40-second schedule that had served as a rich alternative during training. The degree of this preference would depend on inter-response time distributions produced by the subject during testing.

forcement probability functions. Therefore, momentary maximizing, like molar matching, predicts indifference in the Belke probe trials.

Of the three rules of thumb being considered in this chapter, only the active-time model predicts choice distributions of the type observed by Belke. Figure 5.6 illustrates the logic that yields such a prediction. Recall that the active-time model assumes different switching functions, depending on whether a stimulus is associated with a rich or a poor VI schedule. Presumably, during training under the concurrent VI 20 VI 40 schedule of reinforcement, Belke's birds formed a switching function typical of a "poor" schedule. Similarly, in relation to the VI 40 stimulus paired with the VI 80 stimulus, Belke's birds would have formed a switching function typical of a "rich" schedule. Given these assumptions, which are based on data from real birds (Cleaveland 1999), figure 5.6 shows that the active-time model predicts a probe preference qualitatively similar to that reported by Belke. Whether an active-time mechanism might produce a more quantitative fit remains to be seen and would depend on the actual form of the switching curves as well as the response rate during probe trials.

Conclusion

This chapter has considered three rules of thumb that pigeons might use when behaving under concurrent VI VI schedules of reinforcement. These were melioration, momentary maximizing, and the active-time model. Table 5.2 summarizes the qualitative fit produced by these three mechanisms to four data sets. Only the active-time model provided a qualitative fit for all four data sets.

Table 5.2
Summary of three rules of thumb in relation to four data sets.

	Melioration	Momentary maximizing	Active time
Controlling stimulus	Response rate	Comparison among multiple IRTs	Most recent single IRT
Generate matching?	Yes	Yes	Yes
Fit molecular choice structure?	No	Yes	Yes
Fit run-length data?	Yes	No	Yes
Fit Belke data?	No	No	Yes

Throughout this chapter, I have used the behavioral ecology phrase "rule of thumb" instead of the more behavioristic "controlling stimulus" in reference to the choice mechanisms considered. Some might consider this a sort of blasphemy. After all, does it not encourage anthropomorphism, mentalism, and a host of other evils? In my opinion, no. As the introduction of this chapter hopefully made clear, optimality considerations, currencies, and rules of thumb imply different time scales of stimulus control that psychologists would do well to always keep in mind. Certainly, the active-time model is but one rule of thumb that might structure a pigeon's behavior during concurrent VI VI schedules, and the experimental context will shape and select among these mechanisms. Heyman and Tanz (1995), for instance, showed that stimulus conditions can influence whether overall choice behavior by pigeons is better fit by overall reinforcement rate or by the matching law, and Schwartz (1980, 1982) showed that pigeons use different response units under different conditions. To reiterate, the task of the psychologist and the behavioral ecologist is the same: to elucidate the mechanisms that produce behavior and the local environments under which those mechanisms are operative.

Appendix: The Simulations

The simulations of melioration, momentary maximizing, and the active-time model were conducted with the following general assumptions:

1. IRT generation was independent of the choice mechanism. In practice, this meant that an IRT was calculated before a decision rule was applied.
2. Response rate was programmed to be 1 peck per second, using an exponential function of form $(-\ln(n) + 0.2)$, where n is a random number drawn from the range 0 to 1.
3. The time to switch from one alternative to another was set at 0.5 second.
4. Rewards were programmed to occupy 2.0 seconds.
5. Two separate clocks programmed reinforcer deliveries. When a reinforcer occurred at one alternative, the clock for that schedule was reset and did not resume until the reinforcer period was finished. However, the schedule clock at the non-reinforced alternative continued to run.
6. No changeover delay was simulated.

Melioration

1. Local rates of reinforcement were calculated by creating an array of the last n (10, 20, 30) instances of each of three variables: the VI choice, the IRT that had been generated just before the VI choice, and whether that choice resulted in a reinforcer. Local rates of reinforcement were then calculated by dividing the total number of reinforcers assigned to each choice within the array by the sum of the IRTs assigned to each choice within in the array.

2. When local rates of reinforcement were equal to one another or equal to zero, the simulated bird chose either alternative with a probability of 0.5.

Momentary Maximizing

When calculating momentary reinforcement probabilities (equation 4), the minimum switch time of 0.5 second was added to background schedule IRTs but not to the active schedule IRT. This addition was "hypothetical" in the sense that if the simulated bird chose the active schedule, the switch time was not added to the actual background IRT that the program was keeping track of.

Active Time

The active-time probability functions were obtained by averaging those of three actual birds that experienced a concurrent VI 30-second VI 60-second schedule of reinforcement, using a changeover key procedure at the Universität Konstanz (Cleaveland, unpublished data). Averages were rounded to the nearest 0.05. For the VI 30-second VI 60-second schedules switch probabilities were (for 0.5-second, incrementing time bins) (0.6 | 0.8), (0.7 | 0.9), (0.55 | 0.9), (0.4 | 0.9), (0.2 | 0.9), (0.2 | 0.9), (0.2 | 0.9), (0.25 | 0.9), (0.25 | 0.9), (0.2 | 0.9), and (0.2 | 0.9).

Acknowledgment

The author would like to thank Juan Delius for helpful comments. The work was supported by grants from the Deutsche Forschungsgemeinschaft to Juan Delius.

II Memory, Time, and Models

6 Choice and Memory

Daniel T. Cerutti

... what escapes our vision we must grasp by mental sight ... [we] must have recourse to reasoning....

—Hippocrates, "The Science of Medicine," 400 B.C.E. (Lloyd 1978, p. 145)

What is needed is not a mathematical model, constructed with little regard for the fundamental dimensions of behavior, but a mathematical treatment of experimental data.

—Skinner, "Methods of Behavioral Science" (1988, p. 514)

A comprehensive and parsimonious theory of choice has been hard to pin down. Some obstacles are obvious. First, it is easier to engage in *empirical* curve fitting than to generate models with *deductive* validity. Second, theoretical simplification is compromised when a multitude of findings are accommodated by empirically adjusting a model's parameters. A third reason is that natural selection may have produced a multitude of different esponse systems, each with its own dynamics, appropriate to different sets of ecological constraints (Zeiler and Powell 1994). If so, simplification in behavior analysis will be frustrated in ways unanticipated by other sciences—we will have to accept a mixture of mechanisms. Choice may not reduce to the operation of a single simpler process. Finally, our models must ultimately be able to deal with both immediate and remote historical reinforcement effects, and these may require different processes (Davis, Staddon, Machado, and Palmer 1993; Dragoi and Staddon 1999; Staddon, Chelaru, and Higa 2002).

Choice, as broadly construed, is an ambiguous concept in that it subsumes many different situations, from the possibly complex calculations involved in picking stocks to the more immediate problem of choosing a restaurant. This chapter is concerned only with the latter kind of choice, but in pigeons, and examines whether and how a primitive memory-trace process (e.g., Wynn and Staddon 1988) can be used to model choice. Memory is implicated in choice to the extent that choosing is guided by previous consequences, but there are many ways that memory processes might contribute to choice. However such a process might work, its adaptive utility for an organism is obvious: return to a recent source of reinforcement, but stop returning (but not too fast) when it stops paying off. In scope, this project is necessarily modest. In this chapter I test the theoretical validity and parsimony of a memory-trace model of choice. There is no attempt to review the choice literature, to model more than just a few phenomena, or to exhaustively compare the present model with those of others.

Memory, Forgetting, and Reinforcement

Memory is invoked when the effects of contingencies persist over time. We remember how to ride a bicycle, arithmetic, and what we had for breakfast. But the concept of memory in these examples adds nothing to the fact that experience produces lasting changes in behavior. Reinforcement, for example, has lasting effects but is seldom cast in terms of memory. To say that a rat presses a lever because it remembers a reinforcement contingency adds nothing but an additional layer of tautology to the original observation that food reinforces the lever press.

Memory is more easily justified by *forgetting*, when response probability decreases as a function of time or other experience. Memory can complement the concept of reinforcement in this sense. For example, in delayed matching-to-sample, a reinforcement contingency establishes the matching performance, but the probability of selecting a correct comparison on any given trial decreases with longer retention intervals (White 1985; Wixted 1990; Wixted and Ebbeson 1991). Memory is also justified by theory. Many models of learning rely on hypothetical memory states (or analogous concepts like response and associative strength, or inhibition) to mediate between an organism's history, immediate experience, and behavior (Malone 1991; Staddon and Bueno 1991). The quasi-dynamic Rescorla and Wagner (1972) model of Pavlovian conditioning, models of choice (Couvillon and Bitterman 1985; Grace 2002; Mazur 1992) and recent dynamic models of habituation and interval timing by Staddon and colleagues (Staddon 1993b; Staddon, Chelaru, and Higa 2002) are examples that defend the need for an underlying memory process.

The prototypical memory forgetting function, rapid initial decline in memory followed by a protracted slower decline, was revealed long ago by Ebbinghaus (1964). Forgetting functions vary in form depending on procedures and organisms (Rubin and Wenzel 1996). For example, Ebbinghaus described his data with a joint hyperbolic-power-logarithm function, whereas matching-to-sample data from animals have been fit with power functions (Wixted and Ebbesen 1991). In general, the best fitting two-parameter functions are logarithmic, but complex functions are superior with almost all data sets (Rubin, Hinton, and Wenzel 1999). The importance of the search for the memory function (or functions) is that it provides the grist for the modeling mill; however, for the qualitative modeling of choice, the precise function may not be critical.

How can a memory process help us to understand reinforcement? There are two major classes of models, *response-strength* models such as the linear operator of Bush and Mosteller (1955; e.g., Couvillon and Bitterman 1985, 1988; Grace 2002; Mazur 1992), and more recent *timing* models (e.g., Horner, Staddon, and Lozano 1997; Killeen and Fetterman 1988; Machado 1997; Staddon et al. 2002). Each type of model reproduces a different aspect of behavior under schedules of reinforcement (e.g., Baum 1993; Zeiler and Powell 1994). Response-strength models represent reinforcement history by increasing stimulus value (or response probability) with reinforcement, and decreasing stimulus value with un-reinforced responses. Memory in the linear-operator family of models can extend just to the previous trial (or time step), or it can integrate events over many events (an intermediate case is the cumulative-impulse model of Horner et al. 1997). Timing models, on the other hand, incorporate memory traces that are attuned in some way to previous inter-reinforcement intervals plus a threshold trace value (a *response rule*) to regulate the onset of responses. In timing models, response rate usually takes a back seat to timing; but they can be computed, for example, by assuming that responses are emitted at a constant rate after a wait has elapsed. (See also Gibbon, Church, Fairhurst, and Kacelnik 1988; Machado 1997.)

Figure 6.1 illustrates a simple timing model based on a single "leaky integrator" (Staddon 1993b; Staddon et al. 2002),

$$V_i(t+1) = aV_i(t) + bX(t), \quad 0 < a < 1,\ b > 0 \qquad (1)$$

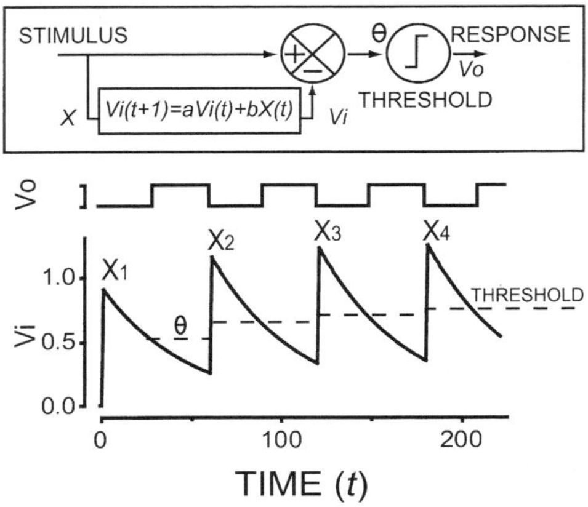

Figure 6.1
A single-response timing model based on one "leaky-bucket" integrator. The model diagram is shown in the box at the top (details in text). The lower-plot trace shows the reinforcement memory trace (V_i) during initial exposure to an FI60 schedule (reinforcers delivered at $X_{1\text{–}4}$. The event record above the memory trace shows the response output (V_o), where θ is the response threshold (horizontal dashed line).

where V_i is the integrated effect of previous reinforcers, a is a constant that determines the rate of memory decay for past reinforcers, and b is a stimulus weighting. The plot of V_i in figure 6.1 shows the effect of reinforcers on a fixed-interval (FI) 60 schedule, where each reinforcer (X_{1-4}) increments the current value of V_i by the quantity bX; between reinforcers, V_i decays exponentially as a function of a.

The onset and offset of responding, V_o, is shown in the event record at the top of figure 6.1. The response-rule threshold is

$$V_o(t) = 1 \quad \text{if } V_i(t) < V_{rft} + \xi$$
$$= 0 \quad \text{otherwise,} \qquad (2)$$

where V_o is the response output, V_{rft} is the trace value at the last reinforcer, and ξ is a constant. After reinforcement, there is a pause in responding until V_i falls below V_{rft} plus ξ, when responding begins again. The constant, ξ, determines the proportion of the interval spent waiting, with smaller values producing longer waits. As in an FI schedule, waiting in this model is proportional to the inter-food interval (IFI), although not exactly. Given a value of a close to unity, this model will approximately reproduce the linear relation between IFI and FI wait in pigeons (e.g., Zeiler and

Powell 1994; the model actually produces a power function with exponent slightly less than one[1]).

Everything else being equal, the post-reinforcement value of V_i in the single-integrator model is determined by the frequency of reinforcement, and the decay plus immediate history determines adjustments to changes in the IFI. This simple scheme does not correctly model adjustments in waiting when changes are made to the FI value (e.g., pigeons show more rapid adjustment in waiting to shorter IFIs: Higa 1996). FI dynamics are better handled by a chain of integrator units in which later units take their input from earlier units, as in the Multiple-Time-Scales (MTS) model of Staddon et al. (2002). But MTS, like the simple integrator model, does not correctly model waiting on variable-interval (VI) schedules. Under steady-state conditions, where the VI value is adjusted parametrically, these models produce a linear relation between average wait times and IFI (as seen in FI schedules); whereas pigeons have been shown to produce monotonically decreasing power functions between wait times and IFI (Baum 1993). There is presently no single model that predicts both FI and VI wait distributions (but see Machado 1997). Because so many choice studies rely on VI schedules, this is a more serious problem for modeling choice than for the modeling of forgetting. Once again, however, qualitative results may not require a precise function.

Memory and Concurrent VI Behavior

Given a good bit of exposure to concurrent VI VI schedules, organisms closely match response rate to reinforcement rates (figure 6.2; Herrnstein 1961). Findings such as these gave rise to the empirical matching relation

$$R_1/(R_1 + R_2) = r_1/(r_1 + r_2), \tag{3}$$

where R_1 and R_2 are response rates and r_1 and r_2 are the corresponding rates of reinforcement on concurrent schedules (Herrnstein 1961, 1970). A minor revision of the equation dealt with the subsequent finding that the relative time spent on two responses (T_1 and T_2) also matched relative VI reinforcement rates (Baum and Rachlin 1969; Myers and Myers 1977; Wearden and Burgess 1982).

But many failures to obtain matching have been found when choices are between schedules other than simple VI VI (e.g., chained schedules),

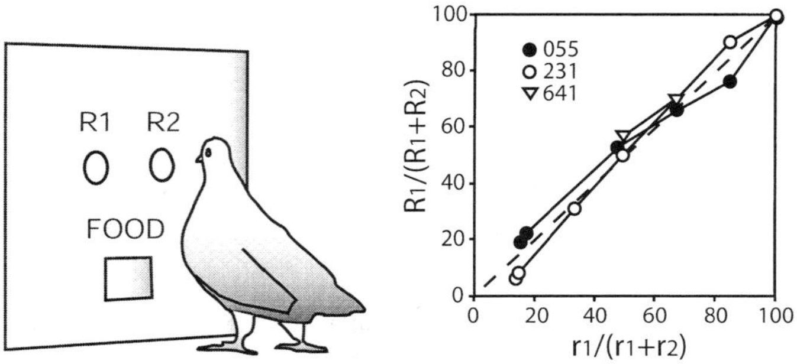

Figure 6.2
The typical two-choice procedure for a pigeon shown on the left arranges food reinforcers for left and right responses (R_1 and R_2). When each response produces food according to independent variable-interval schedules (r_1 and r_2) relative responses match relative reinforcers as plotted on the right (equation 1; Herrnstein 1961).

motivating derivative or innovative formulations. (See Williams 1994.) In even the simplest case of choice between two VI schedules, organisms generally show a small measure of *undermatching,* less preference for the richer VI than predicted by the right side of equation 2 (Baum 1979). The source of undermatching is not completely understood but it can be influenced by the cost of switching from one alternative to the other (i.e., the changeover delay, a reinforcement delay imposed after a switch in responses, reduces undermatching and the rate of switching between schedules; Shull and Pliskoff 1967; Todorov, Souza, and Bori 1993); and it is more likely to be seen in VI schedules employing arithmetic progressions of inter-food intervals than in schedules employing random intervals (an RI schedule (Taylor and Davison 1983). Related to the last result is the finding that pigeons responding on concurrent FI RI schedules show a bias toward the RI alternative (Trevett, Davison, and Williams 1972; see also Killeen 1968). There are many other findings in the choice literature but most rely on concurrent-chain schedule, an elaboration of the simple concurrent procedure (reviews in Williams 1988, 1994). Undermatching and the inter-food interval effect are two molar dependent measures that must be replicated before the problem of concurrent-chain schedules is addressed.

Can we find a simple memory-trace model that predicts these two fundamental molar properties of choice? There are many possibilities. The discussion that follows describes the architecture of a few promising config-

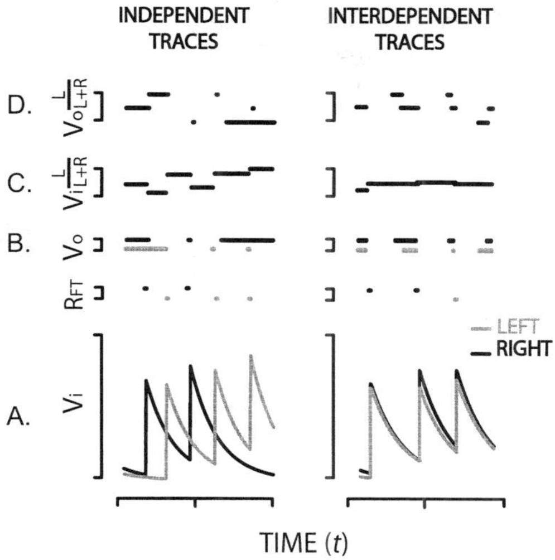

Figure 6.3
A memory-trace model of choice between two VI schedules. Memory traces are generated by single-integrator models. Lower plots (A) are reinforcement memory traces (V_i) for a left VI 60 schedule (black) and a right VI 120 schedule (gray). Response output (V_o) functions (B) are shown directly above memory traces. Upper plots (C and D) show relative trace (V_i) strength and relative response output (V_o).

urations, then presents results from tests that use different combinations of RI, VI, and FI schedules. The reason for describing results of less successful variations is that they document ways that a reinforcement-memory process cannot function. Two types of traces are considered in detail: a *simple-exponential trace*, in which every reinforcer produces an identical forgetting function, irrespective of rate of reinforcement; and a *single integrator* model, that integrates the effect of previous reinforcers so that the height of the trace is determined by rate of reinforcement, but the rate of decay is constant.

The models were evaluated with computer simulations. The approach has less merit than a formal mathematical method, but the dynamical interactions between responses to two random-interval schedules are complex enough to make simulation a faster if not superior test. The simulation program arranged a loop that repeatedly sampled the availability of reinforcement; generated a response, if the response-rule conditions were met; delivered a reinforcer, if one was available and a response occurred;

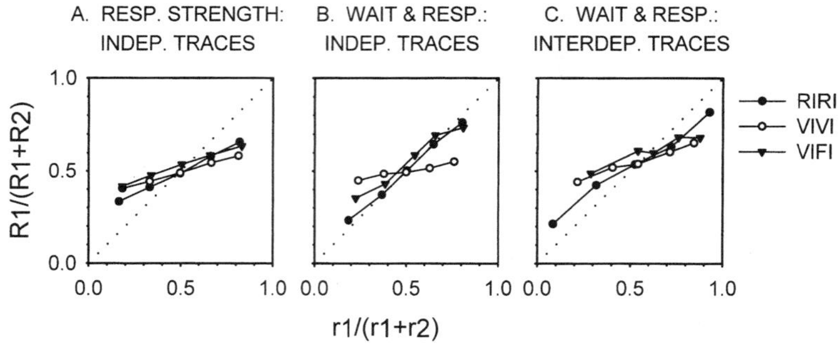

Figure 6.4
Results from three variants of the exponential-decay model ($a = 5$, $T = 100$, $\xi = 1.5$). The fourth possibility, a response-strength model with interdependent traces, produces equal response rates in all conditions and is therefore omitted. Filled circles are results of RI schedules, open circles are results of arithmetic VI schedules, and triangles are results of VI versus FI schedules.

and finally updated the trace on the basis of reinforcement or nonreinforcement. The loop was terminated after the response output showed stability, which was assessed by gathering blocks of 500 reinforcers and quitting once response means of the last three blocks indicated no trends. Points in figures show data means of the last 1,500 reinforcers. Simulations were carried out with five pairs of (RI, VI, or FI) interval schedules: 60/12, 48/24, 36/36, 24/48, and 12/60. RI schedules were arranged by sampling a probability gate with a fixed p at every time step. The concurrent VI schedules (figures 6.4 and 6.6) were 15-interval arithmetic progressions generated as in Catania and Reynolds (1968), and the VI schedules in concurrent VI FI simulations were generated using Fleshler and Hoffman (1962) exponential progressions with 14 intervals (duplicating procedures of Trevett, Davison, and Williams 1972).

Memory Trace Models of Choice

Four simple cases of memory-trace models of choice are illustrated in figure 6.3. The first distinction that can be made between models is shown in left and right plots. Left plots show *independent traces*, where traces are autonomous, timed from their respective reinforcers. Right plots show *interdependent traces*, where each reinforcer affects both traces—simultaneously setting new parameters for the reinforced trace (i.e., a response threshold) and resetting the un-reinforced trace to the value it assumed on the last

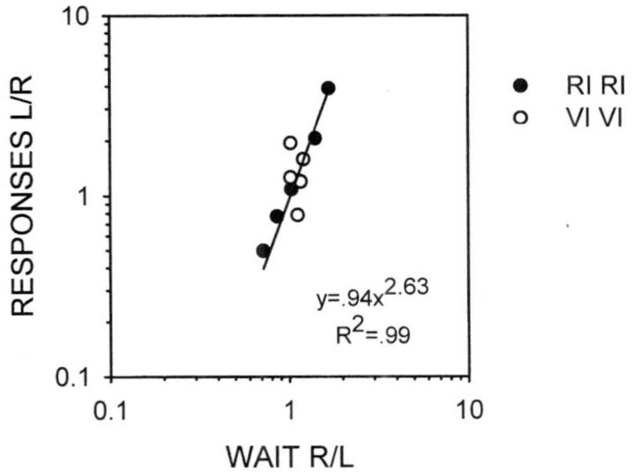

Figure 6.5
Left-right response ratios plotted against right-left wait ratios for concurrent RI RI and VI VI conditions of the simple exponential model (with behavior allocated by a wait-and-respond rule and with interdependent traces: figure 6.5C). Data are plotted on log-log coordinates; data from each data point come from stability sessions. Power function equation and R^2 statistic refer to the line fitted to the RI RI data (filled points).

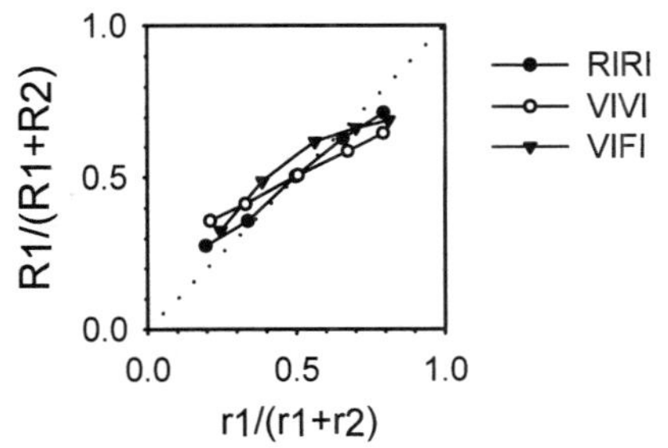

Figure 6.6
Results of simulations with a single-integrator model ($a = 0.95$, $b = 0.5$, $\xi = 0.1$) using a wait-and-respond rule and interdependent traces (independent traces produce identical results). Filled circles are results of RI schedules; open circles are results of arithmetic VI schedules; triangles are results of VI.

occasion of its reinforcement (Staddon and Ettinger 1989). The lower plots show memory traces (V_i) for a rich (gray trace: left response) and lean (black trace: right response) schedule (figure 6.3A). The integrator traces shown in figure 6.3 are incremented by reinforcement and decay with the passage of time (Lea and Dow 1984), but there are other possibilities such as a simple exponential function in which each reinforcer simply restarts the trace at its zero-intercept value (considered below). Directly above the memory-trace plots are plots of reinforcer deliveries, and above them is plotted V_o (figure 6.6B), response output that is regulated by a reinforcement-memory threshold (figure 6.1).

These models can be further subdivided. In a *trace-value model* (Mazur 1992), responses to each alternative are continuously and directly determined by trace value, as in linear-operator models (figure 6.3C),

$$R_L/(R_L + R_R) = V_L/(V_L + V_R), \qquad (4)$$

where responses R_L and R_R are produced in proportion to the relative strengths of memory traces V_L and V_R. The second case is a *wait-and-respond model* based on a timing model, where responses for each alternative begin after a threshold, θ, that is established on the basis of the previous V_{rft} (figure 6.3D). Both models track reinforcement inputs, but the trace-value model produces continuous response output (with response proportions changing after each reinforcer), while the wait-and-respond model allocates responses to one alternative, to both, or to neither. For face validity, wait-and-respond is superior because it can reproduce the post-reinforcement waiting found in the molecular analysis of concurrent schedule behavior (Cerutti and Staddon 2003; figure 6.6 here; Staddon and Cerutti 2003), whereas the response-strength model can only reproduce the molar property of rate on concurrent schedules (i.e., matching).

To summarize and extend these possibilities, a memory model of choice has at least four dimensions, each with at least two solutions:

1. Traces can show *simple decay*, as in linear waiting (Wynn and Staddon 1988), where responses are exclusively determined by the last reinforcer; or traces can be *complex integrations* involving length of training, reinforcement rate, and so on (Staddon et al. 2002; Wixted 1990).

2. Behavior is allocated to alternatives *stochastically* (e.g., probabilistically on the basis of trace strength, as in equation 4); or behavior is allocated

deterministically, in a *winner-takes-all* fashion, with responses allocated to the stronger memory (Davis, Staddon, Machado, and Palmer 1993).

3. Response probability is derived directly from *trace strength* (equation 4 here; see also Couvillon and Bitterman 1985 and Mazur 1992) or responses simply begin after a wait time determined by a *wait-and-respond threshold* rule (Staddon et al. 2002).

4. Traces for each response are *independently* regulated by each response's last reinforcer (the case illustrated in figure 6.3A; see also Couvillon and Bitterman 1985 and Mazur 1992); or timing for both traces is *interdependent*, initiated by each reinforcer, regardless of which response produced the reinforcer, so that each reinforcer produces coordinated waiting on both alternatives (Staddon and Ettinger 1989).

Simple Exponential Models The simplest cases given these model dimensions are probably simple-decay traces with response-strength calculations (see, e.g., figure 6.3C) since it assumes no long-term history effects and require no threshold calculations. Figure 6.4 shows relative responses versus relative reinforcements from simulations employing three variants of one model of this type, a simple exponential-decay model, in which the trace function is

$$V = ae^{-t/T}, \tag{5}$$

where V is the trace value, a is the value of V at reinforcement (i.e., the y intercept), t is time since reinforcement, and T is a constant that determines the rate of decay. The exponential function was chosen mainly because it behaves well at boundary conditions and because it fits many data sets in the memory literature (Rubin et al. 1999; Rubin and Wenzel 1996). In addition, all of the present simulations, including wait-and-respond types, incorporate a stochastic response rule[2] (equation 4) because a winner-takes-all rules produced exclusive choice in all cases (the tautology implied by a stochastic rule is addressed later).

Each plot in figure 6.4 shows three results: concurrent RI RI, concurrent VI VI (Herrnstein 1961; Taylor and Davison 1983; Trevett et al. 1972), and concurrent VI FI (Trevett et al. 1972). The left plot (figure 6.4A) presents results with a response-strength calculation and independently timed traces. The pattern of results is consistent with empirical findings: slight undermatching with concurrent RI RI schedules, more undermatching with concurrent arithmetic VI VI schedules, and a bias toward the VI alternative with concurrent VI FI schedules (linear and power fits are presented in table 6.1). Although the pattern of predicted results is accurate, the best-fitting functions of simulated data are linear, not power functions, as is the case in pigeons (Baum 1979), and the model produces somewhat greater undermatching than pigeons (Taylor and Davison 1983). Not shown in figure 6.4 are results of adding a changeover ratio to concurrent RI RI schedules. Incorporating a changeover delay increased undermatching in all models; this finding runs counter to the effect a changeover ratio has in pigeons (Shull and Pliskoff 1967; Todorov, Souza, and Bori 1993).

The center and right plots in figure 6.4 (B and C) show results of adding a wait-and-respond process to the simple exponential trace. Both of these variants show the correct pattern of results on the three concurrent schedules, albeit with greater variability (data presented in all figures are typical outcomes). The model with interdependent traces has a slight advantage because data show an increased tendency to exhibit power functions (table 6.1) typical of concurrent data (*power matching*: Baum 1979). The variance in response rate with this model is entirely accounted for by waiting. The relationship between waiting and response rate is revealed in yet another power function between left/right response and right/left wait times in the RI RI condition, presented in figure 6.5. The wait versus responses function is very similar to that recently found in pigeons responding on concurrent RI RI schedules by Cerutti and Staddon (2003); however, pigeons show a somewhat steeper slope with exponents between about 4 and 6. Results from concurrent VI VI simulations (circles in figure 6.5) show less variance in wait, consistent with the greater degree in undermatching (figure 6.4C), but empirical data are not available to confirm this result.

It is important to note that the stochastic response rule plays a different sort of role in this simple-exponential model with interdependent traces (right plots in figure 6.3) than that suggested by equation 4. Since left and right traces are identical in height and shape following every reinforcer, all responses are allocated to the first trace that drops below the reinforcement memory threshold, but responses are equally allocated to both alternatives once both of the thresholds are crossed. In effect, response allocation in this model is determined mainly by differences in waiting times.

Table 6.1

Best-fitting linear and power functions for results of simulations.

		Schedule								
		RI RI			VI VI			VI FI		
Model	Function	a	b	r^2	a	b	r^2	a	b	r^2
Simple-Exponential Traces										
Trace strength	Line	0.502	0.245	0.999	0.291	0.348	0.999	0.339	0.359	0.996
w/indep. traces	Power	0.425	0.686	0.975	0.249	0.599	0.969	0.281	0.658	0.992
Wait and respond	Line	0.875	0.064	0.997	0.186	0.406	0.975	0.712	0.186	0.969
w/indep. traces	Power	0.818	0.895	0.993	0.166	0.566	0.955	0.618	0.849	0.967
Wait and respond	Line	0.678	0.176	0.987	0.327	0.374	0.986	0.341	0.402	0.924
w/interdep. traces	Power	0.534	0.789	0.991	0.277	0.666	0.972	0.310	0.720	0.953
Single-Integrator Traces										
Wait and respond	Line	0.760	0.119	0.996	0.497	0.253	0.999	0.635	0.214	0.931
w/interdep. traces	Power	0.700	0.827	0.986	0.448	0.701	0.989	0.630	0.836	0.965

Single-Integrator Models Results from a single-integrator model (equation 1) are presented in figure 6.6. Traces in this model integrate effects over more than just the previous reinforcer, in which larger values of a serve to extend the effect of each reinforcer. This was not the case in the simple-exponential model. Figure 6.6 shows only results of the wait-and-respond model with interdependent traces because response-strength varieties produce greater undermatching with concurrent VI VI schedules, which is counter to behavior seen in pigeons. Independent trace models produce equivalent results to those seen in figure 6.6. Overall, the integrator produces a fair approximation to the pattern of results produced by pigeons on concurrent RI RI, VI VI, and VI FI, although the bias toward the VI in the last case is not as clear as with the simple-exponential model.

The mechanisms that produced these results are clear. In the case of response-strength models, shorter inter-reinforcement intervals produce higher traces. With the wait-and-respond models, shorter inter-reinforcement intervals produce shorter wait times. Each, in turn, leads to higher rates of responding. Given the stochastic response rule, more responses to one alternative means fewer responses to the other. Figure 6.7 illustrates the simple manner in which the arithmetic intervals of the VI VI schedules increased undermatching relative to the concurrent RI RI (data are from the response-strength model shown in figure 6.6). The bottom plots in figure 6.7 show that RI 12 produced more frequent short inter-reinforcement times than the RI 60 up to about $t = 40$, while the arithmetic VI 12 produced shorter intervals only to about $t = 10$. In effect, the RI schedules produced a much larger discrepancy in the number of short IRIs than did the VI schedules. The role of short intervals is equally clear in the case of the concurrent VI FI comparison. Short intervals encountered on the VI side produced responding that precluded responses on the FI side, sometimes even lengthening the FI duration.

Discussion and Conclusion

A memory-trace model of choice, incorporating reinforcement time markers for trace onset and a stochastic response rule, can reproduce at least four qualitative findings in the concurrent literature with a single set of parameters: undermatching as a function of reinforcement intervals, power matching, preference for VI over FI schedules, and a steep power function

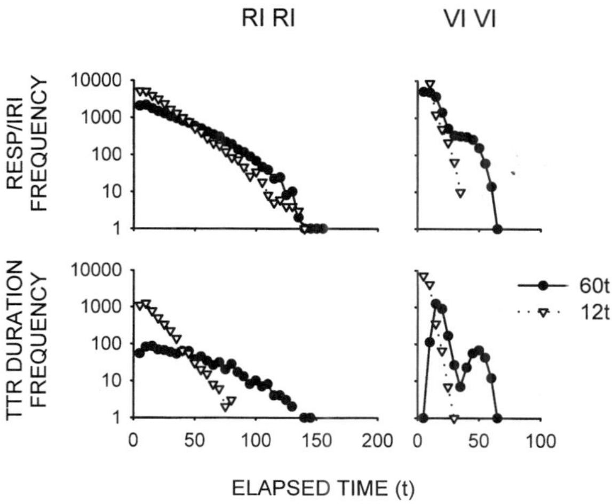

Figure 6.7
Frequency distributions of responses per inter-reinforcement interval (IRI: upper plots) and time to reinforcement (TTR: lower plots) in the concurrent RI RI (left plots) and VI VI (right plots) conditions of the simple exponential model (with behavior allocated by response-strength and with independent traces: Figure 6.5A). Only the RI60 and RI12 schedule performances are shown. Each data point represents a bin of $t = 5$. Frequency is plotted on log coordinates.

between wait and response ratios. The deductive appeal of the model is obvious since it only assumes a memory trace and a response rule. Hence, from this simple molecular process emerges some of the molar subtleties of matching.

Which of the various successful memory models holds the most promise? Two additional considerations point to the wait-and-respond model with interdependent, simple exponential traces (figure 6.4C: henceforth, the WRI model). First, it is the only type that correctly approximated both power matching and the power relation between wait time and responding (figure 6.6). The remaining simple exponential types yield exponents much less than one, and the integrator model yields a negative exponent, both of which are deviations from empirical findings (Cerutti and Staddon 2003). The second reason is illustrated in figure 6.8. Staddon and colleagues have argued that many concurrent chain findings can be explained by some form of proportional post-reinforcement waiting (reviewed in Staddon and Cerutti 2003; Staddon and Ettinger 1989). In a concurrent-chain schedule,

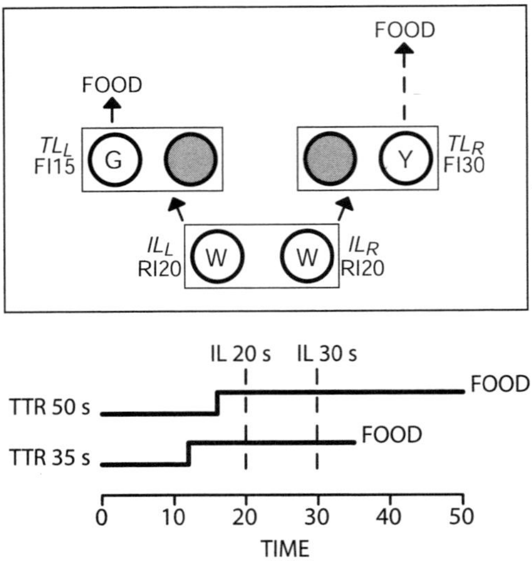

Figure 6.8
The upper diagram shows a typical concurrent-chain schedule programmed on two response keys, with a 50-second time to reinforcement (TTR) on the left and a 35-second TTR on the right. Choices are made on left and right initial-link (IL) keys, each scheduling a corresponding differential terminal-link (TL) schedule according to identical IL schedules. In this example, responses on left and right White RI 20 ILs, lead to corresponding Green FI 15 and Yellow FI 30 TLs. The lower diagram shows the effect on choice of changing the IL schedule values. Two wait-time plots (shown as the step up in the event records) are shown for chains with TTR of 50 seconds and 35 seconds. Waits follow a proportional-waiting rule in which responding begins at 1/3 of the interval. Vertical dashed lines represent mean IL duration for RI 20 seconds versus RI 30 seconds. The effect of lengthening the IL duration, assuming that wait remains a constant proportion of TTR, is to reduce the proportion of responses to the shorter TTR. Adapted from Staddon and Ettinger 1989.

figure 6.8 shows how proportional waiting might explain one of these findings, how given two times to reinforcement, preference for the shorter time increases as initial-link duration is decreased (Fantino 1981; Fantino, Preston, and Dunn 1993). With two fixed times to reinforcement of 50 seconds and 35 seconds, a 30-second initial link yields relative responding of 0.56 in favor of the 35-second delay, while a 20-second initial link yields relative responding of 0.67 in favor of the 35-second delay. In the domain of models considered here, only the pause-and-respond type with interdependent traces can properly model such a finding.

There are several deficiencies in the WRI model. Although there is ample evidence that organisms are sensitive to the immediately preceding reinforcement interval (e.g., Davison and Baum 2000; Dreyfus 1991; Higa 1996; Higa, Thaw, and Staddon 1993; Higa, Wynn, and Staddon 1991; Innis, Mitchell, and Staddon 1993), it is clear that the one-back determination of wait in the simple exponential trace is insufficient; there must also be a longer-term, slower, cumulative memory for reinforcers that would account for history effects such as slower adjustments in responding after longer exposure to training (Davis et al. 1993; Dragci and Staddon 1999; Grace 2002; Mazur 1992; Staddon et al. 2002). The sort of memory dynamics that could reproduce the myriad of history effects now found in the choice literature is unknown, but it is certain to be complex. The model also failed to show overmatching with the addition of a change-over ratio. It remains to be seen if this is a tangential question requiring an elaboration of the model or a deeper flaw in the model. A more serious problem is that the model does not show extinction. A response that is not reinforced retains its previous response threshold. Again, the solution is not obvious, but little is known about how responding extinguishes on concurrent schedules. Additional research, empirical and theoretical, will be required to refine or refute the WRI model.

Despite the absence of a clear quantitative match to data, the success of an interdependent trace, wait-and-respond model, suggests that response rate may be derived, at least in part, from waiting (Staddon and Ettinger 1989). If so, it may be possible to reveal the continuity that must exist between performance on simple schedules, where the relation between waiting and response rate is better understood and their combinations in choice experiments where the emphasis has been only on response rate (Staddon and Cerutti 2003). The lacuna between simple and concurrent schedules must be due, at least in part, to the natural antagonism in science between the need to discover and the need to understand. On the one hand, theory must wait for compelling facts to suggest it; on the other, facts are meager curiosities without a theory to organize them. B. F. Skinner believed strongly in the former proposition: the correct set of facts would eventually lead to a productive theory of behavior. There can be no doubt that facts are primary, but theories have always been the final arbiter in the selection of facts. Only theory can sufficiently distill facts in order to resolve the fundamental dimensions that Skinner sought empirically. In a final analysis, the fundamental dimensions of behavior cannot be decided before a *theoretical validation* (Staddon 1983, 2001).

I would like to end by expressing the great fortune I feel to have John Staddon as a friend and a colleague. Variation and selection are the sine qua non of scientific development, and John has been both a careful listener and a reasoned critic. I have benefited greatly.

Notes

1. Many two-parameter retention functions (review in Rubin and Wenzel 1996) generate respectable approximations to FI waiting under steady-state conditions with this model, but only a logarithmic function will yield a linear relation between FI and IFI.

2. A wait-and-respond model with independent traces, without a response rule that prevents simultaneous responses to each alternative at each time step (i.e., the case shown for V_0 in figure 6.3), will allocate nearly equal numbers of responses to each alternative irrespective of the schedule values if the model also shows (approximately) proportional waiting and a constant running-response rate. (Note that overall rates of responding on different FI schedules are roughly equal; see, e.g., Schneider 1969.)

7 The Spatial Memory of African Elephants (*Loxodonta africana*): Durability, Interference, and Response Biases

Robert H. I. Dale

Women and elephants never forget an injury.
—Saki (H. H. Munro), "Reginald on besetting sins," in *Reginald* (1904)

I am not sure whether the satirist H. H. Munro believed Saki's claim, although it may well be true (at least with regard to elephants). This chapter will examine some characteristics of elephant memory more systematically than did Saki.

In general, it is to an animal's advantage to remember some aspects (usually the stable features) of a situation for long periods and to remember other aspects (usually the unstable features) only temporarily. Consistent with recent arguments questioning the value of cognitive constructs for studying animal behavior (Grau 2002; Staddon 2001a,b; Wright and Watkins 1987), I will use "reference memory" and "working memory" (Baddeley and Hitch 1974; Honig 1978) only as descriptive terms indicating formal task requirements. (See Olton, Becker, and Handelmann 1979.) The stable characteristics of the test situation (such as the shape of the spatial array of food sources) are said to involve reference memory; those features that vary across trials (such as the sequence of food sites visited on a trial) are said to involve working memory. My main goal is to demonstrate that elephants can remember which locations they have visited during a spatial memory test similar to the "radial maze" (Olton and Samuelson 1976). The data will show that elephants rely on memory to solve several spatial problems, rather than relying on their response biases (Dale and Innis 1986) or their excellent olfactory abilities (Rasmussen and Krishnamurthy 2000). In addition, I will describe research showing that performance on the memory task is susceptible to proactive interference and that the retention of reference memory components of the test procedures is durable.

Historical Context

Despite the long history of study and management of both Asian elephants (*Elephas maximus*) and African elephants (*Loxodonta africana*), relatively few studies have been conducted to evaluate their memory abilities (Grzimek 1944; Hediger 1955; Hobhouse 1901; Markowitz, Schmidt, Nadal, and Squier 1975; Rensch 1957).

An analog of the radial maze (Olton and Samuelson 1976) was used to examine the spatial memory of African elephants: In particular, their ability to distinguish locations they had visited during a trial from locations they had not visited. Radial-maze and similar tests have been used to study spatial memory in numerous species. These include honeybees (Brown and Demas 1994), fish (Hughes and Blight 1999), birds (Gould-Beierle 2000), mice (Dale and Bedard 1984), rats (Olton and Samuelson 1976), monkeys (MacDonald and Wilkie 1990), great apes (MacDonald 1994), and humans (Dale 1987). As far as I know, the animals most closely related to elephants (manatees and hyraxes; Shoshani 2000) have not participated in spatial memory tests. However, some of the elephant's closest evolutionary "cousins" (Colbert, Morales, and Minkoff 2001), the odd-toed ungulates, have done so (e.g., horses, Marinier and Alexander 1994; Waring 2002). In addition, many of the more distantly related even-toed ungulates have been tested, including cattle (Bailey, Rittenhouse, Hart, and Richards 1989), goats and sheep (Hosoi, Swift, Rittenhouse, and Richards 1995), and pigs (Mendl, Laughlin and Hitchcock 1997). The present studies extend such tests to another large herbivore, the African elephant (*Loxodonta africana*), a large-brained, long-lived species with a complex social structure and a large home range (Moss and Poole 1983).

Basic Characteristics of Elephant Spatial Memory

The elephants were exposed to a series of progressively more complex test situations to provide a preliminary description of this species' spatial memory abilities. After familiarization with an (empty) food container, a large pot, the subjects were presented with a variety of two-pot tests (Dale, Shyan, and Hagan 1994a). In the first two procedures, choices were not differentially rewarded with food (a "spontaneous alternation" task: Richman, Dember, and Kim 1986). At first, the pots at both locations were empty; in later tests, both of the pots were baited (and refilled between choices). Rats typically alternate choices when no food is involved (as do many other animals), but are more likely to repeat choices ("win-stay;" Richman, et al. 1986) when food is available at both locations. The elephants next received a test where alternation (a "win-shift" strategy; Olton and Schlosberg 1978) was selectively rewarded. The two pots were baited at the start of each two-choice test, but the first pot selected was not re-baited between choices. After the two-choice phase, the subjects were tested with arrays of four, and then eight, food locations. The sequence of choices made during these tests was analyzed to identify response patterns and possible algorithms (Dale and Innis 1986; Yoerg and Kamil 1982) being used by the subjects. In addition, several types of olfactory control tests were administered to eliminate the obvious possibility that the elephants might locate the food by smell (Rasmussen and Krishnamurthy 2000).

General Methods

Subjects

The subjects were five unrelated wild-born female African elephants (*Loxodonta africana*) residing at the Indianapolis Zoo. The animals were maintained on *ad libitum* food and water, except during the test. Their diet consisted of hay, fruit, vegetables, browse, and commercial elephant food and vitamin supplements. The subjects were Cita, 23 years old when testing began, approximate weight 3,450 kilograms; Ivory, 10 years old, 2,150 kg; Kubwa, 16 years old, 2,650 kg; Sophi, 24 years old, 4,350 kg; and Tombi, 15 years old, 2,450 kg. They were managed with a "free contact" technique: The animals participated in a variety of activities each day under the direct supervision of professional handlers (zoo staff). The elephants were housed overnight in three stalls in a large barn. On most days, the subjects were released into a large public exhibit near the barn. On cold days (defined by air temperature, humidity, wind speed, and amount of direct sunlight), the elephants stayed in the barn.

Test Environments

The elephants were given the two-pot tests and the initial four-pot tests inside the largest stall in the barn (with only the test animal in the stall). The stall was 8.3 meters by 7.3 meters, with a concrete floor. It was surrounded on two sides by bars and on two sides by concrete walls. There was a wide variety of visual cues available in the barn. A subject started each test standing with its head above a 0.7 meter by 0.5 meter rubber mat, which served to mark the "start" position. The food was contained in 12-quart stainless steel stockpots with tight-fitting lids. Each lid had a small stainless steel handle, which the elephants used to lift the lids. During tests, each pot was placed on a gray plastic pan, 36 centimeters in diameter, with a rim 6 centimeters high. Black marks on the floor under the plastic pans indicated the goal locations for resetting the pots after the elephants had handled them.

The later four-pot testing, and all of the eight-pot testing, was conducted in a fenced arena, approximately 34 meters by 17 meters, outside of the barn. During testing, this arena was divided in half by a yellow rope hanging at a height of 0.5–1.5 meter, designating a 20 meter × 17 meter test area. The start mat and pots/pans were removed between sessions. The test array was replaced before each test, using fence landmarks to place the start mat, and a large "protractor" and ropes to place the pots at 45° intervals relative to the mat. The absolute positions of the test arrays typically varied by less than a meter across days.

The food reward was one food pellet per pot on the two-pot tests, either one or four food pellets on the four-pot tests (Purina monkey chow #5045, approximately 7.3 grams per pellet), and one Red Delicious apple per pot for the eight-pot tests (approximately 130 grams per apple).

Handling Procedures

The elephants were always tested under the supervision of a handler, at least two handlers were present for each test, and the experimenter/observer manipulated the apparatus but did not interact with the elephants. Each animal was on about five days per week. Since the test procedures were novel, the testing schedule was conservative: It was deemed better to give too many trials on a given procedure than to change procedures prematurely.

Data Analysis

Although the observer recorded the subjects' choices during each test, all trials were videotaped for later analysis. During the four-pot tests, the elephants were tested in an "arc array," with the pots close together in a large stall. The subjects sometimes moved quickly in the confined situation, swinging their trunks near more than one pot during a single choice opportunity. It was difficult for either the observer or the handler to be sure how close an elephant's trunk came to the pots during these choices. In addition, subjects occasionally turned away from a pot without touching the lid, but after moving the trunk to within several centimeters of the pot (or touching it). This happened for both baited and unbaited pots. To reduce the possibility that the subjects were using smell to detect food in the baited pots, the criterion for a choice was conservative: Any approach to within a foot (0.3 meter) of a pot constituted a choice, whether the subject touched the pot or not. A few tests were discarded because a subject selected two pots during the same choice opportunity (a "double choice"), even though the animal may have touched only one (or none) of the pots.

Inter-Observer Reliability

Two trained raters evaluated each videotaped trial, comparing scores using Cohen's Kappa coefficient of agreement (Cohen 1960). This measure describes the proportion of agreements in two raters' observations, corrected for the proportion of agreements expected by chance. For each scoring disagreement between raters, the videotape was re-evaluated by the author, who assigned a value to the disputed observation. A few disagreements were the result of one rater assigning the wrong code to an observation. However, most disagreements resulted from trials on which a double choice may have occurred. The data from such "double choice" trials would have been difficult to interpret, and were not analyzed.

Two-Pot Tests: Assessing Response Biases

Before testing proper began, each of the elephants was familiarized with the stockpot during 4–16 brief exposures to a single empty pot in the large stall. Each exposure ended when the elephant touched the pot or after one minute.

No-Food Test

The key question for this test was whether, during its second choice, the elephant would return to the first pot it had touched or choose the other pot. Each elephant was tested in the large stall with two empty stockpots placed

5 meters apart on the floor, and 4 meters in front of the start mat (figure 7.1). The animal was "released" by a handler's verbal cue and allowed 2 minutes to touch one of the pots. The animal was then recalled to the start position and released again. As a procedural control to disrupt potential body-orientation strategies, the elephant was turned around 180°, to face away from the pots, between choices. To eliminate the possibility of unconscious cueing (the Clever Hans effect), different handlers supervised the first and second choices, and the handlers did not watch each other's part of the test. Each elephant except Kubwa was tested until it had completed both choices on 10 trials (Kubwa stopped responding after a few trials). Because, occasionally, an elephant moved the first pot it touched, leaving mucus on the pot's lid, the observer wiped and replaced the lid of the chosen pot, resetting it in its original position. The observer then touched the other pot, wiping mucus on its lid. These control procedures were used for Tombi starting with the two-pot, "replace-food" condition, and for all testing with the other elephants. On each of the two-pot procedures, subjects were tested twice a day, with 3–4 minutes between trials.

In this condition, the elephants frequently failed to complete a choice in under two minutes. The reluctance to choose was particularly evident for Kubwa: this subject completed only two trials under the procedure. Overall, the subjects failed to complete 31 trials. They made "double choices" on two other trials.

As a group, the four subjects which completed 10 trials exhibited a position preference, choosing the pot to their right on 75 percent of their initial choices during a trial, $t(3) = 5.0$, $p < 0.05$ (table 7.1). The tendency for "spontaneous alternation" was evaluated using a correction for initial response biases (Dember and Fowler 1958): Expected proportion of alternations, $E(\text{alt}) = [1 - (p_L^2 + p_R^2)]$, where p_L = the proportion of initial choices to the left and p_R = the proportion of initial choices to the right. Using the left/right response bias on the first choice of completed trials (table 7.1), an expected alternation frequency was calculated. For example, Cita chose the pot on the right on 8/10 initial choices, producing an expected alternation rate of 0.32. The difference between the actual alternation frequency and the expected alternation frequency was calculated for each subject completing 10 trials. The mean difference score for these four subjects (3.15) was statistically significant, $t(3) = 6.68$, $p < 0.01$, suggesting a tendency to alternate choices in this situation. (Without using the correc-

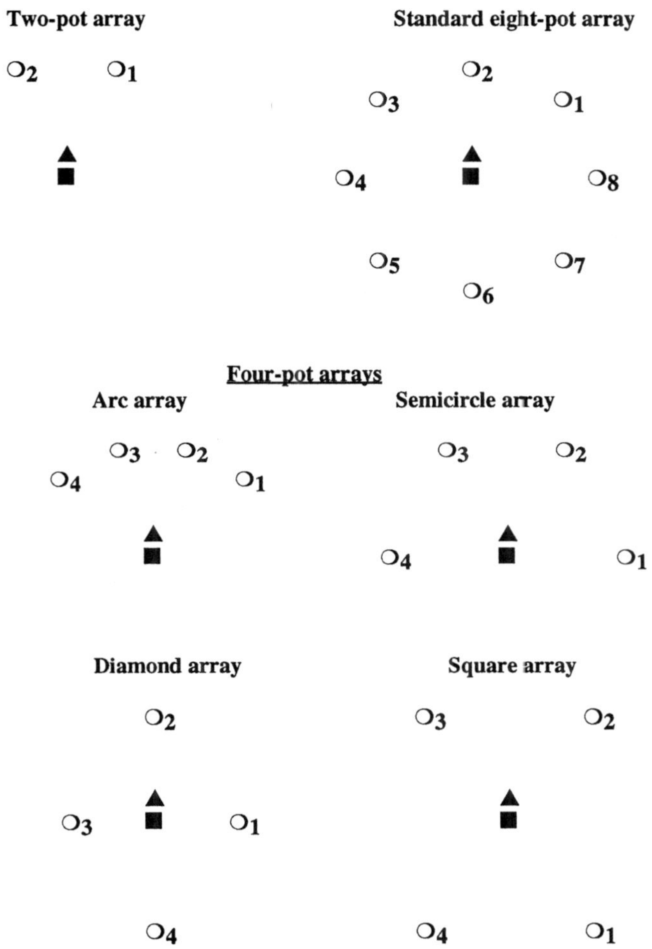

Figure 7.1
The two-pot, four-pot, and eight-pot arrays used in the series of memory tests. The pot locations are numbered as they were for data collection. The diagrams indicate the relative locations of the pots (open circles), the elephant's starting position over the mat (filled square) and the elephant's orientation when released to make a choice (filled triangle). The eight-pot array was rotated 22.5° on some of the later tests, putting four pots in front of the subject and four pots behind it.

Table 7.1
Choice patterns on the two-pot tests. Number of response alternations in ten trials (alternations), number of initial choices to the pot on the right side (right pot), and number of trials discarded before ten trials meeting the criteria were completed. Inter-rater reliability (Cohen's Kappa coefficient) was calculated for each subject over all of the two-pot conditions.

Condition	Subject					
Measure	Cita	Ivory	Kubwa	Sophi	Tombi	Mean (*n*)
No food						
Alternations	7	5	—	7	8	6.75 (4)
Right pot	8	8	—	8	6	7.50 (4)
Discarded	8	3	6	13	3	6.75 (4)
Replace food						
Alternations	7	2	0	0	7	3.20 (5)
Right Pot	10	10	10	10	9	9.80 (5)
Discarded	0	0	0	0	0	0.00 (5)
Not replace food						
Criterion	10	22	20	28	18	19.6 (5)
Right pot (%)	100	48	85	100	83	83 (5)
Discarded	0	1	1	1	1	0.6 (5)
Cohen's Kappa	1.000	0.940	0.950	0.950	0.950	0.96 (5)

tion for initial response bias, these four subjects had only a moderate, non-significant tendency to alternate their choices (67.5 percent of trials; $t(3) = 2.38$, $p > 0.05$).

Replace-Food Test

Before this test, each elephant was given 10–30 opportunities to collect a single food pellet from a closed pot placed on the floor below the animal's head. After this training, all five elephants collected the food pellet rapidly.

In the replace-food test, a food pellet was placed in each pot to see whether adding food would influence the animals' search strategies (Richman et al. 1986). The pot opened on the first choice was re-baited before the elephant's second choice, and both pots were touched and reset by the observer. Each subject received 10–12 trials on this task.

Once food was available in each pot, every subject completed every trial. The initial response bias was even stronger, with the pot to the right being selected on 98 percent of the initial choices (table 7.1). Each of the five subjects exhibited a tendency to choose the pot on the right with its initial choice (binomial test, $p < 0.05$). There was no clear generic response pattern, since two subjects tended toward alternation and three subjects tended toward repetition of their two choices during a trial (table 7.1).

Not-Replace-Food Test

On this test, the elephant chose one of two baited pots, then received a food pellet on the second choice only if it chose the other pot. Subjects were tested to a criterion of eight alternations in ten trials. All subjects learned to alternate within 28 trials (mean number of trials to criterion = 19.6, including the three discarded trials; table 7.1). The response bias toward the pot on the right continued for four of the five subjects (table 7.1: binomial test; $p < 0.05$ in each case).

Inter-Rater Reliability

The Kappa coefficients of agreement for the three types of two-pot tests are presented in table 7.1. The lowest Kappa coefficient was 0.94, indicating a high level of inter-rater reliability.

Conclusions: Two-Pot Tests

Overall, the subjects exhibited a position preference to the right on their initial choices during a trial. This bias was weak during the no-food procedure, but strong for most of the subjects during both the replace-food and the no-replace-food procedures. Similar position preferences have been observed in other large herbivores (Hosoi, Rittenhouse et al. 1995; Hosoi, Swift et al. 1995). It is not clear whether the strong response biases represent hereditary predispositions of the elephants, perhaps related to their foraging styles, or result from the specific life experiences of these animals. Testing with other groups of elephants may clarify this issue.

Because of the response biases, the tendency toward spontaneous alternation was assessed using adjusted scores (Dember and Fowler 1958). There was a statistically significant rate of alternation under the no-food condition, in a manner typical of many other species (Richman et al. 1986). However, this tendency should be studied with forced choice, rather than free choice, procedures (Richman et al. 1986) to control for initial response biases, and with more subjects, before definitive conclusions can be drawn.

Table 7.2
Total number of trials conducted, mean choice accuracy for the last five trials, and inter-rater reliability (Cohen's Kappa coefficient) on the four-pot tests with the arc, semicircle, diamond, and square arrays.

		Subject					
Array	Measure	Cita	Ivory	Kubwa	Sophi	Tombi	Mean
Arc	Trials	11	12	10	12	12	11.4
	Accuracy	3.0	3.6	3.6	3.2	3.2	3.32
	Kappa	0.91	0.94	0.92	0.87	0.87	0.90
Semicircle	Trials	11	11	11	9	11	10.6
	Accuracy	3.8	3.8	3.8	3.6	3.8	3.76
	Kappa	1.00	1.00	1.00	0.96	1.00	0.99
Diamond	Trials	12	10	10	11	10	10.6
	Accuracy	3.0	3.4	3.6	3.2	3.4	3.32
	Kappa	0.94	0.93	0.97	1.00	0.93	0.95
Square	Trials	4	13	10	14	11	10.4
	Accuracy	3.25[a]	3.2	3.8	3.0	4.0	3.45
	Kappa	1.00	0.97	1.00	1.00	0.91	0.98

a. Cita completed only four trials under this procedure.

When food was introduced into the task in the replace-food condition, only two of the five subjects continued to alternate choices. This disruption of spontaneous alternation by the availability of food reward has been demonstrated previously with rats (Richman et al. 1986), although sometimes rats maintain a "win-shift" search pattern on the radial maze when all responses are rewarded equally (Olton and Schlosberg 1978). Ungulates exhibit a win-stay tendency under these conditions (Hosoi, Rittenhouse et al. 1995; Hosoi, Swift et al. 1995).

When the subjects were rewarded for alternating their choices, the "win-shift" strategy was acquired rapidly.

Four-Pot Procedures

Single-Pot Pre-Exposure

Each elephant was given trials on which it was allowed to open a single pot placed in one of four locations in the large stall (arc array, figure 7.1). The four locations were arranged along the arc of a 4.1-meter-radius circle centered on the mat which marked the elephant's starting location. Adjacent locations on the arc were separated by 2.3 meters. On a trial, the elephant was released by the handler and allowed to collect a single food pellet from the pot. The elephant was then called back to the start position. Elephants were tested 2–4 times with each of the four pot locations (a total of 8–16 trials, spread over 2 days).

Arc Array Pre-Training (Barn)

Before the tests in the arena, the elephants were tested with the arc array (figure 7.1) inside the barn. Each subject was tested once per day. For the first 20–25 trials, the reward in each pot was 1 food pellet. The reward was increased to 4 pellets for the next 10–15 trials.

Arc, Semicircle, Diamond, and Square Arrays (Arena)

The apparatus was moved to the outside arena, to determine whether the spacing of the food locations would influence choice accuracy. The spatial separation between food sources (Dale 1982; Douglas, Mitchell, and Del Valle 1974), or between food sources and nearby landmarks (Brown 1992) influences search strategies in other animals. The subjects were tested once per day, 4–5 days per week. The reward in each pot was four food pellets (29–30 grams). The elephants received 10–12 trials on the arc array (figure 7.1). The pots were 4.3 meters from the center of the start mat under the elephant's jaw, and 2.3 meters apart. The subjects next received approximately ten trials on each of three four-pot arrays. To visualize the patterns, imagine the elephant facing forward as being an orientation of 0° on a compass. The first arrangement (semicircle array, figure 7.1) placed the four pots in a semicircle around the elephant, with pots at 60° intervals. The pots were 4.3 meters from the center of the mat and 4.0 meters apart. In the second arrangement (diamond array, figure 7.1), pots were placed directly in front of and behind the subject, and to the subject's left and right. For this test, the elephant stood with the mat beneath its stomach, between the forelegs and the hind legs, between choices. The pots were 4.3 meters from the center of the mat for Tombi, Kubwa, and Ivory. Starting with Sophi's third trial, and for all of Cita's trials, the pots were placed 4.9 meters from the center mat. The larger circle was used for the two largest animals because they would occasionally reach toward the rear pot while they were standing at the center of the circle between choices. The final four-pot array was the square array (figure 7.1), in which the four pots were placed at 90° intervals around the subject, with pots 45° to the subject's left and right. The radius of the array was increased to 6.7 meters for all subjects, in preparation for the eight-pot tests.

The data for the tests with the arc, semicircle, diamond, and square arrays (figure 7.1) are presented in table 7.2.

Inter-Rater Reliability

The inter-rater reliability was high for all subjects. The lowest value of Cohen's Kappa for any subject on any test was 0.87, and the median was 0.965. The inter-rater reliability was lowest for the arc array, possibly because of the close proximity of the pots in this array.

Choice Accuracy

Choice accuracy for this phase of testing was measured by the number of different pots selected in four choices. Because of the strict choice criterion, there were a number of trials discarded during this phase of the experiment. Since an acquisition curve would mean little under these conditions, table 7.2 shows the total number of trials in the arena experienced by each subject and the mean choice accuracy over each subject's last five trials. Generally, the subjects were given 9–14 trials on each four-pot array. The median number of trials was 11. (Cita only received 4 trials on the square array.) The testing order was arc, then semicircle, then diamond, then square arrays. The mean choice accuracy for each subject on the last five (completed) trials in each condition is shown in table 7.2. A within-subjects ANOVA was carried out to compare choice accuracy across the four arrays. There was a clear effect of the Array factor: $F(3,12) = 12.00$, $p < 0.01$. Orthogonal contrasts ($3X_{\text{semi}} - X_{\text{arc}} - X_{\text{diamond}} - X_{\text{square}}$: $F(1,12) = 11.60$, $p < 0.01$; $X_{\text{diamond}} + X_{\text{square}} - 2X_{\text{arc}}$: $F(1,12) = 0.28$, $p > 0.05$; $X_{\text{diamond}} - X_{\text{square}}$: $F(1,12) = 0.83$, $p > 0.05$) indicated that choice accuracy was higher with the semicircular array than with the other three arrays, and performance was equivalent on those three arrays. The subjects' mean choice accuracy was above chance (random choice: 2.734 pots) for each of the arrays: arc array, (3.32), $t(4) = 4.88$; semicircle array, (3.76), $t(4) = 25.65$; diamond array (3.32), $t(4) = 5.75$; square array (3.45), $t(4) = 3.45$ ($p < 0.05$ in each case).

Response Biases and Patterns

Response biases were determined for each array by the distribution of "first choices" during all trials on that array. The distribution of "first choices" on each array was non-random for some subjects on each array. On the arc array, all of the elephants except Cita exhibited a side preference (binomial test, $p < 0.05$): Tombi was biased to turn left (83 percent of all trials: pots 3 and 4) whereas Ivory (83 percent), Kubwa (90 percent), and Sophi (83 percent) were biased toward turning right (pots 1 and 2). On the semicircular array, Tombi again had a "left-turn" bias (100 percent) and Ivory had a right-turn bias (100 percent; binomial test, $p < 0.05$). Kubwa (73 percent) had a non-significant tendency to turn left; Sophi (78 percent) had a non-significant tendency to turn right. With the diamond array, all five subjects showed significant response biases (binomial test, $p < 0.05$). Cita (92 percent), Ivory (100 percent), and Sophi (100 percent) tended to choose pots 1 and 2, whereas Kubwa chose pots 2 and 3 (100 percent) and Tombi chose pot 3 (100 percent). No subject ever chose pot 4 (behind the subject) with its first choice (0/53 trials). Finally, on the square array all subjects tended to choose the two pots in front of them at the start of the test (90.4 percent: pots 2 and 3). Individually, Ivory (85 percent), Sophi (100 percent) and Tombi (91 percent) exhibited significant "forward" biases. Kubwa exhibited a non-significant forward bias (80 percent). Cita (100 percent forward choices) completed only 4 trials under this condition.

Conclusions: Four-Pot Tests

The elephants had above-chance choice accuracies on all four arrays, although performance was best on the semicircular array. Perhaps this array presented the optimal task because the pots were spaced far apart and in front of the subject. Unlike the diamond and square arrays, the subjects were not required to turn around—contrary to their persistent, strong response biases—to obtain food.

Eight-Pot Procedures

The subjects were tested with an eight-pot array (figure 7.1), as an analogue of Olton and Samuelson's (1976) eight-arm radial maze apparatus. The pots were placed at 45° intervals around the perimeter of a 6.7-meter-radius circle, centered on the mat. Before each trial, each of the eight pots was baited with one apple. To begin a trial, the subject was placed in the center of the circle of pots (with its torso over the mat), facing pot 2. It was released by a handler, allowed to choose one pot, then was recalled and repositioned over the mat, facing pot 6 (turned 180°) between choices. The observer then walked around the circle of pots, touching every pot, and replacing the lid on the pot that had been chosen. Any mucus left on the pot lid was smeared on nearby pots. A second handler then took control of the elephant, turned it to face pot 2, and released it for another choice. The procedure continued, with the two handlers alternating, until the subject had made eight choices.

Inter-Rater Reliability

The inter-rater reliability was calculated for all eight-pot trials completed by each subject. Cohen's Kappa was at least 0.97 for each subject, indicating very high inter-rater reliability.

Choice Accuracy

Choice accuracy was measured by the number of different pots chosen during the subject's eight choices on each trial (table 7.3). Random selection under this procedure would produce an expected score of 5.25.

Data are reported for five-trial blocks from the first 25 completed trials for each subject (table 7.3). The numbers in parentheses indicate the number of incomplete (and therefore discarded) trials within each block. In addi-

Table 7.3

Choice accuracy on the eight-pot array: mean number of different pots chosen in eight choices. The number of trials discarded in obtaining each block of five trials is shown in parentheses.

Trials	Cita	Ivory	Kubwa	Sophi	Tombi	Mean
1–5	5.8(1)	7.2(4)	6.6(3)	6.2(1)	6.8(0)	6.52[a] (1.8)
6–10	7.0(1)	7.8(1)	6.8(2)	6.8(0)	6.8(1)	7.04[a] (1.0)
11–15	7.0(0)	7.6(1)	7.4(0)	8.0(0)	7.2(0)	7.44[a] (0.2)
16–20	7.4(0)	7.4(1)	7.6(2)	7.8(1)	7.0(1)	7.44[a] (1.0)
21–25	7.0(0)	7.2(1)	7.4(1)	7.8(0)	7.6(1)	7.40[a] (0.6)

a. Group mean choice accuracy is significantly above chance (random choice of pots), $p < 0.01$.

tion to the 23 incomplete trials, there were five trials on which a subject was faced "backwards," toward pot 6, to start the trial. Data from these five trials are not included. The group mean choice accuracy was significantly above that expected from random choice (5.25) for all blocks of five trials (smallest t value: for trials 1–5, $t(4) = 5.26$, $p < 0.01$). There was a significant improvement in choice accuracy across blocks of trials, $F(4, 16) = 5.80$, $p < 0.01$.

Response Biases and Patterns

The subjects exhibited several consistent response biases during the eight-pot test (table 7.4). All subjects tended to choose the pots in front of them (pots 8, 1–4, figure 7.1) when they were released, only selecting the pots behind them (pots 5–7, figure 7.1) toward the end of a trial. This tendency was assessed with three measures: The percentage of trials with the initial choice made to one of the front five pots; the percentage of the first five choices made to these five pots; and the percentage of errors (repetitions) made to these pots. For a subject choosing pots randomly, the expected value for each of these percentages would be 62.5 percent. The subjects' tendency to choose front pots exceeded chance by each of these measures. The mean percentage of first choices to the front pots was 98 percent; the mean percentage of the first five choices to the front pots was 90 percent; the mean percentage of errors to the front pots was 90 percent (Smallest t value: $t(4) = 11.5$, $p < 0.01$).

The response sequences exhibited by the subjects were evaluated in two ways: by the mean transition size and by the frequency of stereotyped

Table 7.4

Response biases on the eight-pot test: percentage of initial choices, the first five choices, and errors made to the front five pots; mean transition size and percentage of trials with a response pattern involving four or more consecutive choices.

Measure	Cita	Ivory	Kubwa	Sophi	Tombi	Mean
First choice (%)	100	96	96	100	96	98
Five choices (%)	87	90	91	94	90	90
Errors (%)	93	93	95	88	82	90
Transition size	2.07	1.83	2.21	1.81	2.11	2.01
Pattern (%)	56	36	8	44	20	33

choice sequences. The mean transition size was the average distance between the pots selected on consecutive choices, with the distance between adjacent pots being designated as one unit. The minimum transition size was 0 (returning immediately to the pot just selected); the maximum transition size was 4 (choosing the pot in the circle opposite to the pot just selected). A subject choosing pots randomly would be expected to have a mean transition size of 2.00, because each of the eight possible transition sizes (0, ± 1, ± 2, ± 3, 4) would occur equally often. The mean transition size of the five subjects was 2.01, which did not differ from chance, $t(4) = 0.08$, $p > 0.05$. However, the distribution of transition sizes was not random. With random choice, each of the eight transition sizes would have occurred equally often, on 12.5 percent of the transitions. Overall, transition sizes of 4, 3, 2, 1, 0, -1, -2, and -3 occurred on 11.7 percent, 12.2 percent, 10.6 percent, 29.7 percent, 1.6 percent, 13.0 percent, 10.2 percent, and 11.0 percent of the transitions, respectively. In other words, subjects rarely returned to the same pot (transition size $= 0$), whereas choosing the "next pot to the left" was common (transition size $= 1$). The other six possible transition sizes occurred with near-chance frequencies.

To determine whether response algorithms might play a role in determining choice accuracy (Olton and Samuelson 1976), the frequencies of four possible response algorithms were measured: "adjacent" (e.g., 12345678) "alternate" (e.g., 24681357), "every third" (e.g., 14725836), and "opposite" (e.g., 15263748). In 125 trials, there was not a single example of a sequence of seven or eight choices made consistent with one of these algorithms. The criterion for a response pattern was a minimum of four consecutive choices during a trial matching the pattern (e.g., 1234, 2468, 1472, 1526). Adjacent, alternate, every-third and opposite patterns occurred on 26.7 percent, 0.8 percent, 0 percent, and 8.0 percent of all trials, respectively (table 7.4; on two trials, both adjacent and opposite patterns occurred).

The influence of response patterns on choice accuracy was assessed by comparing the mean choice accuracy on all trials with response patterns to that on all trials without such patterns. Although the mean choice accuracy on trials with a response pattern was higher than the mean choice accuracy on other trials, 7.33 vs. 7.07, the difference was not statistically significant, $t(4) = 1.29$, $p > 0.05$.

Table 7.5
Mean choice accuracy on the 8-pot test for the last five trials before, and the first five trials after a 6–8 month interruption of testing. In 1992 there were 4-pot and 8-pot tests. The date for the last test of each type is shown in the table.

	Last 1992 4-pot test	Last 1992 8-pot test	Choice accuracy	First 1993 8-pot test	Choice accuracy
Cita	Dec 12	Dec 9	7.2	June 28	7.8
Ivory	Dec 12	Dec 9	7.2	June 28	7.0
Kubwa	Nov 19	Oct 23	7.6	June 28	7.2
Sophi	Dec 12	Dec 9	7.4	June 28	7.8
Tombi	Nov 19	Oct 23	7.6	June 28	7.0
Mean	—	—	7.40	—	7.36

Conclusions: Eight-Pot Tests

The subjects chose pots accurately from the beginning of this phase of the study, with choice accuracy being above chance even for the first block of five trials. The elephants' choice accuracies were similar to those of other species tested on similar tasks (Olton and Samuelson 1976).

The subjects had a strong tendency to select the five pots in front of them at the moment they were released for a choice. This is not surprising, given that these pots were visible at the time of release and that they could be reached more quickly and (presumably) with less energy expenditure than that required to select the three pots behind the subject. However, the strong tendency to choose the "front-five" pots first implies an asymmetry in the sequence of choices. This asymmetry would reduce the likelihood of long sequences of patterned responses. For example, any sequence of six or more adjacent-pot choices (e.g., 123456) would require choices of some of the pots behind the subject at release (pots 5–7, figure 7.1). This "forward bias" may be why subjects did not show higher levels of response stereotypy. Although the elephants exhibited higher-than-chance proportions of adjacent-pot choice sequences, most of these sequences were only four choices long, as would be expected from a bias toward selecting the pots in front of the animal. The choice patterns which did occur were probably not simple response chains, since the subjects were turned 180° at the center of the circle of pots between choices. Similar adjacent-site choice patterns have been observed in other species (gorillas: MacDonald 1994;

rats: Dale and Innis 1986, Roberts and Dale 1981; pigeons: Spetch and Edwards 1986; pigs: Mendl et al. 1997; Siamese fighting fish: Roitblat, Tham, and Gollub 1982).

Smell-Control Procedures

After the standard eight-pot tests, each subject was given three types of smell-control test: one-choice smell-control (SM1) tests, four-choice smell-control (SM4) tests, and eight-choice smell-control (SM8) tests. Tombi and Kubwa received the eight-choice and the one-choice tests before the four-choice tests. The other three subjects were given the four-choice tests first.

One-Choice Smell-Control Test

Each subject received four SM1 tests inside the large stall in the barn (one test/day). The four pots were arranged in the arc array, with an apple in one pot. (The apple was in a different pot on each of the four trials.) The subject was released at the mat and allowed to select one pot. The elephant was then recalled to the mat, facing forward. The subjects found food on only 3 out of 20 trials (15 percent). This was not significantly different from chance accuracy (25 percent; $t(4) = 1.0$, $p > 0.05$).

Four-Choice Smell-Control Test

All subjects were tested on the arc array in the barn. Four food pellets were placed in each pot at the start of the test. Each subject was given seven standard tests, as described above, interspersed with seven smell-control tests. Before smell-control tests, a monkey-chow-and-water paste was smeared on the lid of each pot, and on the lids of three other replacement pots (in pans) kept in an adjacent room. During the trial, each pot (and pan) that the subject chose was replaced with a new pot (and pan). The observer touched all four pots between choices. Thus, the subject was always choosing among four pots that had not been touched previously, and the lid of each pot was covered with monkey-chow paste. Since Cita only completed five "standard" four-pot tests during this phase of the experiment, the choice scores were compared for each subject's first five standard tests and its first five smell-control tests. The group mean scores of 3.56 on the standard tests and 3.68 on the smell-control tests were not significantly different: $t(4) = 1.18$, $p > 0.05$.

Eight-Choice Smell-Control Test

Each subject except Cita was given six smell-control trials with the eight-pot array in the outside arena. These followed immediately after many standard eight-pot trials for Tombi and Kubwa, and after three standard eight-pot tests for Sophi and Ivory. Before each trial, each of the eight pots was baited with an apple. An "apple sauce" made from the same batch of apples was wiped on the lid of each pot, and on the lids of seven replacement pots (in pans) kept in the barn next to the arena. Between choices, the observer touched all eight pots in the array, replacing the pot and pan that the elephant had just chosen. Thus the elephant was always choosing among eight pots it had not touched, and the lid of every pot was coated with apple sauce. Only those pots in previously unchosen locations contained an apple. Since Ivory only completed three trials under the smell-control procedure, data are presented for each subject's first three smell-control trials, and its last three standard eight-pot trials. The mean scores of 7.67 on the standard trials and 7.58 on the smell-control trials were not significantly different, $t(3) = 1.0$, $p > 0.05$.

Conclusions: Smell-Control Tests

The subjects' mean choice accuracy on the four-choice and eight-choice smell-control tests was above-chance and comparable to performance on the standard four-pot and eight-pot tests. On these smell-control trials, the possibility that the elephants were leaving scent cues on the pots was removed and any scent from the apples (or food pellets) in the closed pots was probably masked by the apple sauce (or food-pellet paste) on the lids of the pots. There is no evidence that these manipulations disrupted choice accuracy. However, we are only beginning to understand the complexities of elephant olfaction (Rasmussen and Krishnamurthy 2000). Thus, we must remain open to the possibility that the food paste or apple sauce on the lids did not smell the same as the reward in the pots and, consequently, may not have adequately masked the scent of the reward. For this reason, the fact that that the subjects chose with chance accuracy on the one-choice test is important. The subjects had the opportunity to detect an apple in one of four pots without any masking cues present, yet did not do so. In combination, the results indicate that olfactory cues were not important during the three tests described above. They are consistent with the results of experiments with other species showing that olfactory cues do not determine performance on spatial memory tests (Dale and Bedard 1984; Suzuki, Augerinos, and Black 1980; Zoladek and Roberts 1979).

Overall, this series of studies extends the demonstration of short-term spatial memory abilities to the African elephant, and suggests that neither response algorithms nor olfactory cues play a major role in determining choice accuracy. These conclusions are similar to those drawn from a variety of other species (e.g., Olton and Samuelson 1976). The data obtained with elephants are similar to those obtained with other large herbivores, especially on the two-pot tests (cattle, Hosoi, Rittenhouse et al. 1995; goats and sheep, Hosoi, Swift et al. 1995).

Long-Term Retention of Test Procedure

Testing was interrupted for 6–7 months (over the winter) then all five animals were re-tested on an eight-pot procedure identical to the standard eight-pot procedures described above. After the interruption, subjects were tested about twice per week. The purpose of the experiment was to determine whether task performance would be retained over the interim period (Dale, Shyan, and Hagan 1994b). Table 7.5 shows choice accuracy on the last five eight-pot tests before the interruption, and for the first 5 tests after the interruption. Since not all of the subjects were treated identically before the interruption, table 7.5 shows the dates of the last four-pot and the last eight-pot test for each animal. The last five tests in 1992 were standard eight-pot tests for Cita, and smell-control tests (SM8) for Kubwa, Sophi, and Tombi. For Ivory, the final eight-pot tests during 1992 included three smell-control (SM8) tests and two standard eight-pot tests. Data presented above suggest that choice accuracy did not differ on standard eight-pot tests and SM8 tests, so that the differences between test procedures can be ignored. Mean choice accuracy before the break (7.40) was not significantly different from that after the break (7.36), $t(4) = 0.17$, $p > 0.05$.

After 5–6 standard eight-pot tests, each subject was exposed to 5–7 trials with a modified (more elaborate) smell-control test. On these "SM8Drag" trials, two heavy chains attached to a 10-foot (3 meters) board were dragged around the center of the circle of pots after every choice. These chains swept the surface of the dirt arena, so that all footprints on a 2.6-meter-wide track of ground inside the circle of pots were eliminated. The chain dragging also distributed any "smell-contaminated dirt" around the circle.

In addition, every pot the elephant chose was replaced with a fresh, empty pot (and pan). The lids of all pots involved in the trial were covered with an apple sauce made that day from the test apples. The apple sauce was "chunky," so that the lid of each pot was smeared with pieces of apple, apple skin, apple paste, and apple juice. These elements should have produced a variety of odors to mask the smell of an intact apple inside the closed steel container. Based on a sample of 4–7 trials per subject in each condition, these precautions produced a small, non-significant increase in the mean trial duration: From 13.1 minutes (standard trials) to 14.5 minutes (SM8Drag trials), $t(4) = 2.48$, $p > 0.05$. The increase in trial duration was not longer because two observers participated in these trials: One to drag the chains and one to replace the pots.

The mean choice accuracy of the 5 elephants dropped slightly during the smell-control trials, $t(4) = 2.99$, $p < 0.05$ (7.44 for 5–6 standard trials/subject; 7.02 for 5–7 SM8Drag trials/subject). However, the mean choice accuracy on the smell-control trials remained far above chance, $t(4) = 9.51$, $p < 0.05$.

Conclusions: Retention Tests

The elephants exhibited high choice accuracy after the 6–7-month interruption, starting with the very first day of testing. This indicates that the reference-memory components of the task are well retained. This is consistent with anecdotal evidence concerning the elephant's excellent long-term memory (Shoshani 2000).

Proactive Interference with Multiple Tests

The elephants were tested on a variant of the eight-pot test—a serial-position test procedure—in 1994 (not reported here), then returned to the standard eight-pot test in 1995 (Dale, Peterson, and Shyan 1995). The elephants were tested on two eight-pot arrays, the standard array, and an array rotated 22.5° clockwise, so that four pots were in front of the elephant at the start of each choice, and four pots were behind it (rotated array).

Initially, Kubwa and Tombi were each tested on 5–6 standard eight-pot trials (mean choice accuracy = 7.36), then on 5–6 smell-control trials (SM8Drag tests: mean choice accuracy = 7.36) Since both did well from the beginning of testing, the other three elephants were started directly on the three-trials-per-session procedure when Kubwa and Tombi were switched to that procedure. Kubwa and Tombi received 15 and 12 sessions, respectively; the other three elephants each received 13 sessions. Cita, Ivory, Kubwa, Sophi, and Tombi completed 11, 11, 13, 11, and 12 trials successfully. Five trials were discarded because of "double touches," two were discarded because of handler error (calling an elephant back before it made a choice), and one trial was discarded because of observer error (stopping a trial too early).

All five elephants were placed on the one-trial-per-session procedure for 4–6 sessions with the standard eight-pot array (figure 7.1), then returned to the three-trials-per-session procedure. Cita and Ivory received 7 and 8 sessions on this procedure, respectively. The other three subjects each received 6 sessions. Only one session was discarded, for Cita, because of a double touch.

Except for the 22.5° rotation, the two eight-pot arrays were identical. The data from both arrays were analyzed in a single two-factor, within-subject ANOVA, using the mean choice scores on the first (rotated) array and on the second (standard) array. The analysis was a 2 (arrays) × 3 (trials within a session) design (table 7.6). There was a significant effect of trials, $F(2,8) = 6.22$, $p < 0.05$. Neither the array factor, $F(1,4) = 7.31$, $p > 0.05$, nor the trials × array interaction, $F(2,8) = 0.92$, $p > 0.05$, produced significant effects. *Post hoc* orthogonal contrasts indicated that choice accuracy on trial 1 was higher than the average choice accuracy on trials 2 and 3, $F(1,8) = 11.59$, $p < 0.05$, but that there was no difference in choice accu-

Table 7.6
Choice accuracy when the elephants were given three trials within a session: number of different pots selected in eight choices during a trial. Data are presented for both the standard array (figure 7.1) and the rotated array.

Array	Trial	Cita	Ivory	Kubwa	Sophi	Tombi	Mean
Rotated	1	6.36	6.18	6.18	6.00	7.09	6.36
	2	6.36	6.27	6.18	5.91	5.91	6.13
	3	6.18	5.73	5.73	5.82	5.73	5.84
Standard	1	6.67	7.33	6.83	7.00	6.83	6.93
	2	6.17	6.33	6.50	7.17	6.17	6.47
	3	6.33	6.50	6.00	7.17	6.50	6.50

racy between trials 2 and 3, $F(1,8) = 0.83$, $p > 0.05$. In other words, the drop in choice accuracy occurred between trials 1 and 2.

Conclusions: Proactive Interference Tests

Despite the major differences in species, apparatus, and procedure, the data indicated a pattern of proactive interference similar to that obtained with rats on a radial maze (Roberts and Dale 1981).

General Conclusions

Captive African elephants exhibited spontaneous alternation and high choice accuracy when selectively rewarded for a "win-shift" strategy on two-pot, four-pot, and eight-pot tests. They did so despite strong response biases and tests that lasted up to 15 minutes. This is impressive for animals that were tested without food deprivation and rewarded with treats. The memory for visited locations was disrupted by giving three tests in rapid succession, but the retention of reference-memory components of the task was long-lasting.

Several types of smell-control tests indicated that the disturbance of olfactory cues had, at most, a minor effect on choice accuracy. The elephants apparently did not depend on food-smell cues or self-generated odor trails to find the food.

Theoretical Model

John Staddon recently defined theoretical behaviorism as "the study of the mechanisms of behavior, where *mechanism* is whatever works to account for behavior" (2001b, p. 143). So far, our research group has demonstrated that elephants search for food systematically, and that the search is guided, in part, by spatial memory. We have presented the "behaviorism" component of John Staddon's theoretical behaviorism, but what about the theoretical part?

I will outline a preliminary, but promising, two-dimensional model derived from a perceptual metaphor: the "Beam" model. (For other uses of perceptual metaphors, see Staddon 1983.) Imagine a beam of light projected by a floodlight (figure 7.2). The bulb itself represents a location in

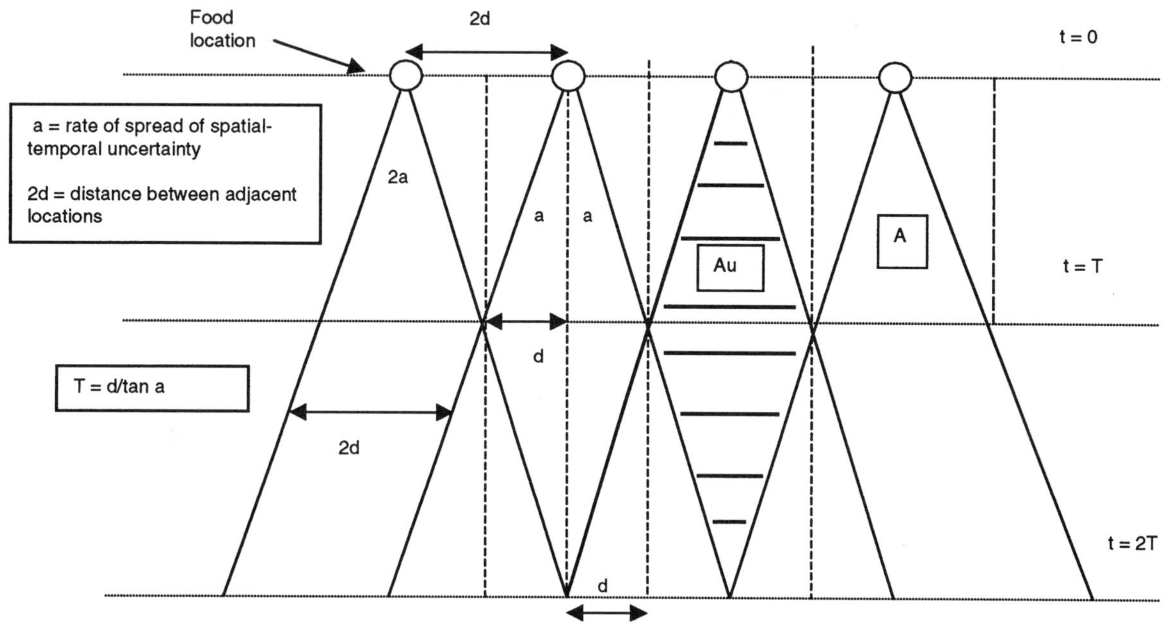

Figure 7.2
The "Beam" model: The uncertainty of the memory for each location increases linearly with time. Assuming equal spacing of the food locations, the memory for each location has a valence, V_i. $V_i = 1$ until time T (i.e., no forgetting/confusion of separate locations). After time T, the memory trace decays in an S-shaped (though almost linear) curve. After time $2T$, the valence decreases as a power function of time. There are two parameters in the model: $2d =$ the distance between adjacent locations and $a =$ an angle representing the rate of increase in spatial-temporal uncertainty. There is a discrimination threshold (DV), above which location valences are distinguishable from 0. $\mathrm{DV} = V_{\max}/k$, where $V_{\max}$ is the maximum possible valence for any of the locations involved and k is a sensitivity constant.

space. The light beam spreads at a constant rate, with the width of the beam representing the subject's degree of uncertainty of the bulb's spatial location. Figure 7.2 depicts four locations and their associated beams of light. The beam from each location expands over time. At first the four beams do not overlap, and each location can be discriminated from its neighbors with complete accuracy. After a time period T, the light beams begin to overlap and the locations can no longer be distinguished perfectly. After a time period $2T$, each light beam is completely overlapped by the beams from adjacent locations.

The valence (V) of the memory trace for each location at time t is determined by the area of the unique or non-overlapping portion of a beam (that is, the initial section of the beam: Au) divided by the total area of the beam at that time (A): $V = Au/A$. Unvisited locations will have valences set at zero. The valence is reset to a value of C when the location is visited—and remains constant for specific period of time (T). T is determined by the rate at which beam spreads ($2a$ = angle of dispersion of the beam) and on the distance, $2d$, between that location and each of its neighbors. In fact, $T = d/\tan(a)$. I will make four simplifying assumptions in my discussion of this model:

1. A location's valence is reset to $C = 1$ whenever it is visited.
2. The valence of each visited location gradually declines from 1 to (almost) 0.
3. All adjacent locations are the same distance ($2d$) apart.
4. The beam spreads at a constant rate ($2a$ = the angle subtended by the beam, in radians).

With these assumptions, the valence of a location at time t after it has been visited is given by the following equations (figure 7.2): For $0 < t < T$,

$$Vi = Au/A = 1,$$

where Au = non-overlapping (unique) area of beam, A = total area of beam, and $T = d/\tan(a)$. For $T < t < 2\mathrm{T}$,

$$Vi = 4T/t - 2T^2/t^2 - 1.$$

For $t > 2T$,

$$Vi = 2T^2/t^2.$$

Although the perceptual metaphor above represents memory in a straightforward manner, it does not translate into a simple mathematical function. The memory trace function has three components: An initial constant value, then a brief S-shaped section, then a power function. The validity of these equations was confirmed graphically—they predicted several values of V $(= Au/A)$ computed from scaled drawings of the overlapping beams.

Several features of the model deserve comment. One is that spatial and temporal dimensions are integrated into a single memory variable (V). At first glance, such an integrated memory trace may seem implausible. However, there is evidence that animals make this type of spatial-temporal integration (Cheng, Spetch, and Miceli 1996; Clayton, Yu, and Dickinson 2003). A second feature is that, at least after time $2T$, valence is described by a power function with two free parameters (a, d). This prediction is consistent with suggestions that numerous and varied sets of memory data are best fitted by a power function (Rubin, Hinton, and Wenzel 1999; Rubin and Wenzel 1996; Sikstrom 2002).

The model also claims that the valence of a location does not begin to decrease until a fixed time T after that place has been visited. Although this feature of the model is driven by the underlying perceptual metaphor, it overcomes one of the major criticisms of previous power-function models—namely, that the function is undefined at time, $t = 0$ (Sikstrom 2002; Wickens 1998). In fact, Sikstrom (2002) has suggested an elaborate connectionist model that—under specific constraints—also generates a forgetting curve that is a power function defined at time 0. Both models suggest a "lag" between the occurrence of an event and the start of forgetting. That two such different approaches—a connectionist model and a perceptual metaphor—result in similar forgetting functions is intriguing. These apparently disparate perspectives may be converging on the same (and perhaps previously ignored) characteristic of memory. It is also quite surprising that the model predicts a sigmoidal memory trace between times T and $2T$. However, empirically speaking, the S-shaped segment of the curve seems almost linear and is short enough that distinguishing it from a power function would be difficult (especially were one not looking for the alternative).

Having discussed the nature of the memory trace for an individual event, I should describe how performance on the spatial memory task is determined. Suppose that the subject compares the valences of all of the food locations before choosing one. The model assumes that the discrimination threshold is a constant proportion of the largest valence of any location relevant to the task. This would seem to be a simple application of Weber's Law to discrimination among memory traces, although the relationship between Weber's Law and timing may be more complex than recently believed (Dragoi, Staddon, Palmer, and Buhusi 2003; Fetterman and Killeen 1992; Grondin 2001).

To predict choice accuracy on the eight-pot spatial memory task, I assumed constant inter-choice intervals (as is often observed). The response/decision rule was that the subject choose randomly among locations with sub-threshold valences, while avoiding the other locations. (Note, however, that one could easily replace the random-choice rule with a specific set of response biases.)

Given these assumptions, the model predicts mean choice-accuracy scores of 6.72 (out of 8) with a valence discrimination threshold of 0.10 (Weber fraction = 1/10) and 7.75 with the valence discrimination threshold set at 0.05 (Weber fraction = 1/20). At the very least, the Beam model predicts choice accuracy in the empirically observed range and has several theoretically desirable characteristics.

In summary, the Beam model provides an alternative perspective from which to describe the behavior of elephants on a commonly used spatial memory task. Professor Staddon's facility and creativity with such quantitative modeling constantly refreshes my respect for him—rejuvenation, if you will.

Acknowledgments

This work was conducted in collaboration with Melissa R. Shyan of the Department of Psychology at Butler University (now at Indiana University East in Richmond) and David A. Hagan, Curator of the Indianapolis Zoological Society's Plains Biome. Preliminary analyses of some of the data presented in this manuscript were presented at the International Elephant Managers Workshops in November 1992, October 1993, and October 1995 and at the annual meetings of the Psychonomic Society in November 1992 and November 1995. Butler University and the Indianapolis Zoological Society provided financial and material support for this research. We wish to acknowledge the collaboration of Zoo employees J. Bolling, D. Collins, T. Csire, I. Kempf, C. Lance, D. Olson, J. Peterson, D. Polk and Butler students T. Couch, A. LaFond, J. Rutherford, T. Solomon, and A. Young.

8 Interval Timing and Memory: Breaking the Clock

Jennifer J. Higa

While working on my dissertation with John Hinson at Washington State University, I began to explore post-doctoral options. The idea of working with John Staddon, Hinson's doctoral advisor in graduate school, was exciting. I had read several of Staddon's papers as a graduate student, and the innovative ideas as well as the range of topics on which Staddon wrote captured and strengthened my interest in theoretical explanations of learning and behavior. During my time in Staddon's lab, I learned much more about quantitative approaches to learning and methods for simulating models and data, and about trying new experimental techniques. Staddon challenged my ideas about behaviorism, philosophy of science in general, and even politics. Conducting research in Staddon's lab was fun and always intellectually stimulating. My post-doc years were among the best years of my academic life.

I spent most of my time in Staddon's lab working on interval timing. Perhaps the most difficult part of preparing this chapter was deciding what material to include. Research on interval timing has a long history and a large database of results and theoretical work, with numerous articles, several conferences, books, and special publications. The present chapter reviews a set of experiments on interrupting the to-be-timed (target) interval by turning off the signaling-stimulus or stopping the timer programming the interval. In these "gap" studies, the location and the duration of an interruption vary within a session. The chapter also presents some data from a study conducted in our labs and discusses the results from a memory approach to timing.

Interval Timing

'Interval timing' refers to a wide range of behaviors that reflect a learned sensitivity to the duration of an event such as a nectar-feeding bout or availability of a prey item. A striking feature is its ubiquity. A variety of animals ranging from rats and pigeons (Harzem 1969; Innis 1981) to captured starlings (Brunner, Kacelnik, and Gibbon 1992) to some fish and turtles (Lejeune and Wearden 1991) show the ability to learn about periods in the seconds to minutes range. What characterizes interval timing from other timing mechanisms is its flexibility: different kinds of events can serve as time markers and control timing behavior (Staddon 1974). On the other hand, interval timing is also relatively inaccurate when compared to other timing processes like circadian rhythms. Indeed, a hallmark of interval timing is increasing variance with increases in the to-be-timed interval. Circadian timing appears to be more accurate in that its variance does not increase much with the average interval (Terman, Gibbon, Fairhurst, and Waring 1984).

The prevalence of interval timing in so many species suggests that the ability to detect, learn, and use temporal information is a basic process of animal behavior and learning. Without a doubt, the time between events—stimuli, responses, and rewards—exerts an overwhelming influence on what associations are made, and how learning progresses. The research on interval timing consists of a set of core results and two principal theories.

Proportional and scalar timing are among the primary results reported in interval timing studies. *Proportional timing* is defined as a linear relation between an independent temporal variable and a dependent measure of behavior. For example, dependent measures such as the time to the first response or peak rate of responding in an interval are proportional to the interval to be timed (Dews 1970). *Scalar timing* occurs when standard deviations of dependent measures of timing are proportional to their mean. Defining characteristics of the scalar property include superposition of response rate functions when normalized along both axes (time within an interval and response rate) and a constant coefficient of variation (ratio between the standard deviation and mean, CoV) across a range of interval values (Gibbon 1977, 1991). Proportional and scalar timing properties have been reported in studies using a variety of timing procedures, including, fixed-interval (FI) reinforcement schedules during which a reinforcer is given for the first response after a fixed amount of time has elapsed (Dews 1970; Richelle and Lejeune 1980; Schneider 1969), a discrete-trial version of the FI procedure in which the target interval is intermixed with long (non-reinforced) probe trials and inter-trial intervals (e.g., peak procedure; see Catania 1970 and Roberts 1981), and differential reinforcement of low-rate schedules during which reinforcement is given for response rates that are at or below a specified level (Staddon 1965).

Theories of Interval Timing

Internal clock models represent a common approach to how animals time and have steered much of the research. The dominant models are Scalar Expectancy Theory (SET; Gibbon 1977; Gibbon and Church 1984, 1990; also Treisman 1963 for an early version) and a Behavioral Theory of timing (BeT, Fetterman and Killeen 1991; Killeen and Fetterman 1988). Briefly, SET consists of three processes—a clock, memory, and a comparison process. On each trial of a timing task, a switch closes and gates a periodic signal (pulses) from a pacemaker to an accumulator that can be incremented and cleared. The content of the accumulator is compared with a sample from a memory distribution of previously reinforced times. The comparison process determines whether the elapsed time has reached some criterion. Specifically, when the difference between elapsed time and a value sampled from memory (or its relative difference) exceeds a threshold, the animal switches from a "no-responding" state to a "responding" state. Variance from any of these processes can affect an animal's estimate of time, and variability in timing behavior such as the scalar property arises from variability in these processes (Gibbon 1991; Gibbon, Church, and Meck 1984).

A competing, alternative theory to SET is behavioral expectancy theory (Fetterman and Killeen 1991; Killeen and Fetterman 1988). According to BeT, behavior itself serves as a cue for the passage of time and mediates time discrimination. BeT is based on a well-established finding that periodic reinforcement produces time-related activities that occur at different points during an IRI. The activities are also referred to as *collateral* behaviors or interim and terminal responses (Roper 1978; Staddon and Simmelhag 1971). What causes the flow of behavior? BeT assumes that each behavior is associated with an underlying state (n), and that pulses from a Poisson pacemaker produce the transition between states. Pacemaker speed depends on the rate or probability of reinforcement in a given context, according to a positive linear function (Fetterman and Killeen 1991). In this way, behavior can serve as a discriminative stimulus for upcoming responses. For example, when discriminating between a short and long interval stimuli (e.g., 5-second vs. 15-second tones) early behaviors in an interval are associated with reinforcement of short intervals; later behaviors are associated with longer intervals. Scalar timing is explained by having pacemaker speed depend on reinforcement rate. For example, during a 30-second interval there may be *n* states associated with reinforcement. When the interval is doubled to 60 seconds, it still takes *n* states to reach reinforcement, but the duration of each state is longer because the overall reinforcement rate in that context is reduced and the pacemaker is running slower.

These models as well as a multiple-oscillator version of SET (Church and Broadbent 1991) and a continuous-time version of BeT (Machado 1997) have been tested under a wide range of timing procedures and they all provide good fits to some of the data (Bizo and White 1994; Killeen and Fetterman 1993; Leak and Gibbon 1995). This is perhaps not too surprising since they share several common features. For example, they all consist of a pacemaker system, a memory component, and a decision process. (For a review, see Church 1997.) Another procedure, which has received less attention, involves interrupting the target interval by changing the cue signaling the interval and/or producing a gap in the program clock keeping track of the interval.

Fixed-Interval Schedules of Reinforcement

The fixed-interval schedule of reinforcement is a relatively simple and reliable procedure for studying timing behavior. On such schedules, a reinforcer is given for the first response that occurs after a fixed amount of time has elapsed since delivery of the preceding reinforcer. Such schedules produce a distinctive pattern of responding between successive reinforcers (called an interval). At the beginning of an interval, following a reinforcer, animals pause or *wait* before responding. Following the post-reinforcement wait time there is either a gradual acceleration in responding (Ferster and

Skinner 1957) or an abrupt change from a low to a high rate of responding called a "break-and-run" pattern (Schneider 1969) as the end of the interval nears. The point in an interval at which rates of responding change (i.e., the "break point") is about two-thirds of the FI requirement (Schneider 1969). Wait time, defined as the time to the first response in an interval, is generally a smaller fraction of the interval requirement, ranging from one-fourth to one-half the interval duration depending on the species and range of intervals studied (Lowe and Harzem 1977; Shull 1970a,b; Wynne and Staddon 1988).

Although some results raise questions about the generality of scalar timing in rates of responding and wait time during long interval durations (Gibbon, Malapani, Dale, and Gallistel 1997; Zeiler and Powell 1994), performance on FI schedules usually follows scalar and proportional timing rules (Dews 1970; Schneider 1969).

Results from "Gap" Procedures

FI schedules and their variants provide a useful method by which to answer questions about the timing mechanism. One set of studies consists of interrupting the timing process by arranging a break or gap in the target interval. What do results from gap studies tell us about how animals time?

Effects of Changing the Stimulus

In one of the earliest gap procedures, Dews set out to test the idea that a chaining of responses produces the scalloping pattern of responding during FI reinforcement schedules, or "time curves" (1962, p. 369). If a chaining of responses determines responding on FI schedules, then, disrupting the chained behaviors should also disrupt the orderly increase in response rates during the interval. Dews first exposed pigeons to an FI 500-second schedule (signaled by a houselight, the keylight remained on throughout the interval) with a 250-second inter-trial interval (during which the chamber was dark). Later, during test trials, he turned the houselight on and off at different 50-second periods in the interval. Figure 8.1 illustrates the procedure. The program clock timing the FI interval continued through the houselight-on and houselight-off segments. Dews reported that pigeons' rates of responding during the stimulus-on segments increased as the time

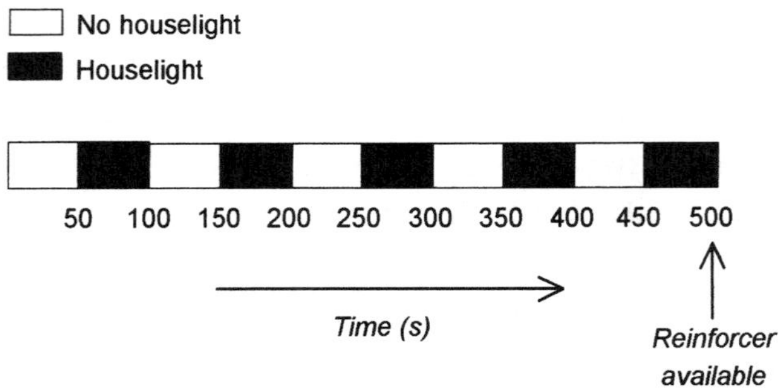

Figure 8.1
Illustration of the procedure used by Dews. A FI 500-second reinforcement schedule during which the houselight turned on and off during an interval. The keylight remained on throughout. Adapted from Dews 1962.

to reinforcement neared and approximated the FI scallop observed under conditions with no stimulus change (Dews 1962, 1965). Variations in the number, duration, and location of the interruptions did not change the overall scalloping pattern in response rates during an interval (Dews 1965, 1966). Furthermore, signaling the interval with or without a visual stimulus did not alter the FI "time curve" (Dews 1962).

If not a chain of mediating responses, what, then, explains the maintenance of timing behavior when disruptions in the stimuli occur during the interval? Dews's results point to the involvement of two processes: *stimulus control* and *temporal control* of behavior (i.e., interval timing). That overall rate of responding was lower when the houselight was off (S^{Δ}) than when the houselight was on (S^{D}) shows that behavior was partly under stimulus control (i.e., houselight on vs. houselight off). That the rate of responding during the stimulus-on periods depended on the location of the stimulus-on segment indicates that behavior was also under the control of temporal relations provided by the schedule. To explain the temporal control of behavior Dews argued that that the scalloping pattern might be the result of a decrease in the delay between responding and reinforcement as the interval progresses, or a "declining retroactive rate-enhancing effect" (1962, p. 373) as the time between responding and reinforcement increases along the lines of delay-reduction theory (Fantino 1969; Fantino and Davison 1983).

Effects of Varying the Operation of the Program Clock

Subsequent studies show that the effect of a gap may depend on additional factors, including what happens to the program clock timing the interval. In rats, response rates following a gap are generally higher when the clock continues to run during a gap than when the clock stops (Church 1978; Meck, Church, and Olton 1984; Roberts 1981; Roberts and Church 1978). Pigeons with extensive training on long FI schedules show similar effects when the program clock continues to operate during a gap in the interval (Dews 1962).

Effects of Varying Gap Duration

Dews (1965) showed, using an FI procedure and pigeons, that although overall rate of responding decreased with longer gaps, the FI pattern was not disrupted. Still, Dews varied both gap duration and the FI requirement and it is unclear whether temporal performance depends on the absolute or relative duration of the gap. Subsequent studies with the peak procedure show that gap duration does change performance. Roberts (1981) reported that in rats increasing the duration of gap (signaled by a blackout) did not change the overall pattern of responding during probe trials. However, the location of peak times within the interval increased by an amount approximately equal to the gap duration. Cabeza de Vaca, Brown, and Hemmes (1994) reported similar results with pigeons. Nonetheless, altogether, the results from gap studies indicate that there is a complex relation between gap duration and location.

Effects of Varying the Location of a Gap

The effects of gap location are mixed. Dews (1962, 1965, 1966) showed in several studies that response rate after a gap was higher the later the gap occurred in an interval, such that the overall pattern was similar to that during intervals without gaps. In other words, it appeared as if the birds continued to time during a gap. Roberts and Church (1978) also showed that gap location does not disrupt the overall timing process. Using a choice procedure, they trained rats on a temporal discrimination task of light durations ranging from 4 seconds to 22 seconds. Responding to one lever was reinforced after presentation of durations less than 12-second ("short") intervals; responding to another lever was reinforced for durations greater than 12-second ("long") intervals. Once discrimination was established, the program inserted gaps during some of the training stimuli. The breaks were either short (2 seconds) or long (4 seconds) and were located either early (2 seconds) or late (4 seconds) in an interval. For example, if the target interval duration was 8 seconds and the trial contained a 2-second gap located 2 seconds after the start of the trial, the rat would be presented 2 seconds of light followed by a 2-second gap (light off) and 6 seconds of light. Overall, gaps shifted the psychometric functions (relating the probability of classifying a stimulus as "long"), such that the probability of calling an interrupted interval "long" (e.g., 2 seconds of light, a 2-second gap, 6 seconds of light) approximately equaled the probability of calling an interval "long" when that interval did not have a gap (e.g., 8 seconds of light only). This result did not depend on when the gap occurred—either early or later during the interval.

In contrast, other studies show that the location of a gap matters. Farmer and Schoenfeld (1966) reported that gaps in the signaling stimulus had minimal effects on the pattern of responding in pigeons when the gap occurred early in an interval. However, later interruptions caused a decrease in response rates, to levels lower than those observed during non-interrupted intervals. Interestingly, after an initial decrease during a gap, post-gap response rate increased rapidly and approached levels normally observed at the end of an interval. More recently, Cabeza de Vaca et al. (1994) concluded that the location and duration of a gap combine to have an effect on temporal performance that differs from previous reports. Using a peak procedure, they trained pigeons to time a FI 30-second interval, signaled by a houselight. A subset of non-reinforced probe trials consisted of breaks in the presentation of the houselight signaling the interval. Gaps were of different durations and occurred at different points in the interval. Of interest was the location of the maximal rate of responding (peak time) during a probe trial. Generally, shifts in peak time varied non-linearly with gap duration. Shorter gaps produced shifts that were closer in amount to the duration of the gap. Longer gaps produced shifts that were longer than that accounted for by the time before the gap and gap duration; however, the location of a shift was not so great as to suggest that the pigeons treated the gap as a marker indicating the start of a new trial. That is, peak time was less than the amount represented by the time that elapsed before the gap, the gap duration, and the target interval duration altogether. On the other hand, shifts in peak time varied linearly with the location of the gap location. The later a gap occurred in an interval, the later was the peak time.

Internal Clock and Memory Models

The gap procedure has produced a mixed set of results that are usually interpreted in the framework of an internal clock model for timing. First, finding that gaps do not disrupt the overall pattern of responding in an interval suggests that animals appear to *continue timing* during a gap (Dews 1962). In other cases, a gap in the interval may *reset* the timing process so that rates of responding after a gap resemble what is observed during the start of a new trial and peak time shifts by an amount equal to the target interval duration plus the duration of the gap and the time elapsed before the gap (Brown, Hemmes, and Cabeza de Vaca 1992; Buhusi and Meck 2000; Roberts, Cheng, and Cohen 1989). There is also some evidence that the timing process *stops* and then resumes, seen as a shift in peak time approximately equal to the gap duration (Roberts 1981; Roberts and Church 1978). In an intermediate case, gaps produce an effect that is somewhere in between a stopping and resetting process (Cabeza de Vaca et al. 1994). Second, the effect of a gap depends on what happens to the program clock timing the interval. Animals appear to stop timing during the gap when the program clock stops (Roberts and Church 1978) and continue to time through the gap if the program clock continues to run (Dews 1962). Third, the effect of a gap on temporal performance depends on its location under some conditions (Cabeza de Vaca et al. 1994) but not other conditions (Roberts and Church 1978). Fourth, results from other timing procedures point to several non-temporal factors that influence timing, including filled vs. unfilled (empty) intervals, stimulus saliency, and attention. For example, pigeons (Mantanus 1981) and humans (Allan 1992) judge filled intervals as being longer than unfilled intervals (e.g., the filled-duration illusion, Gomez and Robertson 1979). Humans (Goldstone, Lhamon, and Sechzer 1979), pigeons (Kraemer, Randall, and Brown 1997) and rats (Kraemer, Brown, and Randall 1995) also judge brighter lights as being longer in duration than dim lights. Moreover, Lejeune, Macar, and Zakay (1999) showed that like humans, pigeons underestimate the duration of a stimulus when they are also required to simultaneously perform a non-temporal task (e.g., pecking a key for food on a VR reinforcement schedule). These non-temporal factors may also have a role in timing under gap procedures.

Can the current theories of timing explain the overall pattern of results from gap studies? The results challenge behavior-based theories such as BeT (Killeen and Fetterman 1988). The maintenance of FI performance despite a general disruption to overall levels of the instrumental response suggests that timing is not entirely dependent on a cascade of behavior in the sense suggested by BeT. Although, it is possible that behavioral states—other than those involved in generating the instrumental response—may serve as discriminative stimuli for telling the animal when to respond. In fact, there is some recent evidence showing a positive correlation between mediating behavior and time estimation in rats (Fetterman, Killeen, and Hall 1998). That is, adjunctive behaviors were better predictors of the rats' discrimination of a short and long interval, than was the passage of time in the trial.

SET can potentially explain the overall pattern of results, but with some modifications (Church 1978, 1984). For example, SET assumes that the switch component of the clock process closes with the onset of a signal (or start of a trial) and gates pulses to the accumulator. A gap in the interval (when the signal is turned off) opens the switch and the accumulator retains the number of pulses collected so far. Turning the signal back on closes the switch and pulses in the accumulator obtained after the gap add to what was collected before the gap. Some researchers have argued that the stopping and restarting of the timing process imply that the system may retain (in the case of stopping) or empty (in the case of resetting) the contents of working memory. Others propose that these effects are not only based on the properties of the clock process, but also on attentional processes that are sensitive to stimulus (non-temporal) attributes in the timing situation, such as the saliency of the signaling cues (Buhusi and Meck 2000; Lejeune 1998). For example, in the standard gap procedure, animals stop timing during a break if it is a relatively short and non-salient event. On the other hand, in a reverse-gap procedure where the absence of a cue signals the interval, the onset of a signal during a gap may be salient enough to explain why the timing process resets (Buhusi and Meck 2000).

Taken together, it is possible to modify internal clock models to fit the data gathered so far from gap procedures. However, given the limited number of studies, the results of which are mixed, and the lack of a coherent theoretical account of the gap effects (e.g., how a timing system recognizes the start or end of an interval, an inter-trial interval or a gap), a search for better methods and different theoretical frameworks seems warranted. For example, some researchers have focused on developing a memory-decay process. Cabeza de Vaca et al. (1994) discovered shifts in peak time (with a peak procedure) that were not indicative of a simple resetting or stopping mechanism. Working in the framework of SET they proposed the following. At the start of an interval, a switch closes which allows pulses from the pacemaker to flow into an accumulator. At the onset of a gap, the switch opens and the clock process stops accumulating time. During the gap, the content of the accumulator is gradually lost, according to an exponential decay. The addition of a memory decay process to SET provides a better account of the non-linear and linear shifts in peak time as a function of gap duration and location, respectively. (For a neural network timing model of the memory decay process, see Hopson 1999.)

Furthermore, recent challenges to pacemaker models (Donahoe and Burgos 1999; Staddon and Higa 1999; Zeiler 1999), suggest it is time to consider models that do not have a clock as their primary mechanism. Our effort at developing a pacemaker-free model is based on the idea of an integrator, originally proposed in a model for the temporal properties of habituation (Staddon and Higa 1996). According to a multiple-time-scale (MTS) model, timing is the result of learning the reinforced and non-reinforced values of an animal's memory for an event or "time marker" (Staddon and Higa 1999). Different kinds of stimuli can serve as time markers and control timing behavior (Staddon 1984, 2001). Food reinforcement on periodic schedules is a typical time marker, although other stimuli such as lights and tones may also serve as time markers. The effectiveness of a stimulus depends on its ability to signal upcoming events and they are susceptible to other effects, such as interference among time markers (Staddon 1983).

Briefly, the MTS model states that reinforcement produces an event trace (a short-term memory) that decays according to a negatively accelerated function as time in the interval elapses. A chain of integrators, each set with its own time constant, determines the rate of decay. Placing a threshold on the output of each integrator, and having earlier units have shorter time constants than later ones, produces a trace that is not fixed, but depends on the system's history of reinforcement. The value of the trace and a threshold determines responding. Memory dynamics of this sort has proven to be a useful principle and is found in other models such as Spetch and Wilkie's (1983) trace-decay model for the choose-short effect in delayed-matching-to-sample procedures, Staddon's (1984) model for stimulus saliency, and Wixted and Ebbesen's (1991) model for human memory, just to name a few. The difference here is that the event-dynamics in the MTS model is derived from a model developed for habituation. The MTS model explains several temporal properties of habituation and accounts for a broad range of interval timing results including proportional and scalar timing, reinforcement magnitude effects, discrimination of relative and absolute durations, as well as timing dynamics (Staddon, Chelaru, and Higa 2002a,b), suggesting that the MTS framework has promise as a theory of timing.

However, we have not applied the model directly to the data generated by the gap procedures. As a result, several issues remain unresolved. For example, what property of a time marker or gap—onset, offset, duration or location (or some mixture of these features)—serves as a stimulus for the MTS system? This is a problem for other memory models as well as internal clock models of interval timing and there is not yet agreement on how best to account for these effects. For example, it is not clear what happens to the contents of memory in the absence of a signal (Cabeza de Vaca et al. 1994). Connectionist models such as Grossberg and Schmajuk's (1989) spectral timing model depend on the presence of a signal, and assume that the onset of a signal activates a series of memory "units" with different time constants that persist until the end of a trial. According to the MTS model, the animal's memory trace for a time marker (reinforcement) changes dynamically throughout an interval. In the case of clock models, the switch which gates pulses into the accumulator is assumed to close with the start of a trial and may open during a break in the signal, but may also be controlled by other stimulus and attentional properties (Buhusi and Meck 2000).

Effects of Variable Gaps on FI Performance: Preliminary Results

Together, the findings described above show that many different types of events have a role in controlling the timing process. The gap procedure and the MTS model bring to the forefront the importance of understanding the role of time markers in temporal processing. We next present preliminary results from a set of experiments aimed at developing an improved method for studying gap effects and the role of time markers in interval timing.

With few exceptions (Roberts and Church 1978), gap procedures involve several types of events and intervals that might have a role in timing the target interval. For example, while inter-trial intervals and long probe trials serve the purpose of allowing the measurement of response rates before and after the expected time to reinforcement, they also likely have an effect on temporal performance. For these reasons, we decided to use a standard FI schedule of reinforcement (FI 60 seconds), without inter-trial intervals. Next, the usual gap procedure involves testing animals with the same gap duration or with a gap that starts and/or ends at the same point within an interval for several sessions (Buhusi and Meck 2000; Cabeza de Vaca et al. 1994; Roberts 1981). To minimize the likelihood that animals develop a strategy or pattern of responding that depends on anticipating a break in the interval, we used a method that varies gap duration and location across intervals, dynamically, according to an average value.

We exposed pigeons to a Baseline (FI 60 seconds reinforcement schedule) condition and a Gap condition (21 sessions each), and counterbalanced the order of conditions. Baseline consisted of 40 intervals, programmed according to a FI 60-second reinforcement schedule such that a food reinforcer occurred for the first response after 60-second elapsed since delivery of the previous reinforcer. The Gap condition was similar to the Baseline condition except that the program turned off the keylight signaling the interval during a subset of intervals. We programmed gap durations to have a mean duration of 10 seconds, and calculated the duration of a gap at the start of each interval according to the following equation:

$$d = -\log(i)/(1/10),$$

where d is the duration of a gap and i represents a random number (between 0 and 1) generated by the computer. The actual gap duration ranged

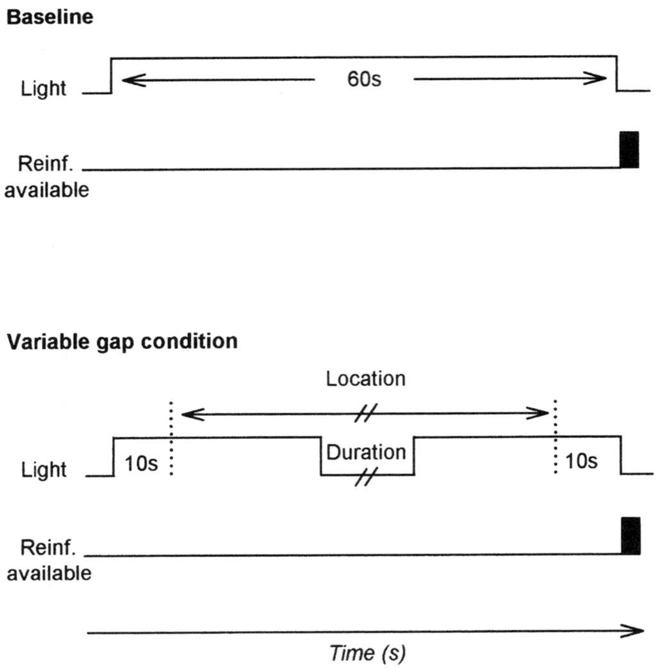

Figure 8.2
Baseline. Intervals were programmed according to an FI reinforcement schedule. The keylight remained on throughout the interval, and a reinforcer was available after 60 seconds elapsed since the onset of a light. Gap condition. Intervals were interrupted by turning off the keylight for a variable duration. The location of the gap also varied, with the constraint that it began at least 10 seconds after the start of an interval and ended 10 seconds before the end of an interval. A reinforcer was available after the keylight had been on for 60 seconds.

from 0.03 to 60.0 seconds. The location of a gap was permitted to vary anywhere during the interval with the limit that it began after at least 10 seconds since the start and ended 10 seconds before the end of an interval (figure 8.2). Because of the variable locations, the 10-second limit provided a minimum time before and after a gap in all intervals, over which we could measure response rates. During gap intervals, the program clock stopped so that the total time before and after an interruption remained equal to the programmed baseline interval duration.

Figure 8.3 presents the average rate of responding throughout the 60-second interval of the Baseline condition. Many of the subjects exhibited

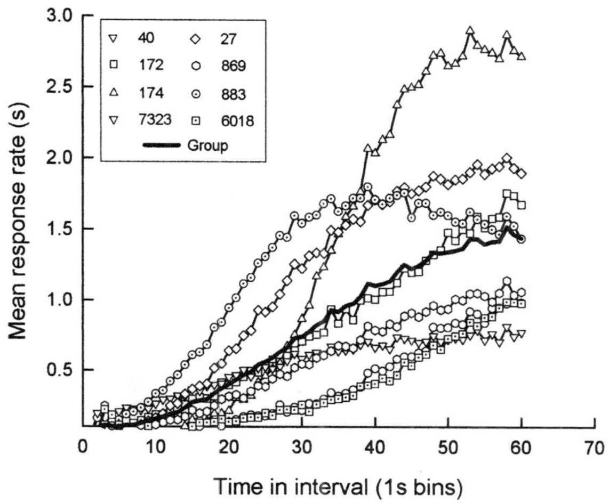

Figure 8.3
Results from the Baseline (uninterrupted FI 60 seconds) condition. The figure shows, for each subject, mean rate of responding (1-second bins) within an interval. Data were based on all sessions of training. The mean for the group is shown as a solid line.

the patterns of responding characteristic of FI schedules: Increasing rates of responding characteristic of a FI "scallop," with peak rates of responding near the end of the interval. Only bird 883 shows a peak in response rates at a point earlier than the time of reinforcement. Thus, the behavior of the subjects appeared to be under the temporal control of the FI schedule.

Figure 8.4 shows some of the data generated by the variable gap procedure, specifically mean rates of responding during the 10 seconds preceding and following a gap in the signaling stimulus. Because both the duration and location of a gap varied randomly across intervals, we analyzed the results from all intervals and classified gap durations as small (0 to ≤10 seconds), medium (>10 to ≤20 seconds), or large (>0.20 second). Gap locations were classified as early (>10 to ≤20 seconds), middle (>20 to ≤30 seconds), or late (>40 to ≤50 seconds), depending on the onset of the gap in an interval.

When examining the effect of gap duration by averaging across the different locations (top panel, figure 8.4), response rates before a gap gradually increased and there were no differences across the different gap durations.

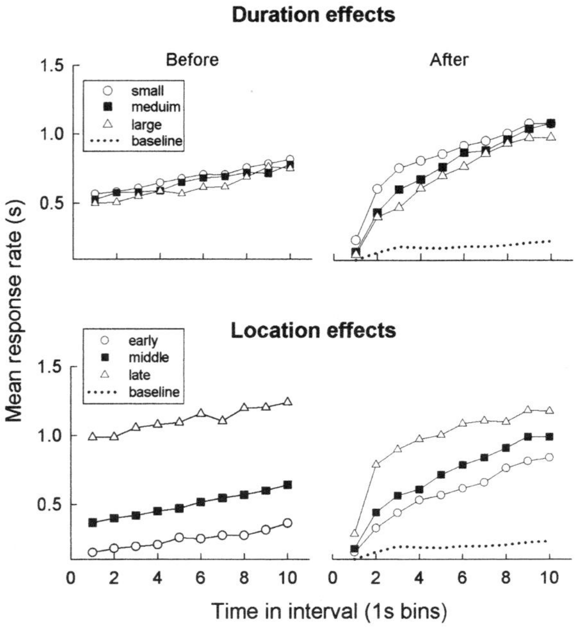

Figure 8.4
Results from the Gap condition. Data shown are mean response rates during the 10 seconds before and the 10 seconds after a gap, and are based on all subjects and sessions. Top panels: Effects of gap duration, classified as small (0–10 seconds), medium (10–20 seconds), or large (>20 seconds). Bottom panels: Effects of gap location, classified as early (10–20 seconds), middle (20–30 seconds), or late (40–50 seconds), depending on the onset of a gap since the start of an interval. The dashed lines show rates of responding during the first 10 seconds of an interval from the Baseline condition.

Rates of responding immediately after a gap were lower than those observed before a gap and increased as the interval elapsed. Furthermore, overall response rates during all gap durations were higher than those observed during the first 10 seconds of intervals without gaps (baseline, shown in the figure). There appears to be some difference in the level of responding across conditions—higher after small gaps and lower after larger gaps, although these differences appear to hold only during the first few seconds of the post-gap part of the interval.

In contrast to duration, the location of a gap produced clear differences in responding. First, rates of responding before a gap were higher the later the gap occurred in an interval. This effect likely represents overall increasing response rates as the interval elapsed. Second, rates of responding after a gap decreased to levels lower than those observed before a gap, then increased as the interval elapsed. Unlike duration, however, the location did make a difference. The earlier a gap occurred in an interval, the lower the overall post-gap level of responding.

A notable result in figure 8.4 is the pattern of responding after a gap. The pattern suggests that the timing process "reset" in the sense that the birds treated the gap as a marker for the end of an interval and the beginning of another. This resetting effect appears clearest for variations in the location of a gap. Generally, post-gap response rates were lower after earlier gaps. However, when comparing the amount by which response rates decreased (measured as the difference between the rates of responding right before and after a gap), the later a gap, the bigger the decrease. However, these are only partial-reset effects when compared to responding during the first 10 seconds of baseline (gap-free) intervals. If the birds treated a gap as a stimulus signaling the start of a new interval, then their pattern of responding should look similar to that observed during the first few seconds of an uninterrupted interval. Instead, figure 8.4 shows that rates of responding after a gap were higher than those observed during the first 10 seconds of gap-free intervals. Furthermore, response rates after a gap eventually reach a point higher than that obtained before a gap.

From the view of internal clock models, decay of temporal information in memory may explain the partial-reset result. Cabeza de Vaca et al. (1994) proposed that onset of a gap in the interval may open the switch to the accumulator and that the content of memory slowly decays during the gap. When the gap is over and the signaling cue is back on, the switch closes and the clock resumes. The decay process predicts a pattern of results that falls somewhere between a stop-retain-restart and stop-reset process, depending on the duration and location of a gap. With respect to duration, the longer a gap, the more likely it is that the contents of the clock will have decayed by the end of the gap period. The resultant pattern should look like a reset effect, as if the animal re-starts timing the interval. Less information should be lost during shorter gaps, and the pattern of responding after the gap should resemble a partial reset in the timing process. For variations in location, the later a gap occurs in an interval, the more time will have been accumulated before the gap, but depending on the form of the decay-function, there may be more accumulated time remaining after the gap.

This process explains the effects we observed when location of a gap varied. Rates of responding before a gap should be higher with later gaps because the clock will have accumulated more time. The data in the lower panel of figure 8.4 support this prediction. However, the model does not explain our results from variations in gap duration. We did not find strong evidence of higher response rates following shorter gap durations. There are at least three explanations for why we did not find a duration effect. First, results from a particular duration (e.g., small) represent an average across all possible locations. Hence, location effects may be overshadowing the effect of gap duration. Second, our birds may have treated the gap as an inter-trial interval (ITI). Cabeza de Vaca et al. (1994) proposed that the speed with which the clock mechanism resets might depend on the ITI duration: quick reset with short ITIs, slower reset with longer ITIs. If so, then the gaps in the present study may have served as an ITI, indicating the end of a trial that caused different types of resetting. Third, some have argued that the resetting mode of a clock may depend on the amount of training (Brown, Hemmes, and Cabeza de Vaca 1992). The clock may reset only after extensive training. Studies reporting resetting effects used procedures involving testing animals for approximately 40 (Cheng and Roberts 1989) to 100 (Brown, Hemmes, and Cabeza de Vaca 1992) sessions. In contrast, we used relatively fewer sessions, at least for some birds. Figure 8.4 shows temporal performance after 21 (for birds that began the experiment with the Gap condition) and 42 (for birds receiving the Baseline condition first) sessions of training. Nonetheless, Dews (1962) tested pigeons for 60 sessions and found no evidence of resetting.

From the view of the MTS model, learning and comparing memory traces for events is key. How might we apply the MTS model to the patterns of responding after a gap? One possibility is to use a method similar to one we applied to relative duration discrimination tasks (Staddon and Higa 1999). In the relative discrimination task, pigeons pecked a center key that produced a red light followed by a green light. After the green light, the side keys were turned on and reinforcement was given for pecking the left key if the red light was longer than the green light and pecking the right key if the green light was longer (Stubbs, Dreyfus, Fetterman, Boynton, Locklin, and Smith 1994). The task produces several interesting results one of which is that discrimination accuracy depends on the order that two durations appear, holding constant the ratio between the long and short duration signals. For example, discrimination is easier after a 4-second light followed by a 1-second light than the reverse. According to Stubbs et al., discrimination is poorer when the short signal appears first because memory for the short signal is weaker after the longer signal. In this situation, the MTS model assumes that an animal bases its response on comparing differences between (memory) traces of the onset of the trial and onset of the green stimulus during a trial, at the time of a choice (a detailed analysis of the results appears in Staddon and Higa 1999).

In the case of the present procedure, we could assume that animals are also comparing memory traces. There are, at least, three events in the procedure of the present study that could serve as potential time markers and generate event traces: onset of an interval, onset of a gap, offset of a gap. Let us focus on explaining the pattern of responding after a gap, and assume that responding after a gap depends on comparing the trace produced by the onset of an interval and onset of a gap. Both traces decay according to a power function (as we used for the Stubbs et al. 1994 data) and the greater the difference between the values of the traces, the greater the response strength. In the case of variations in gap location, at the end of an early gap, there will be a small difference between the trace for the onset of the interval and onset of the gap. Hence, response rates should be relatively low after an early gap. In comparison, after a late gap, the trace for interval-onset will have decayed more relative to that for gap-onset, producing a greater difference. The results should be a higher rate of responding. In short, the later a gap occurs in an interval, the higher should be the rate of responding after a gap, which is what we observed (lower panel, figure 8.4).

What does the MTS model predict would happen with different gap durations? When a gap is over, the trace for gap-onset after a small gap will be higher than that after a long gap because less time has elapsed during the gap. The trace for interval-onset will be the same at the end of either gap duration. Hence, the smaller a gap, the larger the difference between traces, and the higher the overall response rate when the gap is over. Our results are in general agreement with this prediction: Overall, response rates are generally higher after a small gap and lower after larger gaps (top panel, figure 8.4). However, the differences are relatively small and only hold for the first few seconds of a post-gap period. Allowing the gap duration and location to vary within a session may have reduced the effect of gap duration (and location).

A question for future studies is how pre-gap and post-gap responding depend on procedural factors such as variable versus fixed gap durations and locations. The MTS model also underscores the importance of analyzing the role of time markers (Staddon 1974, 1984, 2001a). For one, different events serve as time markers of varying efficacy (Roberts and Holder 1984; Staddon and Innis 1969; Starr and Staddon 1974). In the present study, food reinforcement as well as the onset of a gap within an interval may have served as effective time markers. The location of a gap, while variable across trials, provides some predictive value about reinforcement because it occurs in the context of the elapsing interval. Higher rates of responding after "late" gaps than after "early" gaps suggests that the amount of time that elapsed since the start of the interval still had some effect on controlling temporal performance. In contrast, the duration of a gap may have been a less effective time marker because it changed across intervals and a particular duration did not occur at the same point in the interval.

In summary, a key characteristic of interval timing is its flexibility. Gap studies have generated a complex set of results showing that animals are able to track several intervals and that different kinds of events can serve as a time marker and have an effect on timing behavior. This very flexibility on the one hand allows an animal to organize its behavior and judge duration in a variety of situations, and on the other challenges our understanding of how interval timing is accomplished. Until recently, clock-based models served as the primary theoretical framework. Pacemaker-free models, such as the MTS model, provide an alternative view. Rather than focus on properties of a presumed internal clock, the MTS model emphasizes memory processes, and points out the importance of determining what an animal remembers and learns about during an interval of time. The gap procedure provides a method for evaluating the MTS and other models of timing by distinguishing between memory-based, attention-based, and clock-based processes.

Acknowledgments

Portions of this chapter were presented at a meeting of the Psychonomic Society in November 1999 and at a meeting of the Association for Behavior Analysis in May 2004. The research was supported by grants from the TCU Research and Creative Activity Fund.

9 Learning Mechanisms in Multiple-Time-Scale Theory

Mircea I. Chelaru and Mandar S. Jog

Working in John Staddon's laboratory was, for one of the authors (M. I. Chelaru), being in the right place (Duke University) at the right time (1997). At that time, a seminal paper on multiple-time-scale (MTS) theory was submitted. MTS provoked quite a passionate debate: the paper was published accompanied by many commentaries (some of them quite extended) and by the authors' reply (Staddon and Higa 1999; Staddon, Higa, and Chelaru 1999)!

Why was MTS so provocative? Until its publication the timing domain was largely dominated by Scalar Expectancy Theory (SET), which assumes that time is represented linearly, and uses a simple mechanism for producing intervals: a pacemaker-accumulator system together with a resetting mechanism (Gibbon 1977, 1991). SET is conceptually simple and supports the findings from a large class of timing experiments. Since SET was successful in explaining behavior in so many experiments, many attempts were made to explain the neurobiology of timing by finding biological counterparts of the pacemaker, the accumulator, and the ratio comparator in the brain structures considered to be responsible for timing in animals and humans. But success was far more modest in this endeavor than for using SET in experimental psychology (Gibbon, Malapani, Dale, and Gallistel 1997).

In contrast to SET, MTS theory does not use a linear representation of time and its generator, the pacemaker. In MTS, time is represented nonlinearly, tuned to the learned interval, a concept less "intuitive" than a simple, fixed linear time representation. MTS has the same principle of functioning as SET: a time variable signal is compared with a "reference" signal and, depending on the comparison result, a response decision is made. Both theories succeed in providing a reinforcement-response mapping having the main properties of an interval learning process: proportional and scalar timing. Nevertheless, the internal structure of the two theories is completely different: MTS uses a non-linear, interval-tuned, decaying signal for time representation and a difference comparator, while SET uses a fixed, linear, increasing signal for time representation and a ratio comparator. For both theories, reference memory is acquired by sampling the time variable signal before reinforcement.

At first glance, MTS might appear to be a more complicated theory, serving the same purpose as SET. Why would one use a non-linear, apparently complicated, time representation when a simple linear time representation could do the job? An important reason for using MTS is its ability to adapt its time representation so that the main properties of timing are supported. In contrast, the scalar property is forced in SET by injecting scalar noise in different points of the model. The proportional property is obtained by using a ratio comparator. Finding biological counterparts of a controlled pacemaker-accumulator and a ratio comparator seems to be a formidable challenge. MTS explores possibilities offered by pacemaker free timing theories permitting a better insight into the biological mechanisms of timing.

Subsequent research, accompanied by mathematical developments dealing with internal learning mechanisms, showed that MTS can deal with experimental data from the peak procedure and from dynamic reinforcement schedules. These findings have recently been synthesized into a tuned-trace theory of interval dynamics, which proves that MTS is not only useful for predicting performance on fixed reinforcement schedules, but also for a large class of dynamic schedules (Staddon, Chelaru, and Higa 2002a).

This chapter discusses the learning mechanisms of MTS. Two basic mechanisms exist: tuning the shape of the time signal with the interval, and learning through reinforcement memory. The former is essential for the proper functioning in fixed schedules, while both are important for dynamic schedules. Reinforcement memory helps for fast wait-time tracking, while tuning of the time signal with the interval assures slow wait-time tracking.

The possible neurobiological correlations of time perception with MTS theory are also discussed within the context of potentially validating the theory, while explaining the brain's internal timing mechanisms.

A Timing Structure for Steady-State Responding

After sufficient training on fixed-interval (FI) schedules of reinforcement, subjects respond at a very low rate in the first part of the interval, then change abruptly to a high rate and continue responding at this rate until food (reinforcement) delivery (Schneider 1969). This type of behavior is approximated as a binary response (0 for low-rate responding, 1 for high-rate responding) in both MTS theory (Staddon and Higa 1999) and SET (Gibbon 1977).

Information processing in both theories can be explained by using the structure shown in figure 9.1. The structure has three processing units: short-term memory, RF (reinforcement) memory, and a comparator. The system input is the reinforcement (RF) signal, which is a pulsed binary sequence (1 at the time of reinforcement and 0 otherwise). The system output is the response sequence that approximates steady-state responding with a binary sequence (1 for high-rate responding, 0 for low-rate responding).

The generation of the short-term memory output (STM) starts at the time of reinforcement. STM is non-linearly decreasing for MTS and linearly

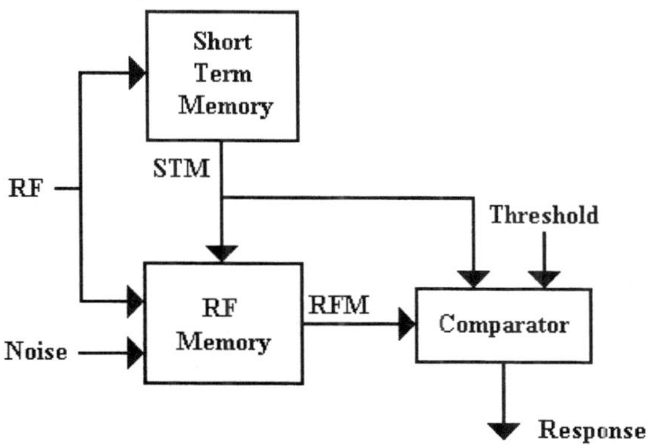

Figure 9.1
A timing structure for steady-state responding in fixed-interval reinforcement schedules. Reinforcement sequence (RF) is binary (1 at reinforcement time, 0 otherwise). Response sequence approximates the steady-state response of the animal with a binary sequence (1 for responding, 0 for not responding). A response is given when short-term memory approximates reinforcement memory.

increasing for SET. The STM signal is compared with the reinforcement memory output (RFM), which is, in both theories, the value of the STM sequence at the time of the previous reinforcement. Depending on the values of STM, RFM, and a threshold, the comparator makes the response decision.

Both theories, MTS and SET, have the same functioning principle for interval timing: a time-varying signal is compared with a fixed value, and, depending on the result of the comparison, a binary response is generated. But the similarities end here since the units' computation equations are entirely different.

For well-trained subjects, the interval timing process has two main properties: the average time of maximal responding is proportional to the interval to be learned (proportional timing) and the standard deviation of the response time is proportional to its mean (scalar timing) (Gibbon 1977). Any good timing theory must support these properties.

The proportional and scalar timing-type behavior of MTS is the result of the internal learning mechanism of the model, which is, perhaps, the most appealing feature of MTS. At first glance, it is surprising that a time-decaying process is able to reflect proportional and scalar timing for intervals in the order of magnitude of 1,000:1. The learning mechanism of MTS is the key to this behavior, as will be demonstrated.

For SET, the predominant timing theory, proportional timing behavior is a direct result of the linearly increasing STM signal and the ratio comparison between STM and RFM signals. To deal with scalar timing (Weber's law), in the simplest implementation of SET, an interval time-driven noise is added to RFM. This special kind of noise, *scalar noise*, has dispersion proportional to the mean. On the other hand, for MTS no special noise is needed. A normally distributed process, with zero mean value and constant dispersion is enough to deal with Weber's law.

Why do we need different timing theories if the end result, that is the properties of responding, is similar? We think that the answer is biological plausibility. After all, interval-timing models should improve our understanding of how time intervals are learned by organisms. A possibility of getting a better insight into the time-learning mechanism is to start with a time-learning model which approximates well an input-output mapping, in our case a reinforcement-response mapping, and try to find processing equivalents in the brain. Despite its theoretical dominance, little progress has been made in identifying the components of SET—the pacemaker, the accumulator, or the ratio comparator—in animal or human brain (Gibbon et al. 1997; Meck 1996). Considering these results, a useful approach is to modify the timing model processing units, and look back to the neurophysiological data for a better fit. MTS is such an attempt.

Short-Term Memory Implementation

The short-time memory unit uses the binary reinforcement RF sequence as input. The short-term memory (STM) signal is obtained by processing the RF sequence (figure 9.1). The STM signal plays the role of the animal's time representation. The STM signal is a non-linear decaying signal, having the largest values at the time of reinforcement. A specific non-linear decaying signal is required for the STM role. The STM signal should be tuned to the interval: it must adjust its shape with the learned interval in such a way that the main interval-timing properties are supported.

The STM signal is produced by using a chain of a particular kind of cell, namely habituation cells (Staddon and Higa 1996, 1999). Every cell has an input, X_i, and two outputs: V_i (used for the computation of STM) and X_{i+1} (used as input by the next cell in the chain). The input of the first cell X_1 is the reinforcement signal (RF), which is one at the time of reinforcement and zero otherwise.

The cell equations are

$$X_{i+1}(n) = \begin{cases} X_i(n) - V_i(n-1) & \text{if } X_i(n) > V_i(n-1) \\ 0 & \text{if } X_i(n) \leq V_i(n-1) \end{cases} \tag{1}$$

and

$$V_i(n) = a_i V_i(n-1) + b_i X_i(n), \tag{2}$$

where $X_1(n) = RF(n)$, n is the index of the discrete time, and the coefficients a_i and b_i are constant real numbers, $0 < a_i < 1$, $0 < b_i < 1$, $i = 1, 2, \ldots, M$.

The STM signal of the MTS model is computed as the sum of the cell outputs V_i:

$$STM(n) = \sum_{i=1}^{M} V_i(n), \tag{3}$$

where M is the number of habituation cells.

Coefficients a_i must be selected in ascending order (the left cells in the chain should have the smallest coefficients) in order to get the proper timing behavior of the model (Staddon and Higa 1996, 1999). All b_i coefficients could be equal without affecting the timing properties.

Computing the a_i coefficients with an exponential law,

$$a_i = 1 - \exp(-\lambda i), \quad i = 1, 2, \ldots, M \tag{4}$$

where λ is a constant, one can ensure a monotonic increase of a_is with the cell index i. Using an exponential law for a_is, with $\lambda \in (0.6, 1.2)$, and equal coefficients b_i, $b_i \in (0.1, 0.4)$, one can obtain reasonable performances for FI, the peak procedure and for some dynamic reinforcement schedules (Staddon, Chelaru, and Higa 2002a,b; Staddon and Higa 1999; Staddon, Higa, and Chelaru 1999).

In contrast to MTS, the STM signal is fixed in SET theory (Gibbon 1977, 1991). The STM signal is a linearly increasing signal, obtained by accumulating the impulses of a pacemaker. For an FI schedule, STM is set to zero at the beginning of the inter-reinforcement interval, and increases linearly until reinforcement, when it is returned to zero.

Reinforcement Memory

The reinforcement memory (RFM) signal is computed in MTS theory as

$$RFM(n+1) = RFM(n) + RF(n)[STM(n-1) + \eta z(n) - RFM(n)], \tag{5}$$

where n is the discrete time (number of iteration), $z(n)$ is a Gaussian distributed noise with zero mean and unitary dispersion, and η is a constant.

At the time of reinforcement, when $RF(n) = 1$, RFM is set to the value of STM before reinforcement, plus a noise term. For the rest of the time, when $RF(n) = 0$, RFM(n) remains constant.

For an FI schedule, the normally distributed stochastic RFM signal has an almost constant mean, related non-linearly to the interval of reinforcement T (as we will see later), and a dispersion equal to constant η from equation 5.

Where are the intervals learned in an MTS system? This is a natural question, because in FI schedules the mean RFM for MTS is almost constant with the interval, for a large range of values. In MTS theory, RFM plays the role of a reference signal, being an indication of the STM signal's lower limit. The comparator uses the RFM signal to establish the time to start or stop responding. As we will see, the interval is learned through the adaptation of the STM signal, which changes its shape, according to the interval value. In brief, the STM signal stops decaying around the same value, the RFM level, having its decay rate controlled by the interval.

In the simplest form of SET, the RFM signal is a normal random variable having the mean m proportional to the interval T, and the dispersion σ proportional to the mean m:

$$m = E[RFM] = k_1 \tau T, \quad \sigma = k_2 m \tag{6}$$

where k_1 and k_2 are constant factors, τ is the clock period, and T is the time of reinforcement (Gibbon 1977). This special kind of distribution (scalar noise) defined by the interval to be learned, is used in SET to deal with Weber's law in timing (Gibbon 1991). The mean RFM signal sets the upper limit of the STM signal, being directly proportional to the reinforcement interval. This means that the intervals are learned by the reinforcement memory in SET, with a precision depending on the interval length.

Comparator

A MTS system starts responding on an FI schedule (Response = 1) when

$$STM(n) < RFM(n) + \theta, \tag{7}$$

where θ is a positive constant (Staddon and Higa 1999). Since STM has the largest values at reinforcement, the response is zero until the (start) condition in equation 7 is met. Then, the MTS system continues responding until the next reinforcement, when it stops responding.

For the peak procedure, the MTS input signal is the stimulus signal, and the RFM signal is computed using the reinforcement signal, with equation 5. If no reinforcement is given after the learned interval elapses, as in some non-food intervals in the peak procedure, the MTS system stops responding when

$$STM(n) < RFM(n) - \rho, \tag{8}$$

where ρ is a positive constant (Staddon, Higa, and Chelaru 1999).

Equations 7 and 8 are good enough to deal with experimental data, not only for FI and peak procedures, but also for some variable interval schedules (Staddon, Chelaru, and Higa 2002a).

In a SET system responding occurs (Response = 1) when

$$|[RFM(n) - STM(n)]/RFM(n)| < \delta, \tag{9}$$

where δ is constant (Church, Meck, and Gibbon 1994). Otherwise there is no response. A SET system starts responding when STM is greater than $(1 - \delta)$RFM and stops responding when STM is lower than $(1 + \delta)$RFM.

Both MTS and SET compare the values of STM and RFM in order to approximate, with a start-stop response sequence, the behavior of well-trained animals in experiments employing FI schedules or the peak procedure. Although, the end response is the same for both theories, the means of achieving this are completely different due to the different representations of time. In SET, the fixed linear representation of time, through the linear STM signal, imposes a ratio comparator to obtain the proportional property of timing. Also, in order to deal with Weber's law, it is necessary to "inject" scalar noise into the SET system. In other words, we must look for a biological structure using a ratio comparison, and for biological memories with scalar behavior. By contrast, the non-linear, adaptive representation of time in MTS needs a difference comparator and a constant noise to deal with proportional and scalar timing (Staddon, Chelaru, and Higa 2002a; Staddon and Higa 1999; Staddon, Higa, and Chelaru 1999).

Is the organism's internal representation of time non-linear, variable, and adapted to the interval to be learned, or is it linear and fixed? We have (at least) two systems, MTS and SET, showing that both types of time representations could be used in order to get a proper mapping between reinforcement and response in different temporal schedules. Finding the biological counterpart components of SET has had only moderate success. For example, none of the biologically inspired computational models of time learning uses a ratio comparator (Gibbon et al. 1997). On the other hand, a difference comparison, like that used in MTS, is very common in neural networks theory (Haykin 1999; Houk, Davis, and Beiser 1998).

As MTS theory is relatively new, few attempts have been made to find counterparts of MTS in internal processing in brain functioning (Staddon, Chelaru, and Higa 2002b). We will discuss later the possible existence of MTS-like processing in basal ganglia, nuclei considered to be responsible for timing in the seconds' range, the range of most animal timing experiments.

Learning Mechanism of MTS

The first response after a fixed time has elapsed is reinforced on an FI schedule. After the interval is learned, subjects respond in advance of reinforcement, making reinforcements occur (almost) periodically. As a result, the reinforcement signal of the structure from figure 9.1 is periodic. This periodic behavior, referred to as steady-state functioning in the following, gave us insight into the learning mechanism of MTS (Staddon, Chelaru, and Higa 2002a).

Short-Term Memory in Fixed-Interval Schedules

In the steady-state phase of an FI schedule, the STM signal is periodic, having a period equal to the FI duration. Considering that the system entered into steady-state regime after k_s reinforcement cycles of an FI of length T, the STM signal can be written as a weighted sum of exponential functions (here is the origin of the term "multiple-time-scale") with base a_i

$$STM(kT + n) = \sum_{i=1}^{M} U_i(T)a_i^n; \quad n = 0, 1, \ldots T - 1, \quad k > k_s \tag{10}$$

where the weights $U_i(T)$ are the values of the outputs V_i at the times of reinforcement, $U_i(T) = V_i(kT)$, $k > k_s$. Equation 10, as well as a detailed mathematical analysis of the steady-state regime, can be found in Staddon, Chelaru, and Higa 2002a.

The weights $U_i(T)$ are constant in time, but dependent on the length, T, of the interval to be learned. Since the coefficients a_i are constant for any T, the weights U_i are responsible for the tuning of the STM signal to the interval T. In fact, the interval is "learned" by MTS through the weights U_i. Figure 9.2 shows the evolution of the weights U_i with interval T, for a MTS system with 10 cells, $\lambda = 1$ (see equation 4) and all $b_i = 0.2$. Figure 9.2 (top) shows the weights U_1–U_5 for the range FI 5–300 seconds. Figure 9.2 (bottom) shows the weights U_6–U_{10} for the range FI 5–2,500 seconds.

In general, a weight U_i starts with a zero value, increases to a maximum value, and then decays to an asymptote equal to b_i. Below a certain time, T_i, the cell i does not participate in the creation of STM, since the weight U_i is zero. The leftmost cells are activated for short intervals, while the rightmost cells become active for long intervals (e.g., U_6–U_{10} in figure 9.2 (bottom)).

Why are the cells activated only when the interval exceeds a certain value? This happens because the input X_i of the cell is zero below a specific interval length. Since U_i is the value of the positive V_i cell output at reinforcement, according to equation 2, we have a null U_i for a null cell input.

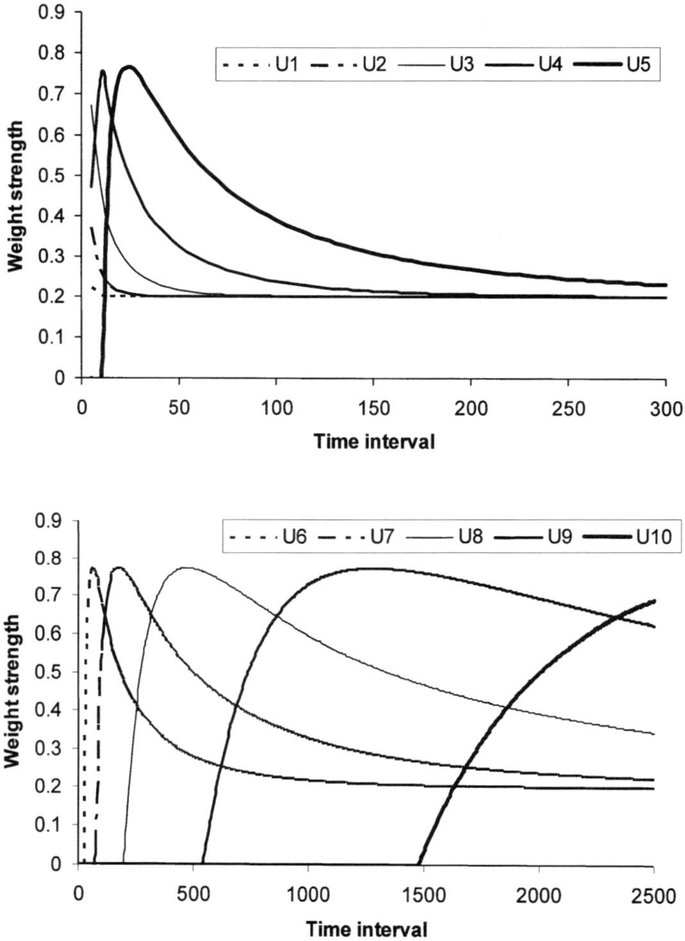

Figure 9.2
Short-term memory is a weighted sequence of exponentials. The weights of the exponentials are constant in time but depend on the length of the learned time interval. At the top, weights U_1–U_5 are shown as a function of time interval, for FI 5–FI 300. The leftmost habituation cells of the MTS system (10 cells, $\lambda = 1$, all $b_i = 0.2$) are activated for short intervals. At the bottom weights U_6–U_{10} are shown as a function of time interval for FI 5–FI 2,500, for a MTS system with 10 cells, $\lambda = 1$, and all $b_i = 0.2$. The rightmost habituation cells become active for long intervals.

How can a cell-input be null? If the memory V_i of a cell is larger than the cell input X_i, the output X_{i+1}, transmitted to the next cell, is zero, as can be seen from equation 1. Thus, the next cell is not active, for the current interval. If a cell is not active, all the following cells in the chain are not activated, because every cell sends a null output X to the next cell.

The STM signal has the same dynamic for a large range of intervals: first STM decreases rapidly then decreases slowly. Because the leftmost cells have the smallest a_i coefficients their contribution vanishes first. This is why STM decreases rapidly after reinforcement Then STM decreases significantly more slowly, and almost linearly, due to the contribution of the rightmost cells, with larger a_i coefficients.

For short intervals, only the leftmost cells are involved in producing the STM signal, which means that the sum from equation 3 has a number of terms less than M. On the other side, all the cells are active for long intervals. Still they do not contribute in the same way to the creation of STM, as one can see from figure 9.3: the leftmost cells contribute with constant weights, equal to b_i, while the rightmost cells contribute with larger weights. It is as if the responsibility of producing STM for longer intervals is delegated to the rightmost cells in the chain, in a smooth manner.

For FI schedules, the learning mechanism of MTS is based on the variation of the weights U_i with the interval: for every interval there is a specific distribution of weights, which support the production of a tuned STM signal. In contrast to SET, in MTS theory knowledge about the interval is not stored in RFM, but in the integrators of the habituation cells. Then what is the role of RFM in MTS?

Reinforcement Memory in Fixed-Interval Schedules

In MTS theory, the RFM signal is obtained by adding a Gaussian distributed noise to the STM signal prior to reinforcement (equation 5). In the steady-state regime of an FI schedule, the cell outputs V_i before reinforcement, $V_i(kT - 1)$, $k \geq k_s$, are constant in time, and non-linearly related to FI duration. They are called "cell memory" and denoted as $M_i(T)$. Their dynamics with respect to the interval T is quite similar to the dynamics of the weights U_i, except for the fact that their horizontal asymptote is equal to zero.

Cell memory, M_i, is a good measure of cell activity before reinforcement. There are two kinds of cell non-activity: when the cell has no input (figure

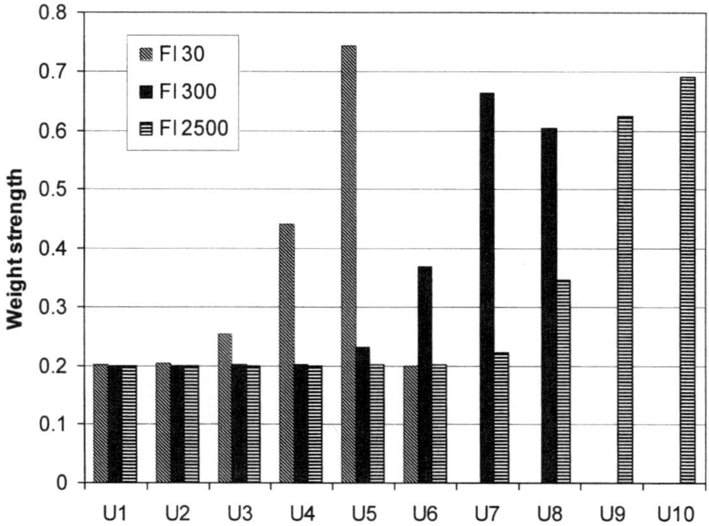

Figure 9.3
Short-term memory weights U_1–U_{10} for FI 30, FI 300, and FI 2,500. The MTS system has 10 cells, $\lambda = 1$, and all $b_i = 0.2$. The leftmost cells contribute with constant weights (equal to b_i) to the creation of STM, while the rightmost cells contribute with bigger weights.

9.2) or when the cell is active but its V_i value is very low. Cell memories (M_is) are a good indication of the second kind of non-activity, as one can see from figure 9.4, where the cell memories for FI 30, FI 300, and FI 3,000 are shown. The MTS system has 10 cells, $\lambda = 1$, and all $b_i = 0.2$. The leftmost cells, with small time constants, have very small cell memories before reinforcement. But the rightmost cells, with large time constants, are still actively contributing to the reinforcement memory.

In the steady-state phase of an FI schedule, the mean value of the RFM signal is equal to the sum of the cell memories M_i:

$$E\{RFM(n)\} = \sum_{i=1}^{M} M_i(T). \tag{11}$$

Considering the behavior of the cell memories, it is not surprising that their sum is almost constant, for a large range of intervals. Figure 9.5 shows the variation of the mean RFM with interval T, in the steady-state regime. A MTS system with 11 cells, $\lambda = 1$, and all $b_i = 0.2$ was used. The range of intervals for which RFM is computed is 5–5,000.

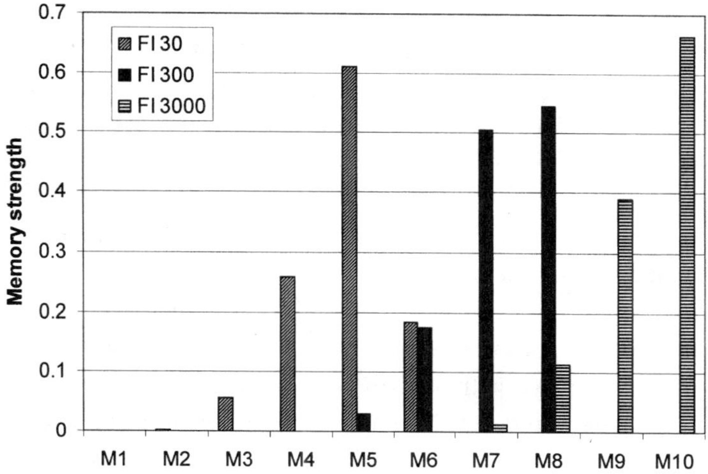

Figure 9.4
A cell memory represents the activation of a cell before reinforcement. The sum of the cell memories is the estimate of reinforcement memory. Cell memories M_1–M_{10} versus time interval are shown for FI 30, FI 300, and FI 3,000. The leftmost cells are active (create RFM) for small intervals, while the rightmost cells are active for bigger intervals. A MTS system with 10 cells, $\lambda = 1$, and all $b_i = 0.2$ is used.

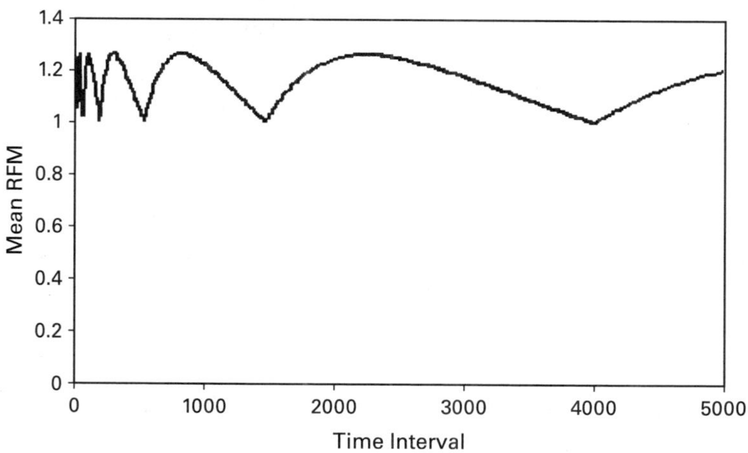

Figure 9.5
Sum of cell memories (mean RFM—see text) as a function of the time interval for FI 5–FI 5,000. The MTS system has 11 cells, $\lambda = 1$, and all $b_i = 0.2$. The mean RFM is almost constant, for a large range of time intervals, due to the STM signal adaptation with the time interval.

In contrast with a SET system that has a mean RFM proportional to the interval T, the MTS system has an almost constant mean RFM, for a wide range of intervals. This is a good argument against the view that an MTS system is not able to deal with long intervals (Gallistel 1999). Using proper time constants (that is, suitable λ in equation 4), and a large enough number of cells, MTS is able to deal properly with wide ranges of intervals.

So, in an MTS system, for FI schedules, the integrators of the habituation cells share the memory of the interval duration. RFM only memorizes the (almost constant) lower limit of the STM signal, having the role of a reference signal for the next reinforcement interval: RFM value plus a constant threshold value is compared with STM in order to decide on the response pattern. In a SET system, the RFM remembers the upper limit of the STM, before reinforcement. Since this limit is close to the interval duration (within scalar precision) one can say that the interval is learned by RFM. For large intervals, large values of RFM must be stored, which could raise questions of biological plausibility.

The variation of the mean RFM signal is much more significant in dynamic reinforcement schedules, where the time of STM signal sampling could be very different between reinforcement trials. This could lead to quite different values of the RFM signal, which are in fact responsible for the fast tracking of the schedule dynamics, as we will see later.

Proportional Timing

Experiments with pigeons have shown that steady-state responding on FI schedules can be described by a two-state behavior pattern: immediately after reinforcement subjects respond at a very low rate and then switch to a high and almost constant rate until reinforcement is delivered. The ratio between the durations of these two states is almost constant. Subjects wait about two thirds of the FI and then rapidly switch to the high terminal rate (Schneider 1969).

The timing structure of figure 9.1 approximates the low responding behavior with zero response and the high responding behavior with unitary response. The time between reinforcement delivery and the first response is called *wait time* (Wt). Experiments have shown that the ratio of wait time to FI duration is almost constant for a wide range of FIs (animals are able to learn intervals of 3,000 seconds; Dews 1970), a property called *proportional timing.*

Proportional timing results in SET from the linearly increasing shape of the STM signal, combined with the ratio comparison between STM and RFM.

Due to the non-linear nature of a MTS system, proportional timing is not an obvious property, as it is in SET. But this property exists; the ratio Wt/T has the same dynamics with interval duration as the RFM signal has in figure 9.5 (of course the mean values are different). What can produce the proportional timing property in a non-linear system like MTS? The answer is the tuning of the STM signal to the interval. The slope of the STM signal is lowered with increasing schedule length T. This slope-tuning feature is illustrated in figure 9.6, where the difference between STM and RFM is shown, on a normalized time scale (proportion of T), for FI 30, FI 300, FI 1,500, and FI 7,500. The MTS system has 11 cells, $\lambda = 1$ and all $b_i = 0.2$. The four curves superimpose almost completely in the low decaying region of the STM signal.

Due to the STM slope tuning, a fixed proportion of the interval corresponds to an almost constant value of the difference between STM and RFM, for a large range of intervals. The constant threshold in the MTS comparator (equation 7) forces the switch to responding (from 0 to 1) at a

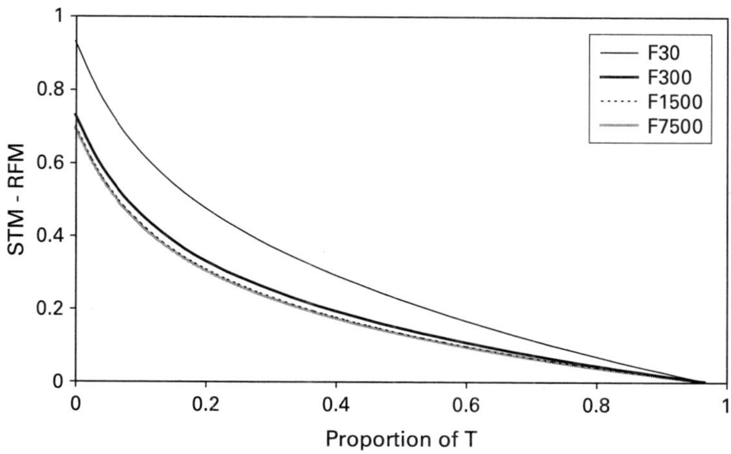

Figure 9.6
STM-RFM variation as a function of the proportion of the interval (T) for FI 30, FI 300, and FI 7,500. The MTS system has 11 cells, $\lambda = 1$, and $b_i = 0.2$ for all cells. The variation STM-RFM has almost the same shape for a large range of intervals, which implies proportional timing.

constant proportion of the FI. This means that proportional timing is a natural property of MTS behavior.

Scalar Timing

Experiments with FI schedules show that the ratio between the dispersion of wait times and the mean of the wait time is almost constant, for a large range of schedules (Catania 1970). This property, called *scalar timing*, is postulated in SET, by adding scalar noise to the RFM signal or to the comparator thresholds (Gibbon 1991). In contrast to SET, in MTS theory scalar timing is a property of the model's behavior. One could ask: why does this difference matter if both theories satisfy scalar timing? Biological memories and ratio comparators with scalar like behavior are the biological equivalent of injecting scalar noise into the SET processing units. By contrast, MTS shows that a certain kind of decaying memory process is able to support proportional and scalar timing. For MTS, it is not necessary to look for scalar-like biological counterparts: it is enough to identify the generator of time-tuned memory activity, because the other components of the model are very common. Thus, the same input-output behavior, but implemented by different means, could suggest completely different ways of getting an understanding of the biological timing process.

In MTS theory it is supposed that the lower end of the STM signal (RFM signal) is represented with an error distribution independent of the interval. This noisy process (RFM signal), with constant dispersion, together with the interval-tuned STM, is good enough for obtaining scalar-timing behavior in MTS systems, for a large range of intervals.

Figure 9.7 depicts the ratio between the dispersion and the mean of wait-time (coefficient of variation—COV) for a wide range of FI lengths. An MTS system with 10 cells, $\lambda = 1$, all $b_i = 0.2$ and threshold $\theta = 0.15$ (equation 7) is used. The noise dispersion η from equation 5 is 0.09. To compute the mean and the dispersion of the wait-time, 1,024 reinforced intervals of steady-state functioning were used, for every schedule. The COV values vary slightly around an almost horizontal line. The corresponding regression line has an almost zero slope, shown by the dashed line in figure 9.7.

The explanation for this scalar behavior is again the MTS adaptation mechanism: for a wide range of intervals, the STM signal adapts its shape in such a way that the STM-RFM differences (figure 9.6) are very close to each other on a normalized time scale. Thus, the comparison between the

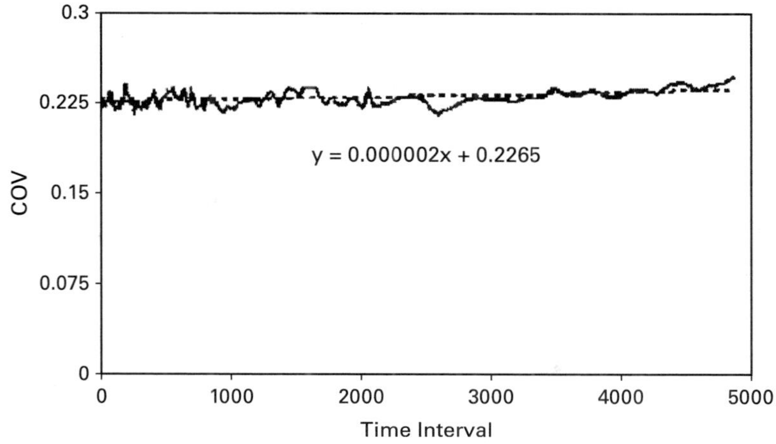

Figure 9.7
COV variation as a function of interval duration for a MTS system with 10 cells, $\lambda = 1$, $b_i = 0.2$ for all cells, threshold $\theta = 0.15$ and noise dispersion $\eta = 0.09$. The mean of COV is almost constant with the length of the learned time interval. (See text.)

sum RFM $+ \theta$ and STM will produce, for different intervals, almost the same wait-time distribution versus the proportion of the interval (Staddon, Chelaru, and Higa 2002b).

MTS and the Dynamics of Interval Timing

Recently, the MTS system was used to simulate animal behavior in some reinforcement schedules which presented changing of interval durations (Staddon, Chelaru, and Higa 2002a,b). These dynamic schedules originated from a response-initiated delay (RID) schedule: After food reinforcement the animal is free to make the operant response. The first response after wait time t turns on a clock, which runs for a schedule-dependent interval, T, at the end of which another food reinforcement is given. By changing T, according to some fixed rule (e.g. pulse, step, sinusoidal) one can get a large class of dynamic reinforcement schedules (Staddon 2001a).

The MTS system was tested for pulse, step, cyclic (sinusoidal), and variable-interval (VI) schedules (Staddon, Chelaru, and Higa 2002a). The behavior of the system was judged through direct comparison with the experimental data. The comparison was not made on a statistical basis:

simply, the MTS system was considered to be a "subject" and the wait time of its response was compared with the experimental wait time shown by different animals. The simulation showed that the model is able to duplicate the experimental data for all the tested schedules, which shows that MTS theory provides not only a good model for steady-state behavior, but is also useful for simulating wait-time tracking in dynamic schedules. However, MTS cannot account for some dynamic schedules: for example, it cannot account for the tracking behavior of rats, when the inter-reinforcement interval (IRI) is changed from a short IRI (120 seconds) to a long IRI (480 seconds) and back to the short IRI. The MTS system tracks these transitions, while the rats do not (Higa and Staddon 1997; Staddon, Chelaru, and Higa 2002a).

How can we explain MTS tracking of wait time in a large class of variable RID schedules? MTS tracking behavior has two major components: fast tracking, as can be observed in pulsed or sinusoidal type schedules, and slow tracking as can be seen in step up/down schedules. Fast tracking is supported by the RFM learning rule (equation 5). For variable schedules the RFM signal is no longer almost constant, as it is for fixed schedules. Since RFM is obtained by sampling the STM signal prior to reinforcement and the IRI varies with time, STM is sampled at different times in its history. This leads to quite different RFM values (especially in pulsed schedules), as opposed to FI schedules. The slow change in wait time in a step up/down schedule is explained by the redistribution of the integrator memories in the habituation cells of the MTS chain. For two different intervals these distributions are different, as was pointed out above. Due to the dynamics of the habituation cells' integrators, an abrupt change (reinforcement is suddenly given earlier/later) is followed by a gradual modification (redistribution) of the weights U_i of the STM signal.

The fast-tracking capability of MTS puts in evidence the second learning mechanism of the model: learning through the RFM signal. The RFM signal is strongly related to reinforcement time. This is why it does not give important information in fixed schedules, because the STM sampling is performed almost at the same time in its history. In contrast, the information from the RFM signal is very important in variable schedules: a change at the time of reinforcement, which forces a change of the RFM memory, is immediately seen on the next trial, and hence fast wait-time tracking is forced by comparator.

MTS and the Neurobiology of Timing

Studies of lesions and synaptic transmission manipulation effects in animal timing tasks, as well as studies of degenerative and/or focal lesion effects on timing tasks in humans, suggest that two brain regions, basal ganglia and cerebellum, are involved in temporal processing. (For a comprehensive review, see Gibbon et al. 1997.) Evidence reviewed by Ivry (1997) suggests that the cerebellum controls durations less than 1 second, while the basal ganglia control longer intervals of the type usually used in animal timing experiments.

The role of the basal ganglia in the neural control of timing was studied partly because of disturbances in rhythmic movement in Parkinson's disease (PD) (Freeman, Cody, and Scahdy 1993; Harrington, Haaland, and Hermanowicz 1998; Nakamura, Nagasaki, and Narabayashi 1978; O'Boyle, Freeman, and Cody 1996). Also, it was shown that time perception in animals is altered when dopamine (depleted in PD) is reduced through pharmacological manipulations (Maricq, Roberts, and Church 1981; Meck 1983, 1996). Dopamine agonists and antagonists produce a temporary distortion in timing accuracy: animals trained ON dopamine agonists and tested OFF show a temporary overestimate of the interval. For dopamine antagonists the reverse is true. Despite these under or over-estimations of the interval, the scalar property is preserved (Gibbon et al. 1997).

These experimental findings were interpreted, from the SET point of view, as pharmacologically induced changes of the clock speed, corresponding to a larger or smaller than normal slope of the increasing STM signal. How can we interpret these findings from the MTS point of view? Since scalar variability is preserved, one can suppose that the interval tuning mechanism, more exactly the functioning of the habituation cells, is not affected by these kinds of pharmacological manipulations. More likely, changing the comparator threshold would affect the timing of the response, while preserving the scalar property.

Manipulations involving lesions or drugs in timing experiments with rats suggest that reference memory of the interval in SET could be linked to acetylcholine function in the frontal cortex, connected by frontal-striatal loops to basal ganglia (Meck 1996). How could these induced memory effects be interpreted within MTS theory? Essentially, the memorized value (RFM) in MTS does not vary with the interval, being mainly a reference of the STM signal lower end, for fixed schedules of reinforcement. For the decision to respond, the difference between STM and this memorized reference is needed. Thus, it is difficult to identify the error source here: variations in the comparator thresholds, or variations of the mean RFM signal? Both of them would force a shift in interval time estimation.

Another source of error in estimating the interval in MTS could be variations of the RFM distribution. This could lead to an increased variability in responding, as was shown in studies of patients with degenerative basal ganglia disease (PD, O'Boyle et al. 1996; Pastor, Jahanashi, Artieda, and Obeso 1992a; 1992b) or Huntington's disease (Freeman, Cody, O'Boyle, Crauford, Neary, and Snowden 1996). Considering the above "memory effects" one could speculate that the location of the biological counterpart of RFM memory is either in the basal ganglia or in the frontal cortex. A constant distributed noisy RFM signal, generated in the frontal cortex, and a variable distributed comparator process, localized in the basal ganglia, can be hypothesized. This could be an explanation for the memory effects produced by induced lesions of the frontal cortex and the increased variability effects produced by diseased basal ganglia.

Basal ganglia could also be the location of STM signal production. This hypothesis is suggested by experimental evidence: time-estimation performance of PD patients exhibits scalar variability when they are ON medication (levodopa and apomorphine) but not when OFF medication (Malapani et al. 1998). The MTS scalar behavior can be affected by changes in the functioning of habituation cells, forced by modifications of the "order" of the cell coefficients (the leftmost cells must have smaller time constants than the rightmost cells for scalar property). Other experiments have shown that striatal neurons are not only involved in detecting and registering stimuli and rewards in sensorimotor tasks, they also show activity indicating expectation of outcome (Schulz, Apicella, Romo, and Scarnati 1998). This activity is small immediately after reward, and then increases until reward is delivered and stops abruptly thereafter. These phenomena might suggest the presence of a short-memory mechanism in striatum.

Much experimental work is needed to elucidate the behavior of the basal ganglia nuclei during timing tasks. To our knowledge, such an attempt has not been made yet. Simultaneous recording of the neuronal activity in different nuclei of the basal ganglia, through recent multi-electrodes techniques (Jog et al. 2002, Jog et al. 1999; Nicolelis 1999), with some well-known schedules of operant conditioning, could be of help in understanding the involvement of these nuclei in internal timing, and also in identifying/validating models of information processing.

Conclusions

The most important feature of MTS theory is its novel way of thinking about temporal memory: memory for a time interval is distributed in cells having different time constants. Different intervals lead to different activation patterns of these cells, which is equivalent to having an interval-tuned time representation. This is a seminal concept, very different from the linear, fixed representation of time in the currently dominant timing theory, SET.

Fixed, linear time representation leads to the "ubiquity of ratio comparisons" together with scalar functioning for clock, RF memory, or comparator thresholds (Gibbon 1992; Gibbon and Fairhurst 1994). On the other hand, the interval-tuned time representation of MTS leads to the use of a difference comparator and a zero mean, constant dispersion noise for scalar behavior. Thus, MTS and SET suggest two completely different approaches to studying the biological timing mechanism: one looks for a biological equivalent of an interval-tuned distributed memory mechanism and a difference comparator (MTS), the other the biological equivalent of a pacemaker-accumulator mechanism and a ratio comparator (SET).

MTS introduces a new kind of learning technique: learning the task is accomplished only by acquiring information into the integrators, since all the coefficients of the model (cell coefficients and comparator thresholds) are fixed. How do MTS cells acquire this knowledge? How does MTS reach a steady-state? Starting with null information in the integrators (null V_i), a number of intervals of a fixed length is given (without using the MTS response). After that, the proper (interval-tuned) information is loaded into integrators, such that the shape of the STM is properly tuned with the interval, and the model responding can be considering as a correct timed input for the reinforcement schedule.

MTS theory is in its early stages of development. Presently, MTS shows that a non-linear, interval-tuned representation of time could be as good as a fixed, linear representation, in some fixed operant conditioning schedules. In addition, MTS is at this time the only theory that can duplicate animal behavior in fixed (FI, peak procedure) and dynamic schedules. In its current form, MTS theory has some limitations: it deals only with wait time, and says nothing about the pattern of responding (the response is binary), and cannot deal with concurrent timing of multiple intervals (Staddon et al. 2002a). It is possible that future developments, like a memory mechanism for multiple intervals, a choice mechanism between intervals, or a more "realistic" response instead of a binary response, will enlarge the modeling capabilities of MTS.

10 Mechanisms of Adaptive Behavior: Beyond the Usual Suspects

Valentin Dragoi

Often forgotten in psychology is the great truth that in science, simplicity ... is the royal road to scientific truth. Not that every simple theory is true; experimental test, after all, trumps simplicity. But when two theories are compared, the simpler ... is almost invariably the better one.
—J. E. R. Staddon (2001a, p. 1)

Science does not consist merely of putting experimental results in order, it only advances through what Einstein called the *free constructive element*—the invention and testing of formal models. I first learned of this thesis from my graduate mentor, John Staddon, whose main belief is that the way to understand the laws and causes of adaptive behavior is through the invention, testing, and modification or rejection of simple models. However, over the years, I realized that John's work was guided more by close adherence to empirical data and less by mathematical elegance, and thus I learned that the "principle theory" approach, which constrains possible models on the basis of well-chosen empirical regularities, should be much more important than the "free constructive" approach. Since these ideas have greatly influenced my scientific thinking, I will use here a combination of "principle" and "constructive" theory approaches to help build models of learning and adaptive behavior according to the principled construction.

The idea that simplicity is the *royal* road to scientific truth has always had a great appeal in behavioral sciences. The best-known theoretical tool subordinated to this thesis is black-box modeling, one of the dominant approaches in theoretical psychology. Generally speaking, the black-box approach implies the modeling of input-output relationships between environmental stimuli and responses generated by the animal, or modeling the relationship between successive responses. The black-box approach has deep roots in engineering—we could learn a great deal about the behavior of an electronic device, without having to understand how the internal machinery works, simply by injecting current at the input pin, and then measuring the voltage and current output levels. This type of analogy has inspired behavioral scientists to use black-box models to predict the rules of behavioral operation without having to "break" the system to find out the animal's internal structure.

Black-box approaches are particularly useful tools in psychology because of their ability to provide a compact summary of behavior without requiring too many assumptions. Indeed, through the elaboration of simple black-box models theoretical behaviorists have greatly contributed to the discovery of simple principles of adaptive behavior. A few examples of well-known behavioral principles include response variation, response competition, short and long-term memory. Historically, the systematic investigation of simple behavioral principles has come in response to one of the fundamental questions in behavioral sciences, namely, What are the key variables controlling adaptive behavior? But is the discovery of simple behavioral principles through the use of black-box models sufficient for understanding adaptive behavior?

So far, black-box models have been primarily aimed at examining the effects of individual behavioral principles. There have been, however, very few attempts to explain key features of more complex behavior, an effort that would require behavioral scientists to take a closer look at *combinations* of individual behavioral principles. Indeed, it is generally accepted that complex behavior arises from the organization of sets of behavioral "primitives," or elementary behavioral principles. For example, it is known that the past history of responses generated by the animal and the past history of obtained reward constitute simple variables that can be used in a dynamic model to predict the strength of the operant response. However, to characterize how the animal allocates responses in a more complex situation, for instance during choice, requires additional variables. These variables (e.g., response competition) would be needed to explain how responses followed by high-probability reward suppress responses followed by low-probability reward. On the other hand, understanding how behavior can be temporally regulated would require a completely new set of assumptions, such as internal clocks or pacemakers, that presumably underlie temporal sensitivity. Evidently, understanding complex behavior requires the elaboration of models that unify and connect simple behavioral principles, and, ultimately, have the capacity to explain complex behavior as an *emergent property* of the interaction between elementary behavioral principles. Unfortunately, although substantial progress has been made in our understanding of the fundamental variables controlling adaptive behavior, exactly how simple behavioral principles can be connected to create emergent properties is just beginning to be explored quantitatively (Dragoi and Staddon 1999; Dragoi et al. 2003; Grossberg and Schmajuk 1989; Machado 1997; Staddon 2001; Sutton and Barto 1981).

There is no general recipe for how simple behavioral principles should be connected. However, at least three criteria may be used to constrain the space of possible combinations: generality, parsimony, and biological plausibility. In this chapter I will exemplify how complex behavior emerges from combination of simple behavioral principles by reviewing two dynamic black-box models that explain key temporal and non-temporal properties of operant conditioning. In the first part I will describe a model that we have used to explain static and dynamic properties of operant behavior in both single-choice and multi-response situations (Dragoi 1997; Dragoi and Staddon 1999), and then I will describe how temporal regulation can emerge from the interaction between simple, non-temporal, behavioral principles (Dragoi et al. 2003).

The Dynamics of Operant Learning

One common property of biological systems is history dependence, i.e., the fact that the same set of experimental conditions leads to different performance depending on earlier conditions. How can we characterize history-dependent properties quantitatively? History dependence implies that learning is a global process that integrates information from the remote past (long-term memory) with present conditions when the animal is confronted with an environmental change. However, behavior can also be characterized on shorter time scales to suggest the importance of local (history-independent) dynamics. A local model is sufficient to explain effects which occur within one experimental session, such as acquisition or extinction, but local models are unable to explain many long-term effects of reinforcement, e.g., why responding to a previously reinforced stimulus recovers after a pause following prolonged extinction—spontaneous recovery (Mackintosh 1974; Mazur 1992); why the ability to perform reversals improves with increasing training—serial reversal learning (Davis and Staddon 1990); or why the partial reinforcement extinction effect, PREE (Kacelnik et al. 1987), is reversed (more resistance to extinction following continuous reinforcement) if training is extensive—reverse PREE (Nevin 1988).

Evidently both long and short time scales are important in conditioning. I will describe next a simple dynamic model (Dragoi and Staddon 1999) in which the interaction between variables at short and long time scales accounts for key dynamic features of operant learning. The model defines two variables, short- and long-term reinforcement *expectancies*. The concept of reinforcement expectancy has a long history in psychology, and also has neurophysiological correlates. For example, expectancy of reward has recently been associated in the primate with the activity of dopaminergic neurons whose fluctuating output signals the changes in the prediction of future events (Schultz et al. 1997). Most theories of Pavlovian conditioning incorporate some notion of expectancy (Daly and Daly 1982; Klopf 1988; Rescorla and Wagner 1972; Schmajuk and DiCarlo 1992; Sutton and Barto 1981; Tolman 1932). However, in contrast to these models, we proposed that the operant response is facilitated when the short-term expectancy is greater than the long-term expectancy (reinforcement conditions improve) and the response is suppressed when the long-term expectancy is greater than the short-term expectancy (reinforcement conditions worsen). In short, the model rests on the following behavioral principles (see also appendix 1):

(i) Response competition Operant responses mutually inhibit each other such that the stronger response will have a higher probability of occurring. The idea of response competition is generally accepted; there is disagreement only on exactly how it should be represented in a model. Herrnstein (1970) proposed that response rate in one component of a multiple schedule depends on its rate of reinforcement relative to the rate of reinforcement in the adjacent components, suggesting a process of comparison (competition) between schedule components. Hinson and Staddon (1978)

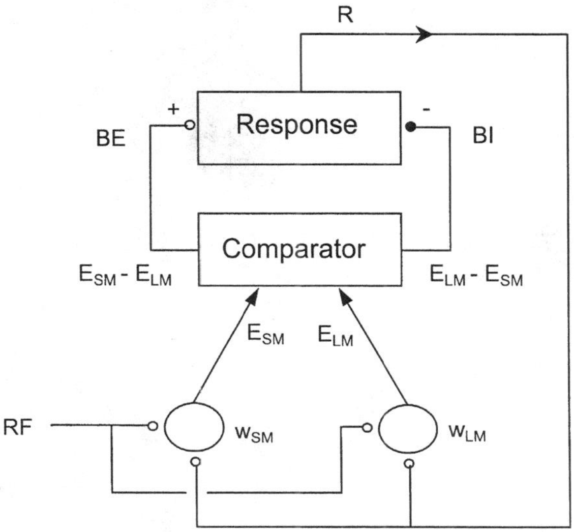

Figure 10.1
Model diagram. The operant response (R) and the reinforcement (RF) build short-term (w_{SM}) and long-term (w_{LM}) memory associations. Responses read out their associations with RF to implement short-term (E_{SM}) and long-term (E_{LM}) reinforcement expectancies. These expectancies are compared to detect changes in the environment. The difference $E_{SM} - E_{LM}$ (behavioral excitation: BE) facilitates responding, whereas the difference $E_{LM} - E_{SM}$ (behavioral inhibition: BI) suppresses responding. Open circles represent excitatory connections; filled circles represent inhibitory connections.

use behavioral competition as a mechanism for schedule interaction. Davis et al. (1993) use a winner-take-all rule to model response selection, also supporting the idea of non-linear response competition.

(ii) Short and long-term memory traces Each response leaves a brief, decaying short-term memory trace (Hull 1943; Sutton and Barto 1981), whereas associations between responses and the reinforcement leave both decaying short-term (w_{SM}) and long-term (w_{LM}) memory traces (figure 10.1). Importantly, these associations increase in strength with the degree of contiguity between responses and the reinforcement.

(iii) Learning expectancy The organism builds short-term and long-term reinforcement expectancies based on recent and remote association memory. Short-term reinforcement expectancy (E_{SM}) is defined as the product

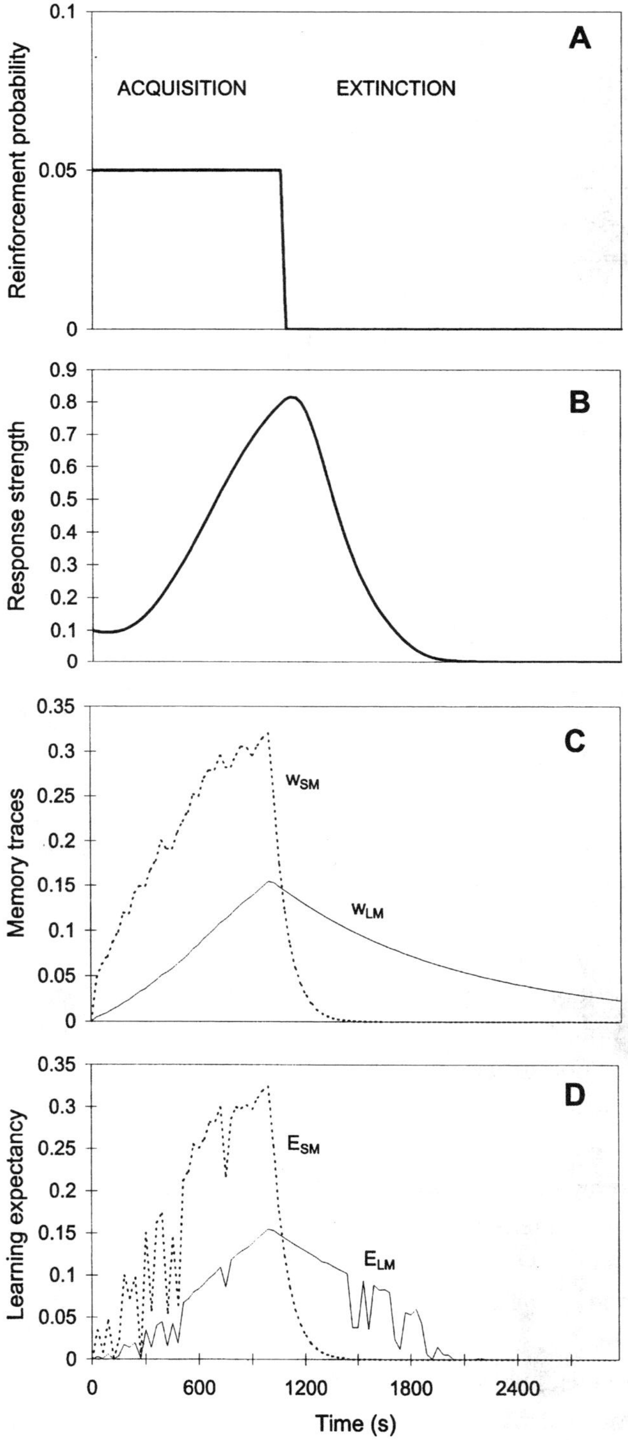

A
ACQUISITION
EXTINCTION
Reinforcement probability
0.1
0.05
0
B
Response strength
0.9
0.8
0.7
0.6
0.5
0.4
0.3
0.2
0.1
0
C
Memory traces
w_{SM}
w_{LM}
0.35
0.3
0.25
0.2
0.15
0.1
0.05
0
D
Learning expectancy
E_{SM}
E_{LM}
0
600
1200
1800
2400
Time (s)

of response and short-term memory traces. Long-term reinforcement expectancy (E_{LM}) is defined as the product of response and long-term memory traces. (See figure 10.1.)

(iv) Expectancy mismatch drives the operant response Long- and short-term expectancies are compared to detect deviations from learned contingency relations (see the comparator in figure 10.1) and their difference controls the operant response. If short-term expectancy is greater than long-term expectancy (reinforcement is under-predicted, reinforcement conditions are improving—if reinforcement increases in magnitude or probability, for example) the strength of the operant response increases. But if long-term expectancy is greater than short-term expectancy (reinforcement is over-predicted, e.g., reinforcement decreases in magnitude or probability) the strength of the operant response decreases.

How does the model work when these simple principles are connected? Figure 10.2 illustrates the model dynamics in a typical operant-conditioning situation in which the reinforcement probability is 0.05 for the first 1,000 seconds, followed by extinction after time 1,000 (figure 10.2, A). The simulation shows that the response strength gradually increases during acquisition and then decreases during extinction (figure 10.2, B). To explain this basic behavior we analyze the dynamics of key variables in the model (figures 10.2, C and D). Successive pairings between the response and the reinforcement ensure the formation of response-reinforcement associations (memory traces) at two time scales, short (w_{SM}) and long (w_{LM}). These associations are formed in parallel; they encode the temporal correlation between the response and the reinforcement. Since w_{SM} has a smaller time constant than w_{LM}, short-term memory traces both increase (during acquisition) and decay (during extinction) at a higher rate than the long-term memory traces.

Figure 10.2
Illustration of model dynamics during acquisition and extinction. (A) Reinforcement probability is 0.05 for times between 0 and 1,000 and 0 after time 1,000. (B) Response strength increases to a maximum during acquisition and decreases to 0 during extinction. (C) Short-term and long-term memory traces for response-reinforcement associations. Each memory trace increases during acquisition and decays during extinction at different time scales. (D) Short-term and long-term learning expectancies are obtained by multiplying the short-term and long-term memory traces by the response trace.

The response multiplied by the short and long-term associations (which act as "connection weights") represents short-term ($E_{SM} = w_{SM}RT$) and long-term ($E_{LM} = w_{LM}RT$) learning expectancies (short-term expectancy is a measure of experienced reinforcement and long-term expectancy is a measure of expected reinforcement; figure 10.2D). As mentioned earlier, one key property of the model is that the mismatch between the short-term and long-term learning expectancies controls the operant response: if the reinforcement is under-predicted (experienced reinforcement is larger than expected reinforcement, i.e., $E_{SM} > E_{LM}$) a *behavioral excitation* signal proportional to the difference between the short-term and long-term expectancies ($BE \sim E_{SM} - E_{LM}$) enhances the response strength; if the reinforcement is over-predicted (experienced reinforcement is smaller than expected reinforcement, i.e., $E_{SM} < E_{LM}$) a *behavioral inhibition* signal proportional to the difference between the long-term and short-term expectancies ($BI \sim E_{LM} - E_{SM}$) reduces the response strength.

Full model simulations and quantitative fits to experimental data have been described previously (Dragoi and Staddon 1999), hence they will not be shown here. However, I note that the model is able to explain key static (steady-state) and dynamic (transient) properties of reinforcement learning in animals. The model has been applied previously to a wide range of operant conditioning phenomena at different time scales: (1) short—assignment of credit (response selection, delayed reinforcement, delayed reinforcement and preference reversal, the effect of non-contingent reinforcement); development of preference in choice behavior (effects of ratio and absolute difference between the reinforcement probabilities); matching; successive contrast effects; behavioral contrast effects; partial reinforcement extinction effect; overtraining reversal effect; effects of context on stimulus preference; and (2) long—spontaneous recovery and regression; serial reversal learning (successive daily reversals and reversals in blocks of days); for details, see Dragoi 1997 and Dragoi and Staddon 1999.

Exploring global models, such as that described in this section, is important because it demonstrates how individual variables, such as short-term and long-term memory processes, can coexist and how their interaction can explain complex behavioral phenomena as emergent properties. History—number of reinforcements and type and sequence of reinforcement schedule—has been neglected in theoretical and experimental work on operant behavior. Emphasis on chronic (i.e., long-term) exposure to fixed conditions of reinforcement has led researchers to equate "history" with "current schedule," ignoring the effects of prior training. However, we have just demonstrated that prior experience can not, and need not, be ignored. Even a simple dynamic theory that allows for multiple time scales can help us to understand how past experience changes the organism and modulates its response to new conditions.

Interval Timing as an Emergent Learning Property

In the previous section I presented a dynamic model that describes how the strength of the operant response can be deduced from the interaction of events at different time scales—this defines what and how strong the response is. However, when an activity occurs is as important as what or how strong the activity is. Yet we know little about the way in which temporal discrimination emerges during learning. Of particular interest in behavioral sciences is interval timing, the learned locating of behavior with respect to a time marker. Mammals, birds, and fish will learn to restrict an operant response for food reinforcement to times when the response has been effective in the past. Two examples: First, on fixed-interval (FI) reinforcement schedules, the operant response is rewarded only after a fixed time since the preceding reward (the time marker). Subjects learn to restrict operant responding to the latter part of the interval. Second, animals will learn to space successive responses in time if such spacing is a condition of reinforcement (Ferster and Skinner 1957—spaced responding), and in this case the average inter-response time (IRT) is proportional to the required minimum.

Traditionally, interval timing was explained by assuming (a) explicit temporal devices, such as internal clocks (or pacemakers) with fixed periods that simply count time (e.g., SET: Church et al. 1994; Gibbon 1977, 1991) or switch between different behavioral states in a certain order (e.g., BeT: Killeen 1991; Killeen and Fetterman 1988), (b) the existence of explicit internal oscillators with built-in temporal properties (Church and Broadbent 1990), or (c) an explicit discretization of time by implementing variables tuned to particular (fixed) time intervals (e.g., Grossberg and Schmajuk 1990; Machado 1977). However, none of these assumptions can be used to explain how dedicated temporal units (internal clocks, pacemakers, or oscillators) emerge during learning to exhibit the temporal properties they have been assigned. Are the temporal regularities in behavior a consequence of explicit internal representations of time or do they stem from processes that have no explicit temporal representation? This question has been rarely asked by researchers of temporal learning. Is it possible that some aspects of timing, at least, might represent emergent properties of other, non-temporal learning processes?

I will argue in this section that the major facts of interval timing can be explained without reference to an internal clock, time scale, or explicit comparison process, in a way that incidentally provides a solution to the resetting problem (the timing process is "reset" by the appropriate time marker), and I demonstrate temporal discrimination in a model that has no pacemaker or fixed internal scale for time and has no comparator beyond the familiar winner-take-all response-competition rule. The model (Dragoi et al. 2003), sketched in figure 10.3, relies on just two assumptions that were elements of the preceding model for non-temporal properties of operant conditioning that we have already explored extensively (Dragoi 1997; Dragoi and Staddon 1999; see also appendix 2):

(i) Variation and selection of responses through competition between response classes There is abundant empirical evidence that three classes of behavior typically occur during different parts of the to-be-timed interval on timing tasks (e.g., Staddon 1977b; Staddon and Simmelhag 1971; see also Dragoi 1997; Dragoi and Staddon 1999; Killeen and Fetterman 1988): (1) elicited responses (behaviors that typically occur immediately after reinforcement, on FI schedules, or before the last response preceding reinforcement, on spaced-responding schedules); (2) interim responses (behaviors that occur in the middle of the inter-reinforcement interval), and (3) the terminal response (the reinforced response, which normally occurs, in the final segment of the inter-reinforcement interval). For simplicity, we combine elicited and interim responses and label them 'other' (O) responses (or behaviors). Terminal responses (e.g., key pecks by pigeons, lever presses by rats) are treated separately and are labeled R responses. These two response classes are the minimum needed for temporal discrimination.

(ii) Competition modulation by the overall arousal level linked to reinforcement rate Specifically, the strength of behavioral competition (which determines the frequency with which the system switches between responses) is controlled by the overall reinforcement rate in the training con-

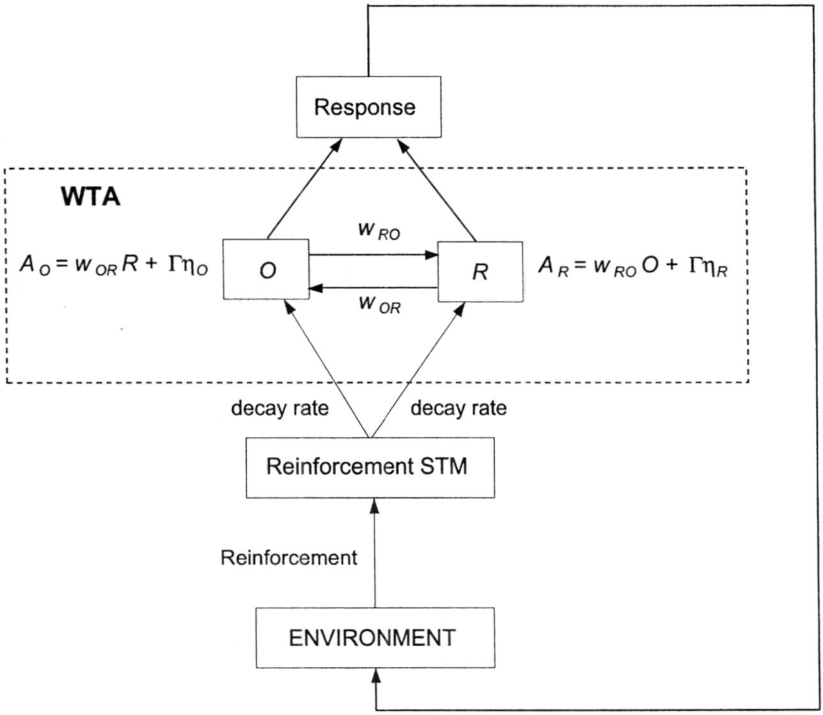

Figure 10.3
Model schematic representation. Terminal (R) and "other" (O) responses compete in a winner-take-all (WTA) fashion; depending on the pattern of responding (the "output"), the reinforcement is obtained at a certain rate and then stored in a short-term memory (STM); the arousal level (reinforcement STM) controls the strength of behavioral competition by modulating the decay rates.

text. It resembles the assumptions of the Behavioral theory of Timing (BeT) that clock rate depends on reinforcement rate (Killeen 1991) and has been applied in a different context by Gibbon (1995) to explain the dynamics of time matching.

Behavioral competition between O and R responses is implemented as a simple two-unit network (figure 10.3), in which associated with each unit are two variables O(t) and $A_O(t)$ for the O unit and two variables R(t) and $A_R(t)$ for the R unit. O(t) and R(t) are output variables that denote the strengths of the O and R responses at time t. Response variation is introduced by using independent noise coefficients, $\eta_O(t)$ and $\eta_R(t)$, added to the two response activations, A_O and A_R (figure 10.3). The response that is generated at time *t* follows a winner-take-all (WTA) non-linear rule—the *response trace* is either set to 1 for the winner unit or it decays at a fixed rate for the loser unit. Importantly, this two-unit system that relies on response competition (winner-take-all rule) is able to generate sequences of the form $O^N R$, which is sufficient for it to act as a timer. (For discussions, see Dragoi et al. 2003.) However, the model behaves like a fixed oscillator which "responds" whenever $R > O$ (the strength of terminal behaviors is greater than that of "öther" behaviors) and "waits" whenever $O > R$ (the strength of "öther" behaviors is greater than that of terminal behaviors).

Behavioral timing is adaptive, however. The terminal response typically shifts with training on any periodic schedule so that it occurs with highest probability in the vicinity of reinforcement. To make the period of the simple oscillator adapt to the temporal regularities in the environment, we have adjusted the rate at which both response units decay after they lose the competition with the other response, by invoking the second principle of the model, i.e., some form of memory for reinforcement should control the strength of response competition. In our model implementation, the overall arousal level, integrated over the recent past (short-term memory for reinforcement, figure 10.3), controls the switching rate of the two types of responses (R and O) by modulating the response trace decay rates. This works in the following sense: higher decay rate means faster forgetting, and, because of the non-linear winner-take-all response rule, faster forgetting means a higher switching rate between the two responses, and consequently a lower period of the oscillator. (Specific mathematical formulations are avoided here but can be found in Dragoi et al. 2003.)

Reset Mechanism

One important feature of the model is that response competition together with modulation of the strength of competition by the recent memory for reinforcement combine to make an effective resetting mechanism that suppresses responding immediately after reinforcement. Suppose that a response (R) occurs and produces reinforcement. If $R = 1$, A_O increases to become greater than A_R. According to the WTA response rule it follows then that $O = 1$, and thus the response is reset. The second principle of our model (modulation of competition strength by the STM for reinforcement) prevents the occurrence of subsequent R-responses that can resume responding before a certain waiting time has elapsed.

Next, I will use the model to address two well-known timing phenomena: spaced responding (differential reinforcement of low rates: DRL), and interval timing (fixed interval: FI), by describing how temporal regulation develops in real time as learning progresses to characterize the dynamics of acquisition and extinction in both DRL and FI schedules.

Spaced Responding

DRL schedules (spaced responding) selectively reinforce inter-response times (IRTs) longer than a specified value. During the initial phase of DRL training animals tend to respond at a high rate. After stable performance is reached, the rate of responding on DRL schedules is directly related to the maximum reinforcement rate (1/minimum reinforced IRT) specified by the schedule and the IRT distribution peaks at or just before the minimum required IRT (e.g., Kelleher et al. 1959; Staddon 1965; Wilson and Keller 1953). Figure 10.4 shows the emergence of temporal discrimination during exposure to a schedule which reinforced responses if they followed either a response or reinforcement by 10 seconds or more (DRL 10). The figure illustrates typical model behavior, both early and late in training. We began the simulations with a high response decay rate, i.e., very brief memory for previous responses, so that the switching rate of the two types of responses, O and R, is very high. (We began with high response decay rates for consistency with experimental evidence (Staddon 1965) that response rates are high during initial training; see figure 10.4A.) However, as training progresses, the decay rate of the two response units starts to decrease to diminish the response switching rate. This is due to the implementation of the second model principle, i.e., short-term memory for reward (that increases with training) modulates the strength of response competition (or the response decay rate). The strength of response competition increases because decreasing the response decay rate means that the trace of the "winner" response decays more slowly, so that it inhibits the competing response for longer (Dragoi et al. 2003). Figure 10.4A also shows that as training progresses, terminal responses become more widely spaced, and this leads to an increased frequency of reinforcement (figure 10.4C) since spaced responding is actually a condition of reinforcement. If training continues

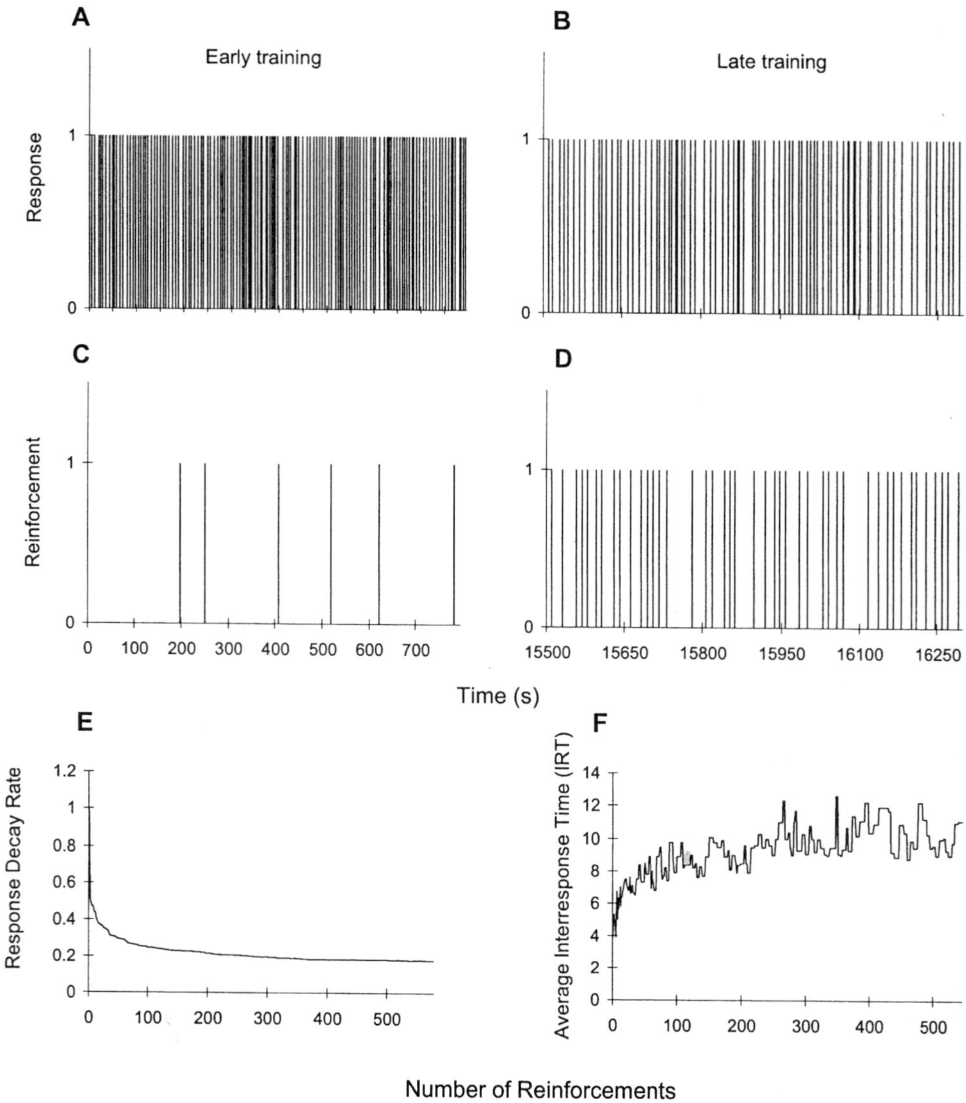

Figure 10.4

Illustration of model dynamics during exposure to a DRL 10-second schedule (early and late training). (A) Response sequence during early training (high response rates). (B) Response sequence during late training (spaced responding). (C) Reinforcement sequence during early training (low reinforcement rates). (D) Reinforcement sequence during late training (high reinforcement rates). (E) The response trace decay rate (α) stabilizes after about 500 reinforcements to a value that ensures relatively fixed response rates. (F) Average inter-response time (IRT) measured over trials.

further, and reinforcements continue to accumulate in short-term memory, the response trace decay parameter stabilizes to a value (figure 10.4E) that ensures relatively constant response rates (in the present simulations the steady state for a DRL 10 seconds is reached after approximately 500 reinforcements; see also figures 10.4B and 10.4D, which illustrate the pattern of spaced responses and reinforcements after 15,500 seconds of training).

Interval Timing

The defining characteristic of interval timing is that animals learn not to respond during the early part of the to-be-timed interval and this *wait time* is usually proportional to the interval (proportional timing). A second characteristic is Weber's law (which is also true of most sensory dimensions), namely that over a considerable range of times, the variability in temporal measures such as wait time is proportional to the mean. Model simulations predict average performance levels for FI schedules (figure 10.5). Panel A represents the total number of responses during each 4-second portion of the interval between successive reinforcements, calculated after the steady state was reached. Responses were considered for the first 300 reinforcements, for each one of FI 32, FI 64, FI 128, and FI 256 schedules. The model is consistent with experimental data in predicting that, on average, the animal pauses immediately after the reinforcement and then, after about two thirds of the interval, the average response rate follows a monotonically increasing curve. One interesting feature of this response pattern is shown in figure 10.5B, i.e., the wait time is proportional to the length of the interval. This behavior is a consequence of the dynamics of the response rate decay parameter that adjusts continuously during learning: Thus, higher reinforcement rates (short FIs) ensure higher values of the response decay rate (figure 10.5D), which produce shorter wait times. After the first reinforcement is obtained, the decay rate of the two response units starts decreasing to reduce the response switching rate. As the reinforcement schedule is made richer (e.g., FI 32 in figure 10.5A), the frequency of reinforcement increases and the response decay rate stabilizes at larger values (figure 10.5D). This means that smaller response decay rates ensure that responses are emitted less frequently and therefore the probability of long O responses ("other" responses or wait time) increases as the reinforcement frequency decreases.

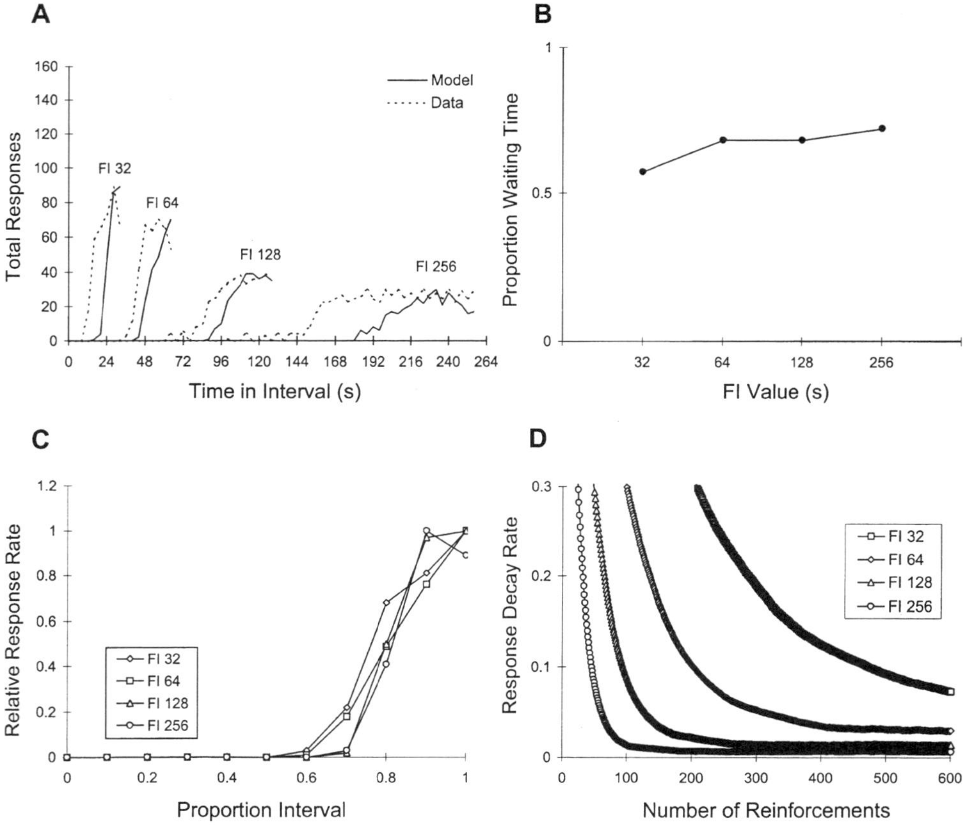

Figure 10.5

Fixed-interval performance. (A) Total number of responses during each 4-second portion of the interval between successive reinforcements, calculated for the first 300 reinforcements after stable performance was reached, for each one of FI 32, FI 64, FI 128, and FI 256 schedules. Data (dashed line); model (filled line). Data are adapted from Schneider 1969. (B) Proportional timing—the ratio between the wait time (response rate less than 10% from the terminal rate) and the corresponding FI value is approximately constant. (C) Relative response rates as a function of relative time in interval for the four reinforcement schedules from panel A. (D) Response trace decay rate as a function of number of reinforcements in each of the four schedules from panel A.

Weber's law is shown in figure 10.5C, which illustrates average response rates relative to the maximum response rate along the (normalized) interval for the FI schedules analyzed in figure 10.5A. For FIs ranging from 32 to 256 seconds, the curves superimpose, illustrating Weber-law timing (the scalar property). Figure 10.5C also shows that as the FI requirement increases, e.g., FI 256, the model predicts that the peak response is obtained just before reinforcement, a deviation from proportional timing. This behavior is a consequence of the way variability is incorporated into the model. When the FI requirement is large, the weight of the additive noise increases relative to that of the response decay parameter (figure 10.5D shows that for long FIs the response decay rate stabilizes at lower values) to degrade the timing performance. This result is not entirely inconsistent with experimental data: for instance, Zeiler and Powell (1994) have shown that the Weber-law property of interval timing does not hold at longer FIs.

In addition to spaced responding and interval timing, the adaptive timing model is able to describe both the steady states and the dynamic properties of acquisition/extinction performance in simple FI schedules, rapid temporal control, and, in some conditions, timing of two intervals (mixed FI-FI schedules). Furthermore, by incorporating familiar learning principles, the model is able to explain basic steady-state properties of temporal discriminations in animals, as well as how temporal regulation develops in real time. The dynamic interaction between two principles, response selection and variation and modulation by overall arousal level, is sufficient to achieve temporal regulation, opening up a promising avenue to a unified framework for "timing" and "non-timing" learning phenomena.

Conclusions

Simplicity is, indeed, the royal road to scientific truth. However, the parsimony criterion has for too long been used by behavioral scientists as a justification for their fierce resistance to the introduction of intervening variables in the study of adaptive behavior. So far, the theoretical arena has been dominated by simple black-box models restricted to the identification of fundamental variables controlling adaptive behavior, but more general aspects of complex behavior have been completely ignored. However, it is time to go beyond testing individual behavioral principles, and explore how complex behavior emerges from the interaction of key learning processes such as memory, competition, or response variation. Although this theoretical effort has already started (e.g., Dragoi and Staddon 1999; Dragoi et al. 2003; Grossberg and Schmajuk 1989; Machado 1997; Staddon 2001; Sutton and Barto 1981), pushing the field away from simple variables and moving it closer to emergent processes will require a massive and rigorous exploration of the theoretical domain in conjunction with experimental testing.

Appendix 1: The Dynamics of Operant Learning

Model Equations

Response Strength

$$\frac{d\mathrm{RS}^i}{dt} = -\alpha_1 \mathrm{RS}^i + w_1 \mathrm{BE}^i (1 - \mathrm{RS}^i) - \alpha_3 \mathrm{BI}^i \mathrm{RS}^i - \alpha_4 \mathrm{RS}^i \sum_{j \neq i} \mathrm{RS}^j$$

STM Response Trace

$$\frac{d\mathrm{RT}}{dt} = \alpha_5 (\mathrm{R} - \mathrm{RT})$$

STM Associations

$$\frac{dw_{\mathrm{SM}}^{\mathrm{R}}}{dt} = -\alpha_6 w_{\mathrm{SM}}^{\mathrm{R}} + \alpha_6 \mathrm{RT} \cdot \mathrm{RF}$$

LTM Associations

$$\frac{dw_{\mathrm{LM}}^{\mathrm{R}}}{dt} = -\alpha_7 w_{\mathrm{LM}}^{\mathrm{R}} + \alpha_7 \mathrm{RT} \cdot \mathrm{RF}$$

Short-Term Learning Expectancy

$$\mathrm{E_{SM}} = \mathrm{RT}(w^{\mathrm{R}} + w_{\mathrm{SM}}^{\mathrm{R}})$$

Long-Term Learning Expectancy

$$\mathrm{E}_{\mathrm{LM}}^i = \mathrm{RT}(w^{\mathrm{R}} + w_{\mathrm{LM}}^{\mathrm{R}})$$

Behavioral Excitation

$$\frac{d\mathrm{BE}}{dt} = -\alpha_8 \mathrm{BE} + \alpha_9(\mathrm{E_{SM}} - \mathrm{E_{LM}})(1 - \mathrm{BE})$$

Behavioral Inhibition

$$\frac{d\mathrm{BI}}{dt} = -\alpha_{10} \mathrm{BI} + \alpha_{11}(\mathrm{E_{LM}} - \mathrm{E_{SM}})(1 - \mathrm{BI})$$

Model variables are as follows: $w^{\mathrm{R}}_{\mathrm{SM}}$ is the STM trace of response R; $w^{\mathrm{R}}_{\mathrm{LM}}$ is the LTM trace of response; $\mathrm{E_{LM}}$ is the long-term learning expectancy; $\mathrm{E_{SM}}$ is the short-term learning expectancy; BE is the output of the behavioral excitation unit; BI is the output of the behavioral inhibition unit; RS is the output of the response strength unit; R and RT represent the response and the response trace; indices *i* and *j* in the equations denote different (competing) response units.

Model parameters are as follows: α_1 controls the spontaneous decay of RS; α_2 controls the strength of excitation from BE; α_3 controls the strength of inhibition from BI; α_4 controls the inter-response inhibition; α_5 is the rate of increase and decay of RT; α_6 controls the rate of increase and decay of $w^{\mathrm{R}}_{\mathrm{SM}}$; α_7 controls the rate of increase and decay of $w^{\mathrm{R}}_{\mathrm{LM}}$, with $\alpha_7 \ll \alpha_6$; α_8 and α_{10} are rate constants of decay of BE and BI; α_9 and α_{11} are rate constants of increase of BE and BI; w_1 is the initial (fixed) level of the connection between BE and RS; w^{R} is the initial (fixed) level of the connection between RT and $\mathrm{E_{SM}}$. Parameter values are as follows: $\alpha_1 = 1 \cdot 10^{-4}$, $\alpha_2 = w_1 = 0.05$, $\alpha_3 = 0.2$, $\alpha_4 = \alpha_6 = \alpha_9 = \alpha_{11} = w^{\mathrm{R}} = 0.1$, $\alpha_5 = 0.5$, $\alpha_7 = 8 \cdot 10^{-3}$, $\alpha_8 = \alpha_{10} = 5 \cdot 10^{-3}$.

Appendix 2: Interval Timing as an Emergent Learning Property

Model Equations

Response Activation

$$\mathrm{A_O}(t) = w_{\mathrm{OR}}\mathrm{R}(t-1) + \Gamma\eta_{\mathrm{O}}(t)$$

$$\mathrm{A_R}(t) = w_{\mathrm{RO}}\mathrm{O}(t-1) + \Gamma\eta_{\mathrm{R}}(t)$$

Response Strength

If $A_R > A_O$ then $R = 1$, else $dR/dt = -\mu\alpha R$

If $A_O > A_R$ then $O = 1$, else $dO/dt = -\mu\alpha O$

STM Reinforcement Trace

$$\frac{dSTM_{RF}}{dt} = \beta_1 RF - \beta_2 STM_{RF}$$

Response Decay Rate

$$\frac{d\alpha}{dt} = \gamma(STM_{RF} - \alpha)$$

Model variables are as follows: A_O and A_R are the response activations; O and R are the response strengths; RF is the reinforcement signal (0 or 1); w_{OR} and w_{RO} are connection strengths between responses O and R; α is the response decay rate; STM_{RF} is the short-term memory for RF.

Model parameters are as follows: Γ is the variability parameter (noise amplitude); $\eta_O(t)$ and $\eta_R(t)$ are drawn independently at each t from a normal distribution between 0 and 1; μ is a proportionality factor; β_1 and β_2 control the increase and decay rate of reinforcement STM; γ controls the rate at which each reinforcement changes α. Parameter values are as follows: Initial values – $\alpha = 1$ and $STM_{RF} = 0$; $w_{OR} = 0.2$, $w_{RO} = 0.15$, $\beta_1 = 0.3$, $\beta_2 = 0.1$, $\gamma = 0.0002$, $\mu = 0.097$. Γ was set to 0.05 for DRL schedules and to 0.03 for FI schedules.

III Behaviorism

11 Varieties of the Behaviorist Experience: Histories of John E. R. Staddon

Clive D. L. Wynne

There is a temptation in a volume of this kind to look back—to recount histories. When did you first meet John Staddon? What is your most striking recollection of him—personal or professional? What do you think is his most enduring contribution to behavioral science?

I certainly would not want to deny anyone the right to talk about histories. Histories of behavior (including possible future histories of behavior) are what make the difference between infatuation and true love (at least according to a recent textbook on behavior analysis: Powell, Symbaluk, and Macdonald 2002). These are important distinctions. I want to talk about histories. But I want to use history of behavior as a tool in understanding Staddon's Theoretical Behaviorism. I want to use history as a means of talking about the future directions that Staddon is forging for behaviorism—not as an excuse to wallow in the past.

Behaviorism, we are routinely advised, is dead, killed by the rise of Cognition sometime between Chomsky's (1959) review of Skinner's *Verbal Behavior* and the awarding of a Nobel Prize to Konrad Lorenz, Karl von Frisch, and Niko Tinbergen in 1973 for founding the field of ethology. Of course a bland uncontroversial Methodological Behaviorism lingers on in an injunction to use objective data in building psychological science. Few psychologists have difficulty accepting this de-clawed behaviorism. But real died-in-the-wool behaviorism—the kind that frightens cognitivists and ethologists alike—survives, so most accounts insist, only among the necrophiliacs who follow Skinner's Radical Behaviorism.

Skinner's behaviorism eschews almost all theorizing. And yet Staddon—a product of Skinner's late lamented Harvard Pigeon Lab—calls his new behaviorism Theoretical Behaviorism. Is this patricide, or even regicide?

More seriously, how does Theoretical Behaviorism relate to Skinner's Radical Behaviorism? Is it an extension from—or a reaction against—Skinner's philosophy of behavior? And more generally, what is new about Staddon's New Behaviorism? After all there have been theoretical behaviorisms before—in particular Hull's hypothetical deductive system of behavior. Where does Staddon's scheme fit into this history? An important part of finding the answer to these questions will be to consider histories of behavior.

Questions about Theoretical Behaviorism

Staddon's Theoretical Behaviorism can be summarized in three axioms (Staddon 1999, 2001b):

1. We can learn about an organism only through its behavior.
2. Histories of behavior lead to changes in state variables, which are constructs inside the animal.
3. The purpose of behaviorism is not just to catalog behaviors but also to uncover mechanisms of behavior. These mechanisms are neither cognitive nor physiological but abstract and algorithmic.

Although Staddon started his professional training in the Harvard pigeon lab, it is clear that a major theme in his intellectual development as a behaviorist has been confronting what he views as the limitations of Skinner's too constrained form of behavioral science. Staddon himself tells us that he "never found the atheoretical simplism of Skinnerian behaviorism appealing" (2001b, p. xv).

In an oft-quoted admonition, Skinner forbade "any explanation of an observed fact which appeals to events taking place somewhere else, at some other level of observation, described in different terms, and measured, if at all, in different dimensions" (1950/1961, p. 193). In place of theory all Skinner would tolerate was "a formal representation of the data reduced to a minimal number of terms" (1950/1961, p. 69). Though in a reconsideration of this position 19 years later Skinner (1969) insisted he was not a "Grand Anti-Theoretician" (p. viii), he maintained a disdain for the hypothetical-deductive method which he likened to guessing who is calling on the phone or the pattern on a card, gambling, and body building: "Such performances command attention even when the results are trivial" (p. ix). This limitation of behavioral theory to minimalist data re-presentation is clearly a frustration to Staddon. Staddon argues that theories in the more developed sciences routinely appeal to hypothetical constructs that have different dimensions from the data that inspired them. These theoretical entities are often not measured directly but are only implied through observation of their indirect effects. Indeed those archetypes of "hard" scientists—physicists—are not only happy to work with theoretical entities whose existence is only very indirectly implied by the most subtle measurements, but even, in the case of quantum mechanics, with theoretical entities whose implications for measurement differ according to the type of measurement made. Why, asks Staddon (e.g. 1999, p. 218), should behaviorism be any less sophisticated?

Can There Be Theory-Free Behavioral Science?

Presumably the reason Skinner adopted such a restrictive view of useful theory in his behaviorism was because of his concern to maintain the independence of behavioral science. From Skinner's perspective the independence of psychology was under continual threat on two fronts: on the one hand the almost unstoppable tide of mentalism; and on the other the encroachment of ever more sophisticated physiological explanations. I think of psychology as like one of those Pacific islands under continuous threat of drowning in rising sea waters, or a small European country in danger of being absorbed by its bigger neighbors. Psychology—the Luxembourg of science.

If behaviorism permitted theoretical constructs at some other level than the behavioral, what would remain of behaviorism? This is still an active concern. Today's behaviorist not only has to contend with renewed threats from mentalistic and physiological explanations of behavior, but also, in the form of functional brain imaging, with an unholy alliance of these two ugly sisters. Physicists do not have these worries. Physics is under no danger of being subsumed by anything, except perhaps Eastern mysticism.

If a new behaviorism is going to permit hypothetical constructs that are more than simple behavioral re-descriptions, then it had better be confident that it is not packing psychology off to the mentalists or the physiologists.

Staddon's claim with his Theoretical Behaviorism is that it is possible to have a theoretical language in behaviorism that can be allowed the license to postulate constructs that exist "at some other level of observation" (Skinner 1953, p. 193) than the purely behavioral and yet will not fall prey to mentalism or physiologism.

Before we consider whether Staddon can deliver on this claim it is worth asking whether behaviorism needs theory of the type that Skinner forbade. Can a science of psychology that strives for efficient explanation and control arise only from the inductive observation and efficient description of regularities in behavior? Just because other sciences like physics play with entities they cannot directly observe does not demonstrate that behaviorism must follow their lead—only that it would be in good company if it did so. What does theory do for scientists?

Theory does two things: it permits efficient description, and, by outlining functional relationships, it allows prediction and the control that successful prediction can imply. (Though many natural phenomena can be predicted by deductions from theory, fewer can be controlled—think of the weather, for example.)

Theory as efficient description is the one type of theorizing Skinner could contemplate—the "laws" (such as Weber's) that summarize a behavioral relationship. Weber's law certainly permits prediction and sometimes control. So why should behaviorists desire more? Staddon argues: "Even if prediction and control are our ultimate aim[s], the apparently direct route is not always the best. By aiming directly at controlling nature—at a technology rather than a science—we may miss fundamental laws that will, in the long run, give us more power than we could have dreamed possible." (2001b, pp. 148–149) Staddon goes on to offer Babbage's "Difference Engine" as an example of premature application of an immature technology, and Faraday's discovery of the dynamo and Mendel's of the principle of genetic inheritance as examples of the advantages to be had from a reasoned and better paced theory-driven approach to scientific thinking.

Mendel is a very interesting example in this context. His units of inheritance remained very much hypothetical intervening variables until their biochemical instantiation in DNA nearly a century after he had postulated them. Plant breeders and other proto-geneticists lived with an entirely theoretical construct of inheritance for decades. This did the science of genetics no apparent harm. Furthermore, genetics only gained in stature as its basic theoretical construct was "reduced" to biochemistry. So if we take Mendelian genetics as an example, neither working with a theoretical construct that is not directly observable in the data of plant and animal breeding, nor the identification of this theoretical construct as a real entity in another realm of science seems to have any negative consequences for the development of a science.

But the crux of Staddon's argument with Skinner, I believe, is not so critically whether one believes in a strongly inductive boot-strapping method of scientific discovery (Skinner) or one that steps back a little from the level of the data and permits more deductive reflections (Staddon)—the crux of their argument concerns internal states.

Who Needs Internal States?

Skinner adamantly and consistently rejected internal states as having any role in the explanation of behavior. His reasons for doing so have been rehearsed often and I shall not go back over them here in any detail. (For a particularly clear exposition, see Flanagan 1991.) At its most fundamental, Skinner's objection to organismal variables was that he could not imagine how they could not be either mentalistic or physiological. Consequently he viewed any concession to intervening variables as denying the importance of the behavioral level of analysis.

Staddon argues that Skinner was able to avoid intervening variables and the internal states they imply only by restricting his focus to reversible behaviors. In a classic single-subject Skinnerian operant experimental design, a subject is exposed to each experimental condition for a long time—typically weeks or months rather than days. It is axiomatic in the steady-state operant paradigm that the stable terminal behavior on a given schedule can be recaptured after an intervening schedule condition. The animal is fundamentally ahistorical.

According to Staddon's Theoretical Behaviorism, this ahistorical approach is badly misguided. Animals are historical beings, and we will never be the same again as we are today. Our behavior today might appear indistinguishable from our behavior yesterday or 20 years ago, but our experiences in the interim have changed us so that if we were presented the same challenge today as yesterday or 20 years ago we would respond to it differently.

In developing this argument, Staddon (e.g. 2001b, p. 141) allows that under certain conditions some behavioral histories may be equivalent: certain different patterns of experience may leave the animal inclined to react in the same way. These are called "equivalent histories." In Howard Rachlin's Teleological Behaviorism (e.g., Rachlin 1994; 1999) the matter is left there—in history—so that it can remain outside the organism. Staddon argues, however, that talk of equivalent behavioral histories offers none of the parsimony that we demand from scientific explanations: ". . . this view . . . provides no compression of the raw data, hence no principled way to predict or understand the effects of a particular history" (2001b, p. 141). I'm not sure this is a compelling argument. Who is to say that Rachlin (or some other behaviorist) might not succeed in developing an efficient science of behavioral histories? It does not seem logically impossible. A more potent criticism of Rachlin's position, I think, is that there is a perversity in maintaining the attempt to keep behavioral history outside the organism—a perversity with consequences for trying to understand behavior. If behavioral history does not amount to a state of an animal then what is it? Where does it exist? Histories, in the ordinary everyday sense, can exist in books, documentaries, or the reminiscences of our elders. But insofar as a history can be a variable in a behaviorism, it can exist only *as a function of* an animal.

Suppose we have two experimental animals and expose them to the same sequence of experiences in the laboratory. In one of these animals a subsequent test shows these experiences to have the effect on future behavior that we expected them to have on the basis of past studies. In the other animal, however, no impact of the training can be observed. The only intelligible way to talk about these differences in behavior is to view the behavioral history as having become a property of the animal—as having changed the animal's state. In one animal the behavioral history has had the predicted impact on the animal's behavioral state. In the other individual, for whatever reason, the behavioral training has not led to the expected state. If we refuse to see the behavioral history as having become a function of the animal—as a behavioral state—it is hard to see how we could discuss the difference between these two animals.

Other Theoretical Behaviorisms

Skinner's contemporaries Clark Hull and Edward Tolman—leaders of the other two major schools of behaviorism in the mid twentieth century—both offered forms of what we could call Theoretical Behaviorism. Both were happy to consider as explanatory elements concepts that existed at a level away from behavioral measurement and that were considered as properties of the organism. Tolman (e.g. 1932) leaned toward what we would now call cognitive explanatory concepts, such as expectations, cognitive maps, means-end readiness, and the like. Though one might like to argue for an influence of Tolman on Staddon's Theoretical Behaviorism I do not view the similarities as strong. Most crucially, Tolman's theorizing was completely verbal—a form of theory with which Staddon has little patience. Absent mathematical formalization Tolman's theorizing lacks the predictive edge that Staddon demands.

Hull's (e.g. 1943) scheme has more points of similarity with Staddon's. Like Staddon, Hull allowed for theoretical intervening variables in his behaviorism. Like Staddon, Hull allowed for a deductive process of imagination as well as an inductive process of systematizing observations in the generation of behavioral theory.

Staddon (2001b, p. 13) suggests that he rejected Hull's hypothetical-deductive behaviorism because of Hull's reliance on physiological intervening variables. This may be less of a difference than Staddon suggests. Staddon acknowledges that his Theoretical Behaviorism shares with Hullian behavioral theory the expectation that its intervening variables will ultimately reduce to brain physiology (ibid., p. 142). Rashotte and Amsel (1998) argue that Hull never intended his physiological speculations to be taken seriously as physiology—only as behavioral mechanisms. They cite Hull's having written to Spence "I simply take these equations and go on from there, paying no attention whatever to the physiological suggestions. . . ." (ibid., p. 128) In point of fact Staddon also uses theoretical constructs that are biological in flavor—even if he is careful not to link them to any specific details of physiology. So the distinction here between Hull and Staddon on the issue of physiologizing is not so cut and dried.

But Hull's theoretical behaviorism is a very different thing from Staddon's. Hull wanted a top-down theory, starting as Newton had with a limited set of basic principles from which axioms and ultimately experimental behavior could be derived. But Hull did not have the equivalent of Kepler and Galileo or the other careful observers and experimentalists upon whom Newton could call. His project was absurdly over-ambitious for 1940 and the amount of systematic data that a project like Hull's would require remains a dream even today.

Staddon attempts no such grand scheme. His models are more modest. They attempt to capture the behavior just of particular animals under specific conditions: *C. elegans* habituating to irritations in their water; pigeons receiving small quantities of grain at regular short intervals of time. It is interesting that, though Staddon's theories are generally 50 years younger than Hull's, the more recent theorist is attempting to account for simpler behaviors. If there is an over-arching ambition detectable in Staddon's behavioral models it lurks in the repeated use of a small toolkit of modeling equipment. If there is ever a Staddon coat of arms, it will surely bear a leaky bucket.

Hull's theorizing is strictly Stimulus-Response (S-R) or, given that he had an interest in intervening variables, Stimulus-Organism-Response (S-O-R). In this sense it is primarily a Pavlovian theory. Hull can only account for truly operant behavior by hypothesizing hidden stimuli to initiate behavior. Here Staddon's Skinnerian legacy shines through. His models are primarily ones of operant behavior and operant conditioning. As a follower of Skinner, he is most interested in behavior controlled by its consequences. In fact, I don't think he has ever constructed a model of Pavlovian behavior.

Staddon has consistently kept to the line that it is for neuroscientists to follow along and find the wetware that underlies the software he proposes. A justifiable note of satisfaction was detectable when the journal *Science* reported the existence of units of cortex that had all the properties of leaky-bucket integrators (Glanz 1998; Staddon 2001a).

Another difference between the two theorists lies in how they use mathematical theoretical language. Hull used equations that lacked mathematical sophistication and he attached theoretical names, such as "response potential" and "habit strength" to the variables in his equations. Staddon's mathematics is more sophisticated and he avoids ascribing theoretically laden names to his mathematical parameters. A simple "value" (often with no additional clarity called "V value") or strength variable is typically all that he needs.

In summary, Hull and Staddon share an interest in generating behavioral machinery. Rashotte and Amsel (1999) report that Hull was fascinated by the idea of hypothetical machines that could simulate adaptive behavior. They share the belief that we must make an imaginative leap to postulate theoretical constructs the adequacy of which we can then test by experiment. And they both strive for a mathematical language in which to capture the essence of behavior and the implications of their theories. But that's where the similarities end. Hull attempted a form of utopian behavioral theorizing in which he tried to build a complete theoretical edifice for all eventualities. He did so using theoretical constructs that were at least physiologically plausible (given the physiology of his times) and were expressed in simple math. Staddon creates less ambitious behavioral models which are expressed in more complex math but whose physiological plausibility is a matter of indifference to him. In his summary on Hull, Staddon writes: "Hull's formal skills were modest; the computational resources available to him were primitive; and his between-group experimental method is ill-suited to the discovery of learning processes in individual organisms." (2001a, pp. ix–x)

Whither Behaviorism?

Staddon's Theoretical Behaviorism is Behaviorism's best hope for a future. As an attempt to account for observable behavior without recourse to mentalism or physiology it is clearly a form of behaviorism. But, as an account that welcomes theoretical intervening variables in its explanations, it is just as clearly theoretical.

A consideration of history in the Skinnerian sense of a past pattern of behavior has enabled us to see why behaviorism needs to admit organismal intervening variables. Consideration of history in the everyday sense of a narrative of events in the past has enabled us to place Theoretical Behaviorism in the context of different forms of behaviorism.

The need to recognize that animals are historical beings—beings whose present actions can only be predicted by considering their past experiences—identifies why we need behavioral states as intervening variables in behaviorism. But a consideration of Staddon's intellectual forefathers also helps us to understand Theoretical Behaviorism. In its emphasis on operant behavior Theoretical Behaviorism shows Staddon's debt to Skinner. Staddon's frustration with Skinner's proscription of theorizing can also be clearly detected in Theoretical Behaviorism. In regard to the use of intervening variables Staddon's behaviorism is closer to Hull. However, where Hull sought a grand axiomatic edifice of theory, Staddon's theoretical ambitions are on a more intimate scale. Staddon puts it this way:

"The alternative I offer is also theoretical, but more like watercolor than oil painting. Rather than building up a massive structure step by step, I propose instead a succession of simple sketches, each designed to capture some aspect of the learning process." (2001a, p. x)

Theoretical Behaviorism is the kind of science most other scientists would expect psychology to be. Most scientists know that "pure empiricism is a delusion" (Miller 1959, p. 200). We cannot observe nature without knowing what we are looking for. Skinner's atheoretical approach was doomed to become arid and extinguish. At the other extreme mentalism is not a serious candidate for a scientific psychology.

What Staddon proposes is simply sensible science. Theoretical—yes, but non-mental and not just physiology. As Thomas H. Huxley said of Darwin's *Origin of Species*, "How extremely stupid of me not to have thought of that."

12 Santayana Told Us, or The Prevalence of Radical Behaviorism

John C. Malone and Susan R. Perry

Progress, far from consisting in change, depends on retentiveness.... Those who cannot remember the past are condemned to fulfill it.
—George Santayana (1905)

Santayana (1905) wrote that we need not repeat the mistakes of the past, but if we can't remember the past, or if we are wholly ignorant of it, we are bound to repeat the mistakes of our predecessors. Psychology in the twentieth century is almost entirely a series of awful mistakes. And it is almost entirely mediational—its explanations refer to inferred entities. Radical behaviorism excludes mediators and is constantly under attack for that reason. However, radical behaviorism may be gaining ground in the forums of its adherents we know nothing about. There may be more radical behaviorists outside behavior analysis than within. Radical behaviorism is more prevalent than you might think. For example, who might have authored these statements?

"Mind" is used as explanation when we are ignorant of causes.

As we become more sophisticated, we refer less to mental states.

We progress when we replace mentalist explanations with behavioral ones.

Thoughts are often irrelevant to actions.

There is nothing mental about free will.

Premeditation does not require mental activity.

"Responsibility" is a social phenomenon.

Mentalist views are dangerous.

Others can often understand and predict our actions better than we can.

These are taken from the writings of Richard A. Posner, a judge of the U.S. Court of Appeals for the Seventh Circuit and a senior lecturer at the University of Chicago Law School. His 1990 book *The Problems of Jurisprudence* shows that radical behavioral views are more widespread than most of us realize, extending even to reinterpretations of law and the administration of justice. Posner doesn't cite Skinner nor refer to behavior analysis, but the tenets of radical behaviorism are evident in his writings. We will argue that the constant pressure to fundamentally change the focus of the experimental analysis of behavior (EAB) so as to include mediators of various kinds (i.e., theories) should be resisted. Malone (1987) and others have commented on this pressure, which has been exerted for a very long time. For example, Sam Leigland (1997) wrote that a recent issue of the *Journal of the Experimental Analysis of Behavior* devoted to the nature of reinforcement was rife with papers arguing for recourse to "underlying causal mechanisms." Those are *mediators* and their use is not unusual—indeed they have been the dominant mode of explanation for thousands of years. But this was *JEAB*, one of the very few journals that promote radical behaviorism—indeed, *the* journal that speaks for modern behaviorism. Should the EAB change so fundamentally as to incorporate mediational theories? We will also describe other instances of the radical behavioral view in areas outside the EAB that should give us encouragement. It would be ironic indeed if such a change occurred just as radical behaviorism gains favor in areas outside the EAB. Psychology at the end of the twentieth century is not an object of pride; it is an embarrassment! Contemporary psychology is a shambles, a junkyard, and by no means a pinnacle of achievement, as a glance at our journals and textbooks quickly tells us.

An overview based on the consensus of popular textbook presentations runs pretty much as follows: Psychology is the study of mind and behavior, which are two different things. The mind is almost synonymous with the brain and composed of faculties, or powers, such as attention, memory, and reason, and these are localized in specific brain centers or distributed in specific neural networks. The senses, such as vision, are directly analogous to input channels—sensory information enters and is processed. Seeing and hearing are somehow brought about by nerve cells in the brain. The mind/brain is profitably viewed as a wonderful computer, whether digital or analog.

It is almost impossible to entertain the possibility that this is the best conception of psychology thus far attained. In fact, it is not greatly different from *Plato's* psychology! And whatever you think of Plato as a philosopher, no one can admire his psychology, based as it is on the dualism of mind and body, as well as on the dualism of subject and object.

And what of the public perception of psychology? Consider this description of a bill passed by the New Mexico State Senate in March 1995:

> When a psychiatrist or psychologist testifies during a defendant's competency hearing, the psychologist or psychiatrist shall wear a cone-shaped hat that is not less than two feet tall. The surface of the hat shall be imprinted with stars and lightning bolts. Additionally, the psychologist or psychiatrist shall be required to don a white beard that is not less than eighteen inches in length, and shall punctuate crucial elements of his testimony by stabbing the air with a wand.... Whenever a psychologist or psychiatrist provides expert testimony regarding the defendant's competency, the bailiff shall dim the courtroom lights and administer two strokes to a Chinese gong. (*Harper's Magazine,* July 1995, p. 16)

Need we say more?

Behaviorism: Methodological versus Radical

What exactly is radical behaviorism and what is the evidence that it should be preserved? Radical behaviorism holds that the entire subject matter of psychology can best be treated as activity. This means that life is a movie, not a set of still pictures. It entails a number of collateral assumptions and it is a view that has been around for a long, long time.

While there are as many "cognitive psychologies" as there are cognitive writers, there are really only two "behaviorisms," although a dozen varieties could be derived from the first category. *Methodological* behaviorism is the kind most often described and criticized by outsiders—it has never been characteristic of B. F. Skinner's thinking. Oddly, it is often accepted by applied behavior analysts (Lamal 1998). *Radical* behaviorism is very different and it is the name of Skinner's view and recent derivatives.

In 1945, Skinner published a piece on the operational analysis of terms in which he attacked the prevailing logical positivist philosophy of science, which had produced what he called methodological behaviorism. This is the view that there is a distinction between public and private events and that psychology (to remain scientific) can deal only with public events. This is the arid philosophy of truth by agreement; something is real if at least two observers agree. Methodological behaviorism accepts the mind/body distinction, assumes that "private" means "mental," and leaves the mind to philosophers and the clergy.

Skinner surely didn't deny the existence of private experience, any more than did Watson, but he did deny the mind/body dualism of the mentalists and the methodological behaviorists. Thinking is something that we do, just as walking is something that we do and we do not think mental thoughts any more than we walk mental steps.

We would think it unnecessary to bring this up now, but recent comment makes it clear that many behavior analysts still believe that private events and behaviors are not available to radical behaviorists! However, one radical behaviorist, Howard Rachlin (e.g., 1994), proposed that all of our "private" lives are actually observable by others. We will see that this opinion is shared by a surprising number of writers.

Characteristics of Contemporary Radical Behaviorism

In 1997 Leigland described radical behaviorism well and contrasted it with its nasty counterpart, methodological behaviorism. We choose to characterize radical behaviorism as follows:

- Radical behaviorism involves no dualisms.
- It deals with dynamics, not statics.
- Radical behaviorism accepts no mediators.
- Private experience is included.
- "Mental" is viewed as temporal extension.[1]
- Traditional operant conditioning terms have no special status.
- Traditional operant conditioning terms are functionally defined.

Radical Behavioral Views Throughout History

Though radical behaviorism is a twentieth-century phenomenon, many thinkers have promoted compatible views throughout history. Thus, radical behaviorism is not a transient fad to be dismissed easily or revamped to fit the tastes of the times.

The Milesians of the Sixth Century B.C.: Monism and Dualism, Mental as Temporal Extension

It may seem odd to refer back to Thales, Anaximander, and Anaximenes as proto-radical behaviorists, but they represented a material monism that stood in contrast to the Pythagorean dualism that proved far more popular. *Needless to say, the competing dualism of Pythagoras was passed on through many successors, including Plato, Augustine, and Descartes and is dominant today.* These natural scientists of Miletus believed that we are truly parts of nature and that there is no special "soul substance" that animates us. As part of nature, we are as understandable as is the rest of nature—if the weather and movements of the planets are predictable to some extent, then our behavior and our thoughts are also predictable. The Milesians also believed that constant *change/becoming/activity* was the rule and that we should seek out regularities in this apparent chaos.

Protagoras of the Fifth Century B.C.: But Dualism Won't Go Away

Protagoras of Abdera could be called the William James of ancient times. He proposed that there is no absolute Truth, that "man is the measure of all things," and that epistemology does not involve the taking in of copies. Sensation is a relation between the sense organ and the object sensed, each dependent on the other. The soul is the sum of its objects and no more. A little-known aspect of Protagoras's philosophy is the pragmatism he promoted. While there is no absolute truth, there is a ranking of truths according to the degree to which they promote health and well-being. His contemporary Democritus, also from Abdera, promoted the representational theory of atomism, an epistemological dualism that relies on the taking in of copies as the basis for knowledge. That theory has survived the millennia and remains dominant today.

Aristotle's *Nicomachean Ethics*, Fourth Century B.C.: But Plato Won Out

Aristotle was an epistemological and (almost surely) a metaphysical monist who has often been cast as the major impediment to the progress of western science. And so he was, but the Western Science that his influence impeded was disastrous for psychology; it was the dualistic mechanical science of Galileo, Descartes, and Newton. They relegated sensory experience to the scrap heap of unknowable subjective "mental" states. Aristotle, as a psychologist, followed Protagoras as a radical empiricist, opposed the copy theory, and promoted dynamics or functioning. And Aristotle wrote *Nicomachean Ethics*, a brilliant treatise that led Howard Rachlin (e.g., 1994) to argue that Aristotle understood the conception of history of reinforcement better than did Skinner.

Nicomachean Ethics begins with the assumption that *happiness* does not depend on hedonism—the gaining of pleasure and avoidance of pain. Even a child can feel pleasure, while happiness requires that a *pattern of life* be established. Happiness is not an emotion nor is it a momentary state of mind; it exists only in patterns of activity. Aristotle wrote that "one swallow does not make a spring" and one act does not define happiness, courage, honesty, love, pain, or contentment—these all refer to temporally extended patterns of behavior.

David Hume's Radical Empiricism

Hume questioned the existence of a unitary "self," that is born, lives, and dies or is reborn. His radical empiricism was essentially the same as the later version introduced by William James. And he knew that our feeling of free will is only a feeling. We may imagine we feel a liberty within ourselves; but a spectator can commonly infer our actions from our motives and character (Hume, Norton, and Norton 2000). Hume is well worth reading for anyone who wants to understand epistemological monism and a clear antecedent to modern radical behaviorism.

Charles S. Peirce

Peirce, the founder of pragmatism, well understood that reification is rampant, long before Skinner argued against it as an attempt to explain unfinished causal sequences:

> In a recent, admired work on *Analytic Mechanics* [by Kirchhoff] it is stated that we understand precisely the effect of force, but what force itself is we do not understand! This is simply a self-contradiction. The idea which the word "force" excites in our minds has no other function than to affect our actions, and these actions can have no reference to force otherwise than through its effects. Consequently, if we know what the effects of force are, we are acquainted with every fact which is implied in saying that a force exists.... (Peirce 1962, p. 117)

This misunderstood genius also defined "reality" for us. In brief, we *think* to remove doubt, a feeling of indecision regarding beliefs that guide our actions. When doubt is removed, we *believe*, meaning that we are dealing with something "real."

William James

William James misinterpreted Peirce's pragmatism, but he understood his version of epistemology. James's radical empiricism is a monism, as he shifted toward a behavioral orientation after 1890. His "positivistic" view was opposed both to the associationism and the "soul/faculty" theory that had defined psychology (James 1971/1879). James viewed mentality and cognition as behavior:

> The theory of evolution is beginning to do very good service by the reduction of all mentality to the type of reflex action. Cognition, in this view, is *but a fleeting moment*, a cross section at a certain point, of what in its totality is a motor phenomenon. (ibid., p. 36)

> We are acquainted with a thing as soon as we have learned how to behave towards it, or how to meet the behavior which we expect from it. Up to that point it is still "strange" to us. (ibid., p. 37)

James also believed that perception does not depend upon copies. As Skinner would argue later, seeing an object not now present does not mean that an "image" must be present:

> The object of which I think ... occupies its definite place in the outer world as much as does the object which I directly see. (1904, p. 11)

> But the interval of time does not transform an object known into a mental state. (ibid., p. 11)

So important aspects of radical behaviorism are not new. Thinkers have long thought of the mind as inseparable from the body and realized that mental copies aren't stored, and feelings aren't mental states, but patterns of activity. But the movement during this century is identified with B. F. Skinner, who, in his insightful early writings, urged us to search for functional units of behavior, and to avoid unfinished causal sequences. Had he only remained true to that position, how different things might have turned out.

Skinner's Contribution and Equivocation

Skinner's insightful papers in 1931 and 1935 defined the reflex as a functional unit, a conceptual expression referring to a kind of correlation between stimulation and responding. The treatment was functional, in that reflexes were to be discovered, not defined in advance. The demonstration of a reflex constitutes an explanation for the behavior involved, since "reflex" meant "orderly relation between environment and behavior." The analysis was extended to respondent and to operant behavior and the way was paved for the discovery of order in behavior at large. Operant behavior may appear at a molecular level, as in the demonstration of operant muscle contractions or reinforcement of specific IRTs (Hefferline and Keenan 1963). But order may also appear at a molar level, as in temporally extended behavior that appears as reliable patterns of responding when a specific reinforcement schedule is in effect or when a chain shows the coherence of a single behavior (Skinner 1931, 1935). The implication of this early analysis is that a thoroughgoing emphasis on molecular units and contiguous causes is a mistake—*order is where you find it.* But molar interpretations are hard to communicate to others and Skinner found it difficult to remember his own arguments (Malone 1987).

As it happened, Skinner may be partly responsible for the "shambles" that he called current psychology (Skinner 1983). He failed to appreciate the obvious implications of his early analysis of the behavioral unit (Skinner 1931, 1935), and he failed to adequately emphasize the difference between his analysis and simple S-R associationism. Thus, when S-R associationism was attacked by the "biological boundaries" advocates of the 1970s and the 1980s, the EAB was assumed to be part of the target. During the same period, the "cognitive revolution" occurred and S-R psychology was attacked further, with the EAB again part of the target.[2]

The confusion of the EAB with S-R psychology was compounded by Skinner's frequent and paradoxical emphasis on molecular behavior and momentary contingencies, a practice which is utterly incompatible with his analysis of the behavioral unit. He inadvertently illustrated that "we are each many selves" or repertoires of behavior, as early as 1938. There he summarized his 1931 and 1935 papers describing the strategy for the discovery of *functional* units—that in the first chapter. However, any reader who had read the previous argument for the behavioral unit would conclude that a chain, once established, is a functional unit—like a single response, since orderly changes occur when we vary food deprivation, the sleep cycle, or other factors. It was only decades later that Skinner modified that view.

Skinner did suggest in 1938 that patterns of responding, such as appear under specific reinforcement schedules, may function as units. But, disappointingly, one searches his writings over the years looking for him to tell us that units emerge—the level may be molecular *or* molar, but order appears and that defines the unit. He did suggest (1938, p. 300) that the pattern appearing during FR schedules may be treated as a unit, but he dismissed this possibility on the next two pages and decided that each response was better viewed as independent, with the series tied together by conditioned reinforcement! Later, he expressed approval of Ferster's and his emphasis placed on the conditions prevailing at the moment of reinforcement!

All of this suggests that Skinner's argument for the functional unit of behavior did not even influence *his* thinking very much! *But he had to be opposed to molecular explanations and contiguous causes,* since they require fillers of temporal gaps—the "cognitions" and "motivational states" that he railed against so strenuously. Thus, the non-dedicated reader must find little to choose between Skinner and mainstream psychology on this point and that is a pity.

Perhaps the unique aspect of radical behaviorism is its molar orientation, which complements its opposition to mediators. This strategy has led to some solutions of basic problems, both within and outside the field ordinarily considered to be behaviorism.

Molar Solutions to Vexing Problems *Within* Behaviorism

The Law of Effect

For 30 years the law of effect has been a molar law. It no longer refers to the S-R-X of textbook presentations. Rather than referring to momentary contingencies and contiguous causes—*current* individual stimuli, responses, and reinforcers, the law has become the *molar* law of effect. Thus, we find that *relative* behavior (over time) matches *relative* reinforcement (over time). "Behavior" may be measured in rate of response, time allocation, or other ways, and "reinforcement" may refer to rate or magnitude or some other aspect. This represents a major advance and has found application in the applied analysis of behavior.

Avoidance Learning

Many textbooks have chronicled the painful history of research in avoidance conditioning, an area which clearly shows the failure of the mediational theories (based on fear) and the molecular approach in general. In 1966, Herrnstein and Hineline showed that a *molar* variable, overall reduction of shock frequency, establishes avoidance responding very quickly. Even when each avoidance response produces immediate shock, responding is maintained, as long as the *overall* frequency of shock is reduced. Again, this shows that behavior *over time* is sensitive to consequences *over time* and that recourse to individual responses tells us nothing.

Conditioned Reinforcement

For decades, reviewers puzzled over the fact that powerful and durable conditioned reinforcement is almost impossible to demonstrate in the laboratory. This in spite of the myriad of acquired reinforcers that daily surround us—money, praise, attention, and more. How do they gain their power except through pairing with already-effective reinforcers? The answer was found in the work of Neuringer and Chung (1967), who showed that tones, flashes of light, and other innocuous stimuli could gain strong reinforcing power when delivered according to the same contingencies that deliver already-potent reinforcers. If an FR 11 schedule produces food 15 percent of the time and a brief flash 85 percent of the time, the flash will act as a reinforcer, increasing response rate dramatically over that occurring with food alone.

Once again, this is a *molar* effect, such that patterns of behavior over time become sensitive to the contingencies in effect—acquired reinforcers gain their power because they are *produced according to the same rule* that produces already-effective reinforcers.

Schedules

Schedules of reinforcement and the patterns of responding they generate constitute powerful evidence for the molar approach. Despite countless attempts to analyze their effects in terms of molecular units and contiguous causes, the patterns of responding on simple schedules remain inviolate. Gradients of reinforcement, chaining, and conditioned reinforcement cannot account for the FI scallop. But there is more.

In a classic presentation, Morse and Kelleher (1977) showed that the effects of drugs and of things usually thought of as reinforcers and punishers may be determined by the schedule according to which they are administered. In a variety of ways, behaviors were established either because they produced food or avoided shock. After long training, conditions were changed so that responses produced only strong shock, which would be avoided under other circumstances. In the simplest example, squirrel monkeys' presses for food delivered according to a fixed-interval schedule, gradually began to result in electric shock. The pressing that initially produced food now produced an "aversive" event, yet responding was maintained. This showed that the contingencies *themselves* could alter the functional relationships among behaviors and consequences—shock maintained responding just as would food; therefore, nothing is inherently reinforcing or punishing under all conditions, as the Premack Principle illustrated years ago.

This is probably the strongest evidence for a molar approach to behavior analysis, and it has been questioned by those who cannot stand to view painful shock as a reinforcer. Thus, since the effect appears only on interval schedules, it has been proposed that it is the punishment of long IRTs by shock that produces an illusory reinforcing effect by increasing the proportion of short IRTs and thus increasing response rate (Galbicka 1997). But, this cannot account for the fact that responding appears in the *patterns* appropriate to the schedule (usually FI) or that responding occurs *at all.*

Radical Behaviorism Outside EAB

Though they may have never heard those words, all reasonable people, given enough education and experience, eventually become radical behaviorists. Thank goodness for the fact that radical behavioral views are becoming influential *outside* the EAB. Thus, we find exemplars in areas outside behavior analysis. We will briefly describe examples in law, social psychology, and cognitive science that seem unknown to most behavior analysts.

Radical Behaviorism and Law

Richard Posner, a distinguished legal scholar and judge, has thought deeply about human thoughts and motives. He understands radical behaviorism and advocates a behavioral approach to the dispensation of justice. Tied in with this is his advocacy of pragmatism, illustrated in his discussion of belief and the causes of action.

As Peirce argued over a century earlier, *action* is the key to *belief* and to *meaning*. A statement has meaning, we believe it, and therefore are prepared to act on it. Without belief and action, words are only words. Posner suggested that even the idea of "mind" has no consequences, and may therefore be dispensed with. Posner's suggestions could have been written by B. F. Skinner:

> Obviously most adults and older children can and do speak without vocalization (that is, can "conceal their thoughts") and form mental images. But this barebones concept of mind, which essentially equates mind to consciousness, is different from the idea that there is a something, the "mind," which is the locus of intentions, the invisible puppeteer, the inner man or woman. It is that idea which may have no consequences for law and should perhaps be discarded, despite the law's emphatic ... commitment to it. (Posner 1990, p. 166)

> ... I suggest that we often use the word "mind" (either in the weak sense of consciousness or in the strong sense of intentionality and control) not to name a thing ... but to cover our ignorance of certain causal relationships. (ibid., p. 167)

That was Skinner's opening argument in 1953, though Posner (1990) cited none of Skinner's works—perhaps Hume and Wittgenstein were enough, or perhaps he was unaware of Skinner's arguments. Posner went on with a Skinnerian analysis:

> One could argue that as law becomes more sophisticated, states of mind should play an ever larger role in liability. Our understanding of the mind may improve—maybe we will learn to read minds. But maybe there is nothing to read, or maybe we are not interested in what the murderer was thinking when he pulled the trigger. If we take seriously the actor's adage that no man is a villain in his own eyes, we can expect to find, if we ever succeed in peering into the murderer's mind, an elaborate, perhaps quite plausible, rationalization for his deed. But so what? We would punish him all the same. (Posner 1990, p. 168)

Finally, though he never cites B. F. Skinner or Howard Rachlin, Judge Posner proposes not only that we lack real "liberty," but that others may understand our actions better than we do. This section is titled "Behaviorism and the Judicial Perspective" and begins with Posner's noting that behaviorism, which relies on external, rather than internal causes, seems antithetical to the "self-conscious" activity of a judge. But there is no inconsistency, he explains, since we commonly predict correctly what another will do without any knowledge of that person's conscious experience. In fact, we often can predict accurately "even when the person himself is undecided" (Posner 1990, p. 187). Can others predict your behavior better than you can? Posner says yes. When the parent or probation officer or psychologist predicts the behavior of another better than does the child, parolee, or patient themselves, it is not because the predictor knows the contents of the individual's mind—that is irrelevant, says Posner. But the expert or parent has information that the individual lacks, either because of lack of training or experience or because of emotional involvement. Perhaps more important, people routinely misrepresent their motives to themselves, pretending to be less concerned with status, money, and other base things than is actually the case. And we think of ourselves as braver, less selfish, and more ethical than we actually are. We recognize the same theme in the works of Bem (1967) and Nisbett and Wilson (1977).

The Nature of Self-Reports: Bem's Self-Perception

In a brilliant analysis of the nature of self-reports, Daryl Bem introduced the theory of "self perception" in 1967. Bem—a social psychologist, but one familiar with radical behaviorism—offered a compelling behavioral alternative to the cognitive mediational theory of cognitive dissonance (CD), which was wildly popular at the time. According to CD theory, dissonant cognitions having to do with our behavior, physiological states, and other beliefs may conflict, giving rise to an aversive drive similar to hunger. We then reduce this dissonance in various ways, often by changing our cognitions so that they do not conflict. For example, subjects induced to engage in counterattitudinal behavior, such as giving a speech favoring Fidel Castro, often show a change in "attitude" toward the disliked topic. In this case, Castro would be rated as less disliked, reducing the dissonance produced by giving the pro-Castro speech.

This is a prime example of a mediational theory, with imagined internal conflicts among imagined cognitions. Bem (1967) proposed that we examine the nature of self-reports and reach a better understanding of "attitude changes." Following Skinner's analysis, Bem argued that we learn to judge the "attitudes" of others through observations of their behavior, so we judge someone's "hunger" by how much we see him eat. Often we apply the same practice to ourselves, as when we conclude "I was not as hungry as I thought." In the majority of CD studies, subjects were asked questions for which they had no ready answer, and so assessed their "attitude" by considering their *own* behavior. I might give you a negative assessment of Castro if you ask me for one and I really have no firm opinion. But if you ask me again, after I have given a pro-Castro speech under coercion that I do not notice, I have more information to go on. Had we known that someone else had given the speech, we would judge his opinion of Castro to be that much more favorable. In judging ourselves, we sometimes do the same thing.

Bem emphasized that this was an account based on "radical behaviorism," but no one seemed to notice. Skinner learned of it at some time or other and wrote a note on it that appeared in his published notebooks. He knew that Bem saw self-perception as a radical behavioral treatment, but for reasons we will never understand, Skinner wrote that he didn't see the connection. Go figure.

Nisbett and Wilson: Telling More Than We Can Know

Richard Nisbett and Timothy Wilson (1977) surveyed data going back to the 1930s in which subjects gave verbal reports to account for their actions. This included studies of esthetic evaluations, phobic reactions, placebo effects, problem solving, PA learning, and dozens of dissonance and attribution studies. They found in the majority of cases, verbal reports were irrelevant and that "the behavioral effects were in most cases stronger ... than the verbal report effects" (p. 235). In cases where verbal report about motive state and behavioral reports about motive state were reported, the correlation "was found to be nil":

> In studies where the data are available, no association is found between degree of verbal report change and degree of behavior change.... (ibid., p. 235)

People have no power to "examine their thoughts" and accurately explain their actions:

> People's reports about their higher mental processes should be neither more nor less accurate in general than the predictions about such processes made by observers. (ibid., p. 249)

Nisbett and Wilson found that people have virtually no knowledge of their mental processes, though they commonly believe that they do. It's a pity that Skinner did not recognize kindred doctrine in this latest form of attribution theory, which shows that verbal reports are just verbal behavior, and that's just more behavior. Verbal reports do not reveal anything.

Piaget's Last Word: Cognitive/Developmental Behaviorism?

The "genetic epistemology" of Jean Piaget is usually construed as a theory of cognitive stages. But in a chapter titled "Piaget's Theory," published posthumously, Piaget specifically criticized cognitive-mediational views and emphasized a monist non-mediational position. He criticized the mediational view:

> In the common view, the external world is entirely separate from the subject ... objective knowledge, then, appears to be simply the result of a set of perceptive recordings, motor associations, verbal descriptions ... producing a sort of figurative copy.... (2000, p. 34)

Action is crucial and the result is not the taking in of copies:

> But this passive interpretation of the act of knowledge is in fact contradicted at all levels of development and, particularly, at the sensorimotor and prelinguistic levels ... in order to know objects, the subject must act upon them ... since objective knowledge ... has its origin in interactions between the subject and objects ... objective knowledge is always subordinate to certain structures of action ... *the subject and the object are fused* ... (ibid., pp. 34–35, emphasis added)

Piaget was not a radical behaviorist, but he was not as much a mediationist as we may have thought.

The "Cognitive Revolution"

Given the accomplishments of radical behaviorism, do we really need to feel envious of mainstream cognitive psychology? Does the discipline that exemplifies *mediation* and *underlying processes* warrant emulation? How well has cognitive psychology and cognitive science, the "creationism" of psychology, done? Where has the cognitive revolution gotten us?

Since the 1960s there has been great pressure to join the "cognitive revolution," due to the perception that great strides are being made by those who "dare to study the mind." In fact, "cognitive science" is a sham, a synonym for "pop" psychology, a field in which the adopting of a vocabulary has been treated as a revolution:

> (Cognitive psychology responds to) every passing breeze of fashion within psychology or criticism from others impatient for day to day demonstrations of social relevance. (Estes 1979, p. 660)

> Memory theorizing is going nowhere. The reason is that it is rooted in mediationism, the doctrine that memory is mediated by some sort of memory trace. (Watkins 1990, p. 328)

Clark Glymour, a worker in cognitive neuroscience, offered the following observation:

> One January a few years ago, shortly after the governor of Arizona had been impeached and the Exxon Valdez had spilled its cargo around Port Arthur, I had one of those uncanny experiences reserved for the people who read old news. Paging through the San Jose Mercury for January 1917, I came upon an article describing the impeachment of the governor of Arizona and a report of a large oil spill at Valdez, Alaska. Nietzsche, it seems, was on to something, the Eternal Return, the no news under the sun, the history repeats itself sort of thing. I have had similar uncanny experiences over the last few years reading bits of the literature of cognitive science as it has emerged in our time, and reading in the same years the literature of physiology, psychology, and psychiatry in the closing years of the 19th century. (Glymour 1997, p. 373)

Another observer correctly interpreted the "revolution" as a continuation of the mediationism of neobehaviorists of the Hullian S-R tradition:

> . . . the high romantic drama and intellectual adventure of revolution making and the joy of breaking behaviorist crockery must have been much more appealing than the day-to-day mundaneness of normal science. I was in graduate school at the University of Illinois from 1970 to 1974 and was told by William F. Brewer that a revolution was going on. The present article started as a dissenting class paper that I wrote for him. (Leahey 1992, p. 315)

Leahey argued that "the history of American psychology is a plausible but dangerous myth" and that there have been no revolutions, aside from Wundt's founding of psychology. The advent of behaviorism in 1913 was "revolutionary only in that it broadened psychology to include animals, children, and the insane," a conclusion also reached by Hilgard (1987).

"Cognitive psychology/science" refers to no one entity, as an examination of textbooks quickly reveals. White (1985) examined the studies cited in seven popular cognitive psychology textbooks, finding that of 3,200 references, only 19 were included in all seven texts. Only 144 were cited in even four of the seven books. White also found that the 3,500 references in eight textbooks on human memory included less than 1 percent that appeared in all the books. A whopping 80 percent (2,800 references) were cited in only one of the ten books.

Best (1995) found the same thing—the citations in second editions of five cognitive psychology books published between 1985 and 1988 included only 19 that appeared in all texts and 80 percent appeared in only a single textbook.

If only 20 percent of the references appear in more than a single textbook, it is difficult to argue that cognitive psychology is a coherent discipline. Endel Tulving, a noted memory researcher, was quoted as follows:

> After a hundred years of laboratory-based study of memory, we still do not seem to possess any concepts that the majority of workers would consider important or necessary. If one asked a dozen or so randomly selected active memory researchers to compile a list of concepts without which they could not function, one would find little agreement among them ... if one compares different textbooks of memory, one discovers that there is little overlap among their subject indexes. It seems that important concepts of one author can apparently be dispensed with by another. (White 1985, p. 117)

Cognitive psychology/science is not a coherent discipline and it is certainly not to be emulated. Rather, it seems to illustrate the horrors of mediationism better than any argument I could make.

Radical Behaviorism since 1990

Applied Behavior Analysis: Controversy

How closely does the applied analysis of behavior follow the tenets of radical behaviorism? Has it remained non-mediational, yet shown an appreciation for private experience as a part of our subject matter? Has the molar perspective exerted any influence? These questions are hard to answer, at least based on the past few years' issues of the *Journal of Applied Behavior Analysis* (*JABA*). Since 1995, the articles chosen by the editors, and placed on the Internet, focus on the treatment of pica, tics, self injury, reading/spelling, and eating. Methods include reinforcement, punishment, effort requirements, and other simple and specific methods. One paper, on habit reversal, reviews the use of competing behaviors in treating "habits," such as tics and nail and lip biting, a method promoted by Edwin Guthrie in the 1930s. Another investigates the membership of self-destructive behaviors in the same or different response classes. Private behavior is not mentioned, nor is assessment of patterns of behavior occurring over time. But at least mediators have not crept in.

Brian Iwata (1994) provides a rare example of a "functional analysis," and this consists of assessing pathological behaviors in different contexts, so as to infer the past contingencies that produced the behaviors. In the case of self-injurious behavior, some subjects showed that a history of attention paid was operating, while for others self stimulation or escape from academic demands was responsible for maintaining (and presumably establishing) the problem behavior.

Does private experience play a part in applied behavior analysis? Interestingly, the answer is difficult, since many behavior analysts are methodological behaviorists. Friman, Hayes, and Wilson (1998) recently proposed that "anxiety" be conceptualized in the terms of behavior analysis and treated as avoidance behavior. Lamal (1998) criticized this proposal as a reversion to mentalism and argued that emotion is a private event and therefore outside the realm of behavior analysis. While methodological behaviorism seems alive in *JABA*, others are using verbal reports as corollaries of private behavior, including emotion, in the way that Skinner always advocated.

Rachlin's Logical Extension: Molar Behaviorism and TEPOOOB

Howard Rachlin proposed that mentalists see only the behavior of others and feel that they must *infer* the person's hidden mental state which "mediates" between the behavior and the environment—but he sees something different:

> For me, as a behaviorist, an observer of another person may actually see that person's mental state—the mental state is an observable pattern of behavior-environment interaction—and must infer the historical pattern of contingencies of reinforcement behind it. Thus, perhaps paradoxically, for the mentalist, behavior is the only objectively and directly observable datum, while for the behaviorist a mental state is directly and objectively observable.... The critical difference between the mentalist and the behaviorist is the point where explanations may stop. For a mentalist, explanations of behavior may stop when they have been traced to a current internal cause ('I ate the spinach because I believed it would be good for me'). For a behaviorist, explanations of behavior (or mental states) may stop only when they have been traced to a previous external cause ('I ate the spinach, and believe it is good for me, because when I used to eat spinach as a child it pleased my mother and when my mother was pleased she was kind'). (Rachlin 1987a, p. 177)

Rachlin extended Skinner's interpretation to incorporate Ryle's arguments against the "category error" and gives us a conception of molar behaviorism congruent with Aristotle's position, particularly as it appears in *Nicomachean Ethics*:

Overt behavior does not just reveal the mind—it is the mind. Each mental term stands for a pattern of overt behavior. This may include such mental terms as 'sensation', 'pain', 'love', 'hunger', and 'fear' (terms considered by the mentalist to be 'raw feels') as well as more complex mental states such as 'belief' and 'intelligence' that are sometimes said to be 'complex mental states' and sometimes 'intentional acts.' Behaviorists differ among themselves as to whether 'raw feels' are overt or covert behavior (Skinner sees them as covert behavior), but the essence of radical behaviorism is the belief that intentional acts are nothing but patterns of overt behavior. (Rachlin 1987b, pp. 156–157)

The language of description/explanation promotes the plausibility of mediational/mentalist/cognitive theories, which therefore seem more "natural":

With regard to plausibility, behaviorism looks worse than any of the other theories. It seems implausible that a mental event such as a 'hope' could originate outside us and that our behavior, rather than being only a sign or indication of what we hope, is itself the hope. We understand very little about mental events such as hopes. Mentalism, with its vague and shaky reliance on introspection, accurately mirrors our current vague and shaky understanding of mental events. This is what lends mentalism its plausibility. The problem is that mentalism imperializes its own vague and shaky understanding; it provides no path to a more coherent model of the mind. (ibid., p. 159)

The Push For Mediation: Staddon's States

John Staddon has long campaigned for the inclusion of *theory* in radical behavioral research, arguing that the concept of "internal state" is necessary, acceptable, and inevitable. In brief, "state" would refer to the product of a specific conditioning history and would allow us to differentiate among cases where the current behaviors of our subjects are indistinguishable but have arisen due to different histories. Brian Iwata (e.g. 1984) has shown that it is possible to distinguish different histories that lead to self-injurious behavior by placing subjects in different contexts and observing their behavior. Similarly, Staddon argues that different histories supporting apparently similar behaviors may exert their influences when conditions change. Such effects cannot be predicted without reference to internal states.

Staddon (1997) showed that habituation in a dish of nematodes required the concept of internal state in order to be interpretable. When stimulation occurred rapidly (short inter-stimulus interval (ISI)) or slowly (long-ISI), habituation occurred more and less rapidly, respectively. Recovery from habituation was a different story—the short-ISI condition, where responding had decreased to a lower value than that for the long-ISI animals, showed more rapid recovery and recovery to a higher level of responding, than was the case for the long-ISI group. Staddon points out this is an unpredictable result, if only observations of responding are available.

In the nematode case, two internal states (integrators of stimulus input) account for the data. The first is a rapid-recovery device that provides input to the second integrator, a slow-recovering device. Whatever biological equipment mediates the habituation of nematodes, we know that two "somethings" are required. The "states," or "somethings," are integrators in the nematode example and Staddon labels them V1 and V2, the variables that define the current state of the model. Staddon explains what they are:

> Behaviorists are often puzzled by these variables: what are they? The honest answer is "I have no idea." They may correspond to some physiological variables, the levels of two chemical reactants, for example. The point of the model is not to say what they are (that's a job for the physiologist), but to say how many of them are needed to account for the behavior—and how they behave (i.e., the structure of the model). The aim of the model is, literally, to define the dimensions of the behavior. Habituation in the nematode is pretty simple; it looks as if two dimensions are enough. (1997, p. 117)

Staddon suggests that "radically behavioristic readers should not get their knickers in a twist" over this proposal to "explain" data. He urges us to "Just say, *explain*" means a formal representation of the data reduced to a minimal number of terms, in a calm voice a few times and the anxious feeling will go away.

What's going on here? Did Staddon forget to wear his knickers? He views his proposal as consonant with the spirit of radical behaviorism—even quoting Skinner's adage on "formal representation of the data." Many radical behaviorists do indeed find this puzzling (personal communications, A. C. Catania and P. N. Hineline), because Staddon wishes that radical behaviorism change in *only* one way. If it doesn't, he predicts that there will be no role left for it. The so-called cognitive revolution has fizzled out and the application of neural networks to psychology is "questionable." The one area of promise seems to be cognitive neuroscience, he concludes, and the relevance of radical behaviorism to that endeavor is nil. And we can't "stick limpet-like to the wishful simplism of radical behaviorism." What exactly do we need?

Staddon says that we need to modify radical behaviorism by incorporating what seems to be its antithesis—we need *theory*, "the postulating of events taking place somewhere else, at some other level of observation (or none) described in different terms, and measured, if at all, in different dimensions" (1997, p. 109). This, of course, is Skinner's definition of "theory," which he argued against in his classic 1950 paper in *Psychological Review*. Staddon has never subscribed to this view and he has stated his opposition many times, drawing adherents and puzzling others.

Staddon's proposal seems at first sight similar to that of the mediational theorists of decades ago—Clark Hull, Kenneth Spence, and many others—who were superseded by modern behaviorism and whose program was essentially continued as the "cognitive revolution," especially in its information processing form. (See Leahey 1992; Malone 1987.) But it differs in one important respect that does make it more amenable to radical behaviorist thinking. And, you guessed it, Staddon's view also has a helluva drawback.

On the positive side, Staddon does not propose a list of postulates or a series of processing stages derived *in advance* from reasonable assumptions about the way that organisms work. This inductive approach distinguishes him from Hull and Tolman. And he does not assume "representations" or other paraphernalia of the cognitivists, who also do their "assuming" in advance. His internal states are to be *inductively* determined and to signify histories of exposure to contingencies. There are to be as few as possible—he cautions against "Erector Set" models and dismisses biological plausibility. Maybe his states *are* appropriately viewed as economical descriptions of the data. But there *is* one drawback.

Staddon's data are drawn from a 1992 article in *Cognitive Neuroscience* describing the reaction of nematodes to taps on the glass jar in which they reside. The orienting response they display consists of "flipping over," and this is shown by varying percentages of the animals, constituting the strength of response on a given trial. This is about as simple a behavior as can be imagined and the changes in response of this group of nematodes are the source of very nice and clean data—really clean data. And there's the rub. To infer internal states in the way that Staddon proposes requires data that are virtually non-existent in the EAB, to say nothing of psychology in general. Open any journal and scan the figures, tables, and verbal descriptions and one quickly sees that nothing like the clarity of data Staddon requires is present. Perhaps that explains his concentration on relatively simple phenomena, such as timing behavior in animals. Even in that restricted area, the complexity is enough to render modeling difficult.

Staddon argues that if internal states are required to explain *even* the simple behavior of the nematodes, as they flip over in response to a tap on the glass, such theoretical states must be necessary to explain more complex behavior. This is the same argument used by Wolfgang Köhler when he demonstrated transposition in chickens and argued that this meant that higher organisms must be capable of such higher-level functions. But, unless applications are presented that involve some kind of behavior more interesting than habituation, Staddon's internal states seem not to apply to what everyone calls "psychology." And if learning, choice, avoidance, imitation, discrimination, generalization, schedule-induced behavior, masochism, depth perception, and the other myriad categories of behavior are to be explained in terms of internal states, will their laboratory analogues need to be so simplified as to be unrecognizable or the models so complex as to be unrecognizable?

Psychology is far from ready for "internal states," and there is still a role for radical behaviorism: to determine what it is that organisms do on a *gross* level. If the fine level of analysis is ever required, internal states will be welcome indeed.

Notes

1. This view is not universally accepted, but it has great merit.

2. The critics of the EAB were in both cases S-R associationists themselves before the scales were lifted from their eyes!

13 The End of Psychology: What Can We Expect at the Limits of Inquiry?

John M. Horner

The opinion which is fated to be ultimately agreed to by all . . . is what we mean by the truth. . . .
—Charles Sanders Peirce (1878)

If we don't blow ourselves up in the next 400 years, then, when all the laws of psychology are known, ...
—John E. R. Staddon (personal communication, 1982)

In a paper titled "How to Make Our Ideas Clear," C. S. Peirce outlines an elegant thought experiment on scientific progress and the notion of truth. Reality (or truth), from Peirce's pragmatic point of view, is what is ultimately fated to be agreed upon at the limits of scientific inquiry. When our experiments are done and we all agree that our theories correspond to the world, Peirce claimed, our theories will then be what is "true." No metaphysical definition of truth is needed. Peirce's object in defining this thought experiment is to articulate a clear notion of truth, but his thought experiment and his operational definition of truth have recently become the center of debate between realists (Boyd 1984; Hacking 1983; Putnam 1978) and pragmatists (Collins 1992; van Fraassen 1989) on the nature of truth. Realists contend that even at the limit of inquiry, our theories might be incorrect. Pragmatist counter, how would you know? More important, who cares, except a bunch of philosophers who will be out of a job otherwise?

John Staddon (1982) offered an interesting corollary to Peirce's thought experiment. For Peirce, truth was found in the dovetailing of inquiry onto a "fated" agreement among observers. How, Staddon asks, will psychology look when science has run its course and our understanding of behavior has reached its limit—when our theories exhaust our understanding of behavior and answer our questions to the degree possible through scientific method? However interesting the debate over what is true or real is to the philosophically inclined, Peirce's thought experiment raises the question that Staddon finally asks: What can we expect from our theories at the limits of scientific inquiry? And specifically for psychologists: What can we expect from a science of psychology at the limits of inquiry? Is it simply, as Peirce says, that we will all agree on our theories, or need we consider what it means to scientifically explain psychological phenomena?

Psychology has a special interest in this question, because much of the debate on methodology in psychology rests upon what will count as a scientific explanation of psychological phenomena. How can we know what the important questions of our field are, if we do not know what constitutes a suitable explanation? The history of psychology is replete with arguments about the appropriate subject and nature of the study of psychology. We turn next to a short, schematic history of psychological explanation as a way of exploring the tensions within the field over what will count as an explanation.

A (Very) Short History of Explanation in Psychology

Immature sciences often postulate a plethora of unobservable entities to explain natural phenomena. Thales talked of the world's being full of gods, but spirits, forms, souls, abstract figures, and even numbers were advanced as the fundamental parts of causal systems in the past. Early psychology too showed a proliferation of unobservable entities to explain behavior. Folk psychology asks that we accept an array of mental phenomena in our explanatory framework. Beliefs, wants, thoughts, desires, and memories are all part of the explanatory matrix of our language that allows us to communicate about our behavior to others. "I want to go to the movies." "I think the store is in this direction." "I don't remember her name." But underlying this language is also an explanation for our behavior: we do what we want, based upon what we know (with some external constraints placed on our behavior). This is a powerful explanatory framework, because it can be used to account for virtually all human (and presumably animal) behavior—after the fact.

Behaviorism (Skinner 1976) was a response to these kinds of explanatory devices in psychology. At the beginning of the twentieth century, psychology could be defined as the study of "mental life," but by the middle of the century, much of academic psychology was strongly behaviorist. The rebellion occurred chiefly because the unobservable entities of early psychology had no formal status; they were "mental" and as such had only limited veridical standing. Except for perhaps phenomenologically, they had no status independent of the explanatory system in which they were used—in the strictest sense; they were free variables for use in any explanation of behavior.

Watson (1913) rejected the use of unobservable entities in the explanation of behavior. For him, there was no mental life, so they could not be used to explain behavior. Skinner's (1963) radical behaviorism attempted to construct an explanatory framework that was equally devoid of unobservables by using only the environment (Skinner 1966a), present and (long or short) past, as the causal factor in an explanatory framework for behavior. Because he relied exclusively on environmental variables to explain behavior, Skinner used a functional explanatory framework rather than a mechanistic or a causal one.

This functional approach raises the question "What was to be explained?" Were the individual muscle twitches or responses to be analyzed, or were more aggregate behaviors the appropriate object of study? Watson (1930) was equivocal on this point, but Hull (1943) sought the basic unit of behavior in reflexes or habits. Tolman (1932) and Skinner (1931, 1935) sought a broader definition of behavior, one that looked for order at a higher (molar) level. Mechanistic explanations tend to focus on basic units, whereas functional explanations are more likely to focus on higher-order measures of behavior. In a functional explanation, the orderly relationships between environmental variables and behavior are the object of study, with little interest in the "underlying processes," so Skinner had little interest in "theory" (Skinner 1950). If behavior could be understood in its relationship to environmental variables, then there was no need for unobservable processes to explain it or, if all the relationships could be mapped out, for theory. Following Newton's treatment of gravity, Skinner wished to posit "no theory" to explain behavior.

This insistence on avoiding unobservables in an explanatory framework was oddly out of step with the rest of science. Over the years, physics, chemistry, and biology had all made productive use of unobservable entities in their explanatory frameworks; only radical behaviorism eschewed their use. This had a twofold effect: one, to restrict psychology to a functional account with little interest in underlying mechanisms; and two, to insulate it and its methods from other fields of inquiry. Psychology was about the orderly relationship between behavior and environment, and nothing more. Thus, its relation to other fields was not essential to its explanatory framework. Indeed, such isolation seemed justified at the time. Psychology as a science was still reeling from the seductive tendency to use "mental" constructs as a way of explaining behavior, and knowledge of the underlying biological substrate of behavior, the nervous system, was in its infancy. Mechanistic appeals to "the brain" as the cause of behavior were still only a convenient repository of our ignorance. Yet the stricture of radical behaviorism seemed wholly out of step with the rest of science and theoretically confining.

The computer changed all that. The computer proved to be a powerful metaphor for mental processes because essentially dumb processes could be designed to do very complex things. The advantage over previous mental models was not so much in terms of their explanatory sophistication, but instead their ability to avoid a homunculus fallacy in a mental mechanisms account. With no little man controlling their behavior, computers were obviously machines; however, they could do complex things—like solve mathematical proofs (Newell, Shaw, and Simon 1958). Therefore, their actions, or more precisely the running of computer programs, could serve as a metaphor for the action of mental process. This insight proved liberating for psychologists, because it meant we could pursue not just unobservable entities to account for behavior, but mechanistic (and theoretical) models of behavior. The cognitive revolution was off and running (Miller 1962; Neisser 1967); the only problem was still the ontological status of mental events. Cognitivists hoped that the mental constructs of their theories would some day find validation in the nervous system.

But the cognitive revolution soon ran into trouble. In the early 1980s, cognitive psychologists began to see their search for mental mechanisms as a sterile and unproductive enterprise (Jenkins 1981; Neisser 1978). Cognitive phenomena were more "contextual" than many psychologists had expected; a human's ability to solve complex tasks seemed to be highly dependent on the situations in which they occurred (Jenkins 1974; Neisser 1982). There seemed not to be any unitary, underlying mechanism, but a host of mechanisms all designed for specific tasks. Memory was not one thing, but many things. The hope for a single unified theory of any cognitive process faded. Some saw the search for mechanism as nothing more than taking the plethora of functional relationships between the environment and behavior as defined by experimental analysis and turning them into mechanistic metaphors for those relationships (Jenkins 1981). Psychologists began to ask "What have we accomplished?" The silence was deafening. Could an analysis aimed at a mechanistic explanation of processing information succeed, or were higher-order relationships the appropriate level of analysis?

Recently, researchers have begun to model psychological phenomena using neural networks (e.g., Rumelhart, McClelland, and PDP Research Group 1986)—simulated nodes not unlike individual nerve cells that make connections to other nodes and thus have computational power (McCulloch and Pitts 1943). This approach is substantively different from cognitive psychology because the unobservable entities are not considered to have the same ontological status as mental entities, but instead are designed to simulate neurons. While many simulated neural networks are biologically implausible, the action of neural networks has proved relatively powerful at mimicking some simple behavioral phenomena. For instance, 25 years of attempting to program a computer to recognize speech proved relatively futile; however, in the past 15 years neural networks have proven remarkably effective at speech recognition. Even if the current algorithms for neural networks have yet to simulate their biological counterpart accurately, the general power of these kinds of systems to perform very complex processes is well established. However, while the new connectionism has proven to be a powerful mechanistic explanatory device, it still looks to psychology for phenomena to explain. It has very little to say about what the important phenomena are, or what kinds of things we should be looking at to explain how animals adapt to their environment.

Explanatory Tensions

What does this short history tell us about the nature of a suitable psychological explanation? Even today, there is no consensus about the aims and methods of psychology. However, there appear to be a number of tensions running through a science of psychology:

1. What is the place of unobservables in psychological explanation? Are theoretical or hypothetical entities necessary, or even useful?

2. What kinds of explanation are appropriate for psychology? Should we try to uncover only functional relationships between environment and animal, or should we seek mechanistic explanations for behavior?

3. What level of explanation should we seek? Should we seek to explain orderly behavior in the aggregate (molar) or should we try to explain individual behavioral events (molecular)?

Peirce and Staddon's thought experiment about the end of inquiry might well help us understand these issues in a way that can be useful in our inquiry today. How these tensions are resolved at the limit of inquiry should tell us something about the most fruitful way to proceed in our study.

Unobservables

Perhaps the use of unobservables in psychological explanation is the most contentious issue in the philosophy of a scientific psychology. The aversion to the use of unobservables as hypothetical entities was the early driving force behind the behaviorist revolution and culminated in the philosophical stance of radical behaviorism. The brazenness of their use helped fuel the cognitive revolution. However, one can legitimately ask whether they are useful in an explanatory framework.

Take, for example, how we account for the effects of the distant past on behavior. Much of psychology, specifically cognitive psychology, assumes that past experiences have an effect on current behavior through the mediation construct of memory. Memories are formed from experience and are stored for later use. Memories are thus representations of past experience. They may decay or suffer interference, but memories are the bridge from the past to current behavior, and are used as the hypothetical construct to account for historical effects on behavior. Skinner (1987) and others (e.g. White 1991) have seen this mediational construct as pointing our investigation away from the real explanation—past experiences and present circumstances—and thus obscuring our understanding of behavior. Instead, we should try to understand how experiences "change" the organism's response to current circumstances. A mediational construct is not necessary. What understanding have we gained from the mediational construct of memory?

But what does it mean to be unobservable? Are just hypothetical constructs unobservable, or can things we could potentially see be unobservable in practice? For instance, Skinner puts all his explanatory variables into the form of potentially observable phenomena, such as historical contingencies. But when providing an explanation of an organism's behavior, in practice how useful is an appeal to the organism's history? Often an organism's history is as unobservable as any mental construct; it has disappeared from our scrutiny. An appeal to historical variables at least has the potential to be observed and manipulated in any experimental treatment of behavior, but often it has been used as yet another free variable in an account of the phenomena of interest.

Skinner was often guilty of this excess by simply translating psychological phenomena into the language of operant conditioning. (For an eloquent presentation of this point, see Malone 1975.) In his 1966 paper on problem solving, Skinner argued that specific past learning experiences shaped our ability to solve problems. Köhler's chimps could solve the banana problem because of the learning experiences in their past. These past learning experiences were, of course, potentially observable, but Skinner was not specific about the kinds of past contingencies that were required for solving a particular problem. In a sense, Skinner's (1966b) explanation is little more than a theoretical account of problem solving, with the free variable of past contingencies to fill the explanatory gaps. It was left to Epstein, Kirshnit, Lanza, and Rubin (1984) to specify what those past experiences should be—for a pigeon. Epstein et al. achieved behavior in pigeons remarkably analogous to that of Köhler's chimpanzees by first training them to peck movable blocks for reinforcement. Once pigeons had acquired this behavior, obtaining access to an elevated food source proved to be a relatively simple matter for these animals to "solve" by moving blocks around their cage by pecking at them, much as Köhler's chimps had solved the problem of moving boxes around the their cages.

And yet we know that hypothetical constructs have proven useful in other fields. For example, in biology the hypothetical construct of the gene has played a major role in the development of that field, if somewhat obliquely. Darwin's theory of natural selection required a mechanism for inheritance. However, Darwin (1896) was convinced of the influence of Lamarckian transmission on the evolution of organism and so tried to incorporate a Lamarckian mechanism, pangenesis, in his theory of heredity.

Darwin hypothesized that each somatic cell submits information about its physical characteristics, both inherited and acquired, via gemmules, to the germ cell. In 1889, de Vries (see Gould 2002), abandoning the need for Lamarckian transmission in his theory of intracellular pangenesis, claimed instead that each cell contains all the particles needed to reconstruct an organism. Johannsen's notion of the gene, derived directly from de Vries's concept of inheritance, gave us the modern mechanism of inheritance. Notice that the proposed nature of the gene is determined by its hypothetical action, and not by any direct observation of it. Is it necessary to account for Lamarckian transmission? If not, the mechanism for inheritance, as Darwin proposed it, is incorrect.

With the rediscovery of Mendel, aided by de Vries, the concept of the gene became a cornerstone of evolutionary theory. Was the hypothetical construct of the gene important in understanding the general form of natural selection? Not at all, since Darwin had the general mode of inheritance wrong, but got the basics of natural selection right. Has the hypothetical construct of the gene been important in the development of modern evolutionary theory? Yes. Not only would the modern evolutionary synthesis of Wright, Fisher, and Haldane have been impossible without the gene concept; long before the physical nature of genes was uncovered by Watson and Crick, Hardy (1908) was able to incorporate the processes of genetic drift and gene flow into evolutionary theory.

The concept of gene allows us to think about heritability in a certain formal and logical way, where the concept of pangenesis would have led us astray. Could female-dominated eusociality in bees, wasps, and ants be understood without an understanding of the unusual genetic inheritance (haploidy/diploidy) of Hymenoptera (Hamilton 1972)? Yet it has only been recently that our technology has given us a means of observing the physical analogs of genes, DNA and RNA. Now our understanding of genetic inheritance at the molecular level can propel our understanding of evolution (e.g., genetic cladagrams). But is natural selection explicable simply through the actions of genes, hypothetical or otherwise? No, Mendel had no insight into natural selection through his work on peas. Indeed, it seems difficult to backtrack from an understanding of the mechanism of inheritance to an understanding of natural selection—arguments to the contrary aside (Dawkins 1978).

In evolutionary biology, as well as in other areas of science, hypothetical constructs cannot long stand alone as explanatory devices without some independent verification. If we postulate an unobservable, its proposed action should be consistent with our expectation about how that thing should act, least it fall to the wayside of useful construct (e.g., gemmules). But if it proves useful, we expect that at some point in the future independent verification of its existence is forthcoming. Imagine if all our new biotechnology had found gemmules instead of genes. Where would we be then?

Often the unobservables in psychology have a separate ontological status that simply does not permit any independent observation. What is a "mental process?" Even if the philosophy of the nature of mental processes were more sophisticated than simply something apart from the physical world, how potentially would it be observed? If there is no way of independently verifying or measuring mental states, then they are relegated to the status of free variables in an explanatory framework. What most cognitive psychologists hope is that their postulated mental processes will someday find a home in the nervous system, yet most cognitive theories, which postulate mental processes, do not take biological suitability into account. If the brain can do anything, then it too becomes a free variable in any explanatory account. In all sciences, unobservables (hypotheticals) must (in the end) have some validity outside the theoretical framework. Otherwise they are just free variables with little or no value, except in adapting *post hoc* explanations. At the end of inquiry, anything that does not have a way of being independently measured outside its explanatory framework will simply be a free variable—which is the reason behaviorists revolted in the first place.

Kinds of Explanations

Generally, psychologists have been concerned with either causal/mechanistic or functional explanations of behavior. Because they have emphasized the organism's adaptation to its environment, behaviorists have usually sought a functional explanation of behavior. Cognitivists and others have used a mechanistic approach because they have sought the underlying processes that guide behavior. In some cases, the proposed mechanism is mental in nature, but appeals to neural or physiological mechanisms are also acceptable in an explanatory framework. These distinctions are never rigid and many individuals who would classify themselves in one camp or another, may be inclined toward the other explanatory framework (e.g., Gibson 1966, 1979; Hull 1943; Jenkins 1974; Neisser 1976; Tolman 1932). But, in general, behaviorists have been most comfortable with purely functional explanations of behavior and others have sought a causal/mechanistic explanatory framework in psychology.

Kuhn's (1970) doctrine of incommensurable paradigms is one of the most overused and misapplied notions in all of the philosophy of science; however, it works well to describe the competing perspectives of behaviorism and cognitive psychology. Much of the difference between their paradigms results from the respective explanatory frameworks that the two have adopted. Often it seems that adherence to one particular kind of explanatory framework in psychology is little more than a dispositional attitude. Radical behaviorists (Skinner 1963) believe that the *only questions* in psychology are those concerning the functional relationships between organism and environment, and that concentrating on mechanistic accounts, be they mental or neural, only detracts from our understanding of behavior. Those on the cognitive side believe that only an explanation of "how" our cognitive apparatus works can account for many of the phenomena in which they are interested. Neuroscientists, on the other hand, point out that the brain must underlie all psychological phenomena, and therefore no explanation is complete without reference to the neural processes involved.

One might well ask which perspective is best? But, for now, let us play the thought experiment of what would happen if these explanatory paradigms were to run independent of each other to the end of inquiry—a functionalist verses a mechanistic approach playing out to the point where they both achieved the same degree of power at explaining psychological phenomena. Let us pretend that the predictions each made matched the observations equally well and gave essentially the same answer. What then might we expect?

Wittgenstein (1961) and others have argued that if two theories (or ideas) do not make different predictions, they are essentially equivalent explanations. Jenkins (1981) argued a similar and more specific point when he claimed that the mental mechanisms proposed by cognitive psychologists are really nothing more than metaphors for the functional relationship between the environment and organisms. Similarly, if an explanation based on neurology could explain the environment's effects on behavior, then the predictions we make about behavior via neural mechanisms would be equivalent to purely functional accounts. If these notions of explanatory equivalence are correct, then at the end of inquiry we might find it possible to map the theories of one perspective onto the theories of the others. The different frameworks might then be collapsed just as Schrödinger did by showing that quantum mechanics was mathematically equivalent to his wave theory of matter. They were two "different mathematical formulations of the same structure" (Heisenberg 1971, p. 71). All sides, having the same explanatory power, would then resolve into mirror theories.

In his paper "On Aims and Methods of Ethology," Tinbergen (1963) outlined four kinds of explanations used in ethology: causal/mechanistic, functional, ontogeny, and phylogeny. According to Tinbergen, each of these perspectives can stand on its own as an explanatory framework. Thus, each perspective constitutes a valid explanation of behavioral phenomena. Tinbergen argued that our knowledge of behavior was not complete without an understanding from all four explanatory frameworks. Our knowledge of these explanatory frameworks was therefore complementary. Like Tinbergen, we might take the middle road and argue that all are necessary, but instead it seems possible that at the end of inquiry, these different frameworks will give roughly equivalent answers to our questions. This leads us to the conclusion that a final understanding will take the perspective of all these explanatory frameworks into account, just as Tinbergen argued. Can we fully understand behavior without understanding the neural mechanisms that underlie it? Can we understand the neural mechanisms without understanding the functional relationships between the organisms and its environment?

Before the limit of inquiry, we might have a more practical problem: which approach is more fruitful? If, as Jenkins (1981) suggests, cognitive mechanisms are nothing more than metaphors for functional relationships, then it is fair to ask whether a mental mechanistic approach is any more fruitful than a straightforward functional account in the first place. Perhaps mental metaphors are easier to grasp and manipulate than functional relationships, making progress in this field faster. Is the construct of memory easier to deal with than the construct of states or equivalent histories? Which is more misleading? Different individuals might respond variously, but most would acknowledge that to date a functional approach has given us very powerful tools in shaping the behavior of organisms. A cognitive-mechanisms approach has had a much more limited range of successes. However, such may not be the case in the future. A cognitive or alternatively a neural-mechanistic approach might gain in explanatory efficacy as our technology advances. While this essay's previous section on unobservables held that any explanatory framework that left hypothetical entities unverifiable would not be viable at the limit of inquiry, a mechanistic approach might become very fruitful, very fast, if those unobservable mechanisms could find independent verification. It seems doubtful that mental mechanisms will achieve that kind of validity, but if the brain is the biological substrate behind behavior, a neural-mechanisms approach will succeed at some point.

Level of Explanation

What do we expect from a scientific explanation? Many philosophers of science (e.g., Kuhn 1970) argue that an explanation's value is derived from the conceptual framework it provides for researchers in which to view a phenomenon. These philosophers hold that if an explanation provides a coherent way of categorizing and organizing related phenomena, so providing a structure in which to do science, it has value and credibility with the practitioners of that field. However, many explanatory frameworks might fit these criteria and yet have varying degrees of credibility at the limits of inquiry. Even if different explanatory frameworks organized their fields' endeavors in comparably valuable ways, at the limits of inquiry their explanatory power can be compared by how well they allow us to predict or control the phenomena in question.

The nature of science is that our theories must to some extent be testable against the observations we make. The testability of our theories demands that they have some efficacy in predicting or controlling phenomena. In many instances, our capacity to manipulate the relevant variables, which would allow us to control a given phenomenon, is negligible. But we can at the very minimum expect that our theories will give us some predictive power over the phenomena of interest. Thus, at the limits of inquiry, we should expect our ability to predict behavioral phenomena to have been maximized. We might then legitimately ask, how much may we expect our psychological theories to predict at the limit of inquiry?

Traditional scientific methods seek to uncover the causal relationships among variables. Thus the scientific worldview is one of determinism—all things have their antecedent causes. Of course, this need not be so. Some things in nature may occur randomly, so some portion of their behavior may not be predictable from knowledge of their antecedent conditions. However, even in cases where our current theories, such as quantum mechanics, propose a stochastic process there is much debate within the field as to whether stochastic processes are really a fundamental property of the phenomena or whether some factors controlling the behavior of the phenomena are unknown—the "God doesn't play dice with the universe" position. However, even if our knowledge of the causal relationships among things were complete, there might still be a failure of our ability to predict phenomena at the limit of inquiry.

In recent years, work in non-linear dynamics (see Holden 1986) has shown that even if a system is purely deterministic our ability to predict that system's behavior is limited. In linear systems, changes in one variable produce easily quantifiable changes in the system; non-linear systems exhibit extreme sensitivity to initial conditions, such that small differences in the starting points can lead to wildly different results. This makes the behavior of such systems often appear random on the surface, even if they are governed by a simple set of equations. Non-linear systems are thus called chaotic. What this sensitive dependency means in practice is that the behavior of a chaotic system is relatively difficult to predict, even if we know all the equations that govern its behavior and have a measure of its initial conditions. Why? Because a measure of a system's initial conditions does not guarantee that we have precisely measured its initial state. Measurement errors, even if small, can lead to widely different outcomes as time passes.

Horner (2002) and others (Palya, Walter, Kessel, and Lucke 1996) have shown that the behavior of organisms may exhibit this kind of unpredictable dynamic. Following Shaw's (1984) work on the predictability of the dripping faucet, Horner (2002) was able to illustrate that the inter-response times of pigeons pecking for grain on a periodic schedule showed many of the characteristics of a chaotic system. First, a discrete Fast Fourier Transform of pigeons' moment-by-moment response rate over time exemplified the kind of red shift in frequencies that is characteristic of chaotic systems. Then, using a measure of information developed by Shaw (1984), Horner was able to show that our ability to predict a pigeon's behavior, at least in terms of inter-response time, deteriorated the further into the future those predictions were extended. In a relatively few responses, the behavior of each animal becomes harder to predict as measured by Shaw's metric.

Horner's (2002) finding suggests that, at least at the level of the individual response, behavior may be chaotic and so harder and harder to predict as we extend our predictions into the future. In truth, this is not a surprising finding. Most psychologists believe that, given the number of possible variables that appear to control behavior and the difficulty of measuring them, prediction of behavior over time would be difficult if not impossible. Still, most appreciate the endeavor of trying to understand the variables that influence behavior. Horner's (2002) finding does not contradict these suppositions, but does provide a further caution. Even if we discover relatively simple relationships between variables, our ability to apply that knowledge will still be tenuous.

Such limitation in the predictability of behavior has a profound effect on what level we may expect our psychological theories to operate. Learning theories have acknowledged a distinction between molar and molecular levels of analysis (e.g., Tolman 1949) that has recently been resurrected (Baum 2002). Molecular analyses are those dealing with individual responses or behaviors, while molar analysis involve more aggregate measures of behavior. One example is concepts of the reflex. A molecular analysis of this concept might define a reflex as involving a stimulus that excites a receptor, and produces a response that is a movement of a muscle group, whereas a molar analysis might define the concept broadly enough that a stimulus could be going to school and the response learning how to read. Of course the dividing line between these levels of analysis can be rather arbitrary, and many authors over the years have suggested different criteria for distinguishing them.

Researchers in the area of learning have long argued over what is the appropriate level of analysis. While many early theorists of behavior confined their explanations to a molecular analysis (e.g., Hull 1943; Watson 1930), others (Baum 2002; Skinner 1931, 1935, 1976; Tolman 1949) argued that a molar analysis is more fruitful and easier to defend theoretically. The level at which a researcher defines his or her task will of course determine the level of analysis at which his or her explanation of behavior should work. If we see our task as explaining molar events, then molar theories will be preferred; if, on the other hand, molecular events were the level at which one wished to explain behavior, then molecular theories would be required.

Horner (2002) shows that at the level of the individual response (i.e., molecular level) there may be an underlying dynamic explaining behavior—there is some predictability and so presumably some deterministic rule that can explain it—but the dynamic for producing individual responses is chaotic, so our ability to predict the behavior of the organism at this level is limited. Therefore, we may be able to discover dynamic laws at the molecular level, but those laws may be of limited usefulness. This seems to indicate that we should abandon our analysis at the molecular level, but it really is only a caution about what we can expect from explanations at this level.

Although complex and difficult to predict, chaotic systems often produce well-ordered behavior. The butterfly shape of Lorenz attractor is a prime example. While the exact trajectory of this kind of system is difficult to predict for long intervals into the future, the overall form the behavior takes is easy to see. Therefore, while we may not be able to extend our predictions at the molecular level, our understanding of the dynamics at this level can tell us something of the overall form of behavior. Thus, we will have to compare the molar predictions of molecular theories in order to test them. The necessity of such comparisons does not rule out a molecular level of analysis or theorizing, but it does limit our expectations of molecular analysis. Instead, dynamic descriptions of behavior at the molecular level will have to be tested at the molar level, and our theories will necessarily only be practical at the molar level.

Horner's (2002) finding also tells us that our current methodologies may not be sufficient to handle the complexity of behavioral phenomena. Linear systems can be more easily broken into parts and then reassembled with each part solved. Such a process allows us to simplify complex linear systems by such methods as Laplace and Fourier transforms, and scientific methods that isolate relevant variables. Non-linear systems cannot be reassembled in the same fashion because addition of each new part does not sum to make the total (Tufillaro, Abbott, and Reilly 1992). Our auditory system may decompose a song into its respective frequencies, but playing two songs at the same time does not produce a coherent whole. Most of our research methodologies in psychology today are based upon linear techniques and we assume that a problem, once decomposed and solved, can be reassembled. However, if the underlying dynamic is non-linear, then this approach to behavior may reveal the important factors in the determination of behavior, but it does not allow us to reassemble that solution into a coherent whole. That would require a different methodology based upon non-linear dynamics.

Conclusion

Peirce's limit of inquiry thought experiment was formulated to provide a pragmatic definition of truth in an empirical context. When all methods of obtaining an answer to a particular empirical question dovetail into an agreement among observers, that agreed-upon answer is accepted as truth. Staddon's corollary to the limit of inquiry is not so much concerned with truth as it is with the state of affairs when all the questions have been sufficiently answered. When we have, in a sense, maximized our understanding of the world and ourselves, what can we expect of our explanations of behavior at the limit of inquiry?

For thousands of years, people have proposed various explanations of behavior, but these explanations have often been more a way of accounting for behavior rather than truly explaining it. An account, in this sense, is to argue that behavior is under the control of certain process, unseen or unobservable, and so contains a number of free variables that can be used to modify the predictions of behavior without having to independently verify either the variables' existence or their measurement. "I did it because I wanted to" is only one of the more egregious and common accounts of behavior. Behaviorism was a rebellion against this type of accounting and it set for itself the task of observing and measuring variables responsible for behavior. Of course, many behaviorists (e.g., Skinner 1987) have made just such an accounting of behavior by appealing to things practically unobservable, if potentially not—historical contingencies.

At the end of inquiry, if all questions are laid to rest, then we may expect no free variables in our explanations. Every theoretical construct will require an independent verification or measurement, or we will go looking for it. Questions will remain. Mental or theoretical constructs, which have questionable ontological status and so may not be verifiable by means independent of their use in a model, will disappear from the explanatory framework in favor of constructs that can find independent verification. This should lead in two different directions; one into biological reductionism and the other in search of functional relationships between the organism and the environment.

But these two directions or kinds of explanation, if they allow equivalent explanatory power, will either collapse into a single explanatory framework, or will be incommensurable at the limit of inquiry. One may hold a certain affinity to a given kind of explanation over another, but even if the first explanatory model proved initially more fruitful than the other and reached the limits of its own inquiry first, would we stop there? In psychology, even if we succeeded in describing all the functional laws of behavior first, would we stop there without knowing how the neural mechanisms that mediated them worked? Even if the limit of inquiry means no more questions, at some point we would have to push on and integrate the two perspectives.

Our ability to predict behavior will be limited. Even if we reach a limit of inquiry and understand all the factors affecting behavior, we will not be able to apply them with infinite certainty to our predictions of behavior. At some level those predictions will break down and we will be left with a degree of uncertainty. For those who have sought the soul, consciousness, or free will in a scientific worldview, I am sure this will eventually be reassuring. What we cannot predict—apparent randomness of behavior—will leave room for variables beyond our models, and so there will always be questions about the adequacy of our models and so too our place in the natural world. But at the limits of inquiry, we may maximize our understanding without achieving certainty. As Bronowski (1974) has pointed out, science—like art—cannot give us a perfect representation of the world, only strengthen our understanding of it. So it will ultimately be with a science of behavior. Our theories, whatever their form, will only give us a broader understanding, not accurate predictions.

But of course, this is only a thought experiment, a fun game, perhaps an interesting paper. Fortunately, we do not live at the limit of inquiry. What would it mean not to have any more questions? Like immortality, such a state sounds dull. But what can this thought experiment tell us about how we should conduct ourselves in a science of behavior?

First, while the history of psychology is strewn with unobservables—in a sense free variables of questionable validity—we should not forsake their use, but instead be cautious of their use. The less in doubt the ontological status of our theoretical constructs the better. Other fields have had remarkable success using theoretical constructs to make their theories fit the observed outcomes of their experiments (e.g., gene, neutron). And so, in many senses has psychology (e.g., synapses, inhibitory processes, receptors, trichromatic visual system, dual-process, etc.). But once we postulate these entities, if they prove useful enough, someone will go looking for them—in whatever form we propose. Whatever happened to the ether (Michelson and Morley 1887)? What will happen to all the dark matter and dark energy in the universe?

Where should we to draw the line over the use of unobservables in our theories? Certainly, where their ontological status is in question. Generally, where their number multiplies beyond the number of phenomena they purport to explain. Probably, where they provide little insight into related phenomena. But in general, if we stick to testing the general forms of our models, our experiments will point us in the way of the most fruitful theoretical entities.

Black-box theorizing may provide a suitable alternative to a purely functional approach in the near term (Staddon 2001a,b). However, black-box theorizing would have to pay off down the road with something more than a translation of functional relationships into a mechanistic explanatory framework. It would either have to pay off with real insights into behavioral phenomena or, more ambitiously, with insights into the structure and function of the underlying neural mechanism. If there is something in the box, then we should find something that corresponds to the proposed mechanism, or other mechanistic explanations will prevail. When we use a black-box approach we should always ask ourselves: Is this just another way to represent functional relationships? Have we gained a real insight? Should we expect to find a neurological mechanism to do what we are proposing? If not, what is the ontological status of the stuff in the black box?

Parsimony of explanation is not always an adequate guide for this approach. Parsimony is a statement of aesthetics in science, not a guarantee that we have hit upon the right answer. We often wonder at the exquisite efficiency of a bird's wing and marvel at natural selection's capacity to produce an optimized form, but evolution is also contingent upon the phylogeny of the species. Thus, evolved forms often express inefficiencies of design based upon historical contingencies (Gould 1980). There is thus no guarantee that the simplest mechanism proposed to account for behavioral data will in fact be the one that evolution has hit upon. Instead, natural selection may have "tinkered" a solution from processes that are already available to solve a particular problem, leaving us with a very un-simple solution. While Ockham's Razor usually cleaves away superfluous theorizing, it may not always be the best tool for cutting psychological phenomena.

Next, as our technology improves, mechanistic explanations may become more fruitful and less distinct from functional accounts. Some might argue this is already the case, but explanatory frameworks that simply located our ignorance in the functioning of the brain still abound in psychology and are no more fruitful than other accounts that utilize free variables. Like our misunderstanding of evolution in its early conception, our current understanding of the brain still does not give us many insights into behavior. Neurologizing, like ethologizing long ago, still seems like a risky approach to a science of behavior. However, strict adherence to a functional explanatory framework may continue to isolate us from the rest of the scientific enterprise. Other fields have found much fruit in the interstices between fields; so too may psychology. Certainly behaviorism's encounter with ethology in the middle of the twentieth century had a profound impact on our study. Neuroscience may prove to be an equally stimulating encounter.

When can psychologists jump in with both feet to try to integrate a functional and a neurological (mechanisms) approach to behavior? Most of us cannot; we are too far down our career paths to ever bridge the knowledge gap—effectively. But our students can, and it is time to start encouraging them to take our already well-developed fundamental understanding of simple behavioral processes to the neurological level in search of mechanistic explanations. Behaviorism's purely functional approach has succeeded, beyond even what we are willing to admit to ourselves; others can now take that understanding beyond our own field and our own explanatory framework to the rest of the scientific community.

Next, a full understanding of behavior will require something beyond the exclusive use of linear methods. Because non-linear systems cannot be reassembled from the analytic methodologies we use today, psychology needs to break out of the experimental methods so touted by our research design textbooks and instead focus on newer analytical techniques (Tufillaro, Abbott, and Reilly 1992).

Lastly, while being able to predict behavior down to the last gram of force applied to a response key may be a noble undertaking, it is probably a futile one. Who really cares? Our theories, whatever their form, should aim at explaining the molar aspects of behavior, not its most intricate detail. And here is where they should also be judged—at the molar level. The theoretical sophistication of psychology is probably greater than any other field in science. And, with enough parameters, even pigs can fly. As Staddon and Horner (1989) illustrated with relatively simple models, parameter setting in models can produce wildly different predictions. So how may we judge them? By their most obvious and fundamental predictions. Our theoretical capacity can far outstrip the fundamental behavioral phenomena we have to account for (e.g., Hull 1943). Thus our theories should at least make sense of those fundamental aspects rather than concentrate on the minutiae.

But here is the rub. As often happens in scientific discourse, the multiplication of assumptions and the concern with minutiae will take preeminence if we cannot recognize our own limits in this inquiry. Our tests require more than just an objective eye; they require a spirit of endeavor. If we are true to science, as opposed to our theories, we should be as critical of our own ideas as we are of others, and be prepared to admit where they do not explain the phenomena we set out for them to address. We need to be honest with ourselves—to have a "disinterested devotion to truth" (J. Staddon, personal communication, 2002)—so that both now, when the future will most likely prove all our theories wrong, and at the limit of inquiry, when as Peirce would argue the truth is known, we may call it a noble endeavor.

As an undergraduate at the University of Tennessee at Knoxville, I took a course from John Malone, then a recently hired student of John Staddon's. What Malone taught was unlike anything I had previously encountered in psychology courses. It was a field of both substance and verve. I asked him where I could learn more about this brand of psychology, and he sent me to John Staddon's lab at Duke. Here along with John were others who were seeking to understand behavior in a rigorous fashion—graduate students John Hinson and Alliston Reid and post-docs Ken Steele and Bob Dale. John Staddon set for us a program in which if we could reduce behavior to a small number of fundamental processes, it could be understood. For me, as a graduate student at Duke, Staddon opened up an enterprise in which behavior could be understood, and taught me that discovering something about it could be one of life's most sublime pleasures. I am grateful to John for having given me the opportunity to participate in one of the noblest things we humans can do: learn about our world. It is a wonderful endeavor.

14 Reflections on I-O Psychology and Behaviorism

John E. Kello

At first glance there would seem to be little intercourse between the traditions of John B. Watson and B. F. Skinner, on the one hand, and those of Hugo Münsterberg, Walter Dill Scott, and Frederick W. Taylor, on the other. Behaviorism as a guiding conceptual framework for the developing science of psychology grew out of the functionalism that characterized American psychology circa 1900, and was most visibly promoted by Watson. "Experimental Analysis of Behavior" (EAB) is familiar terminology for the conceptual and empirical approach to behaviorism as subsequently articulated by Skinner. Its research focus has centered on animal learning in the laboratory setting. Industrial-Organizational (I-O) psychology, quite in contrast, despite the occasional tongue-in-cheek reference to the "rat race," has focused squarely and explicitly on human behavior in the workplace.

So far, the case for intersection looks pretty bleak. Indeed, one could argue that of the various conceptual frameworks that guide the field of I-O psychology, behaviorism by that name, and certainly Skinner's EAB form of behaviorism, have been at best secondary in their impact. Behaviorism has surely been less salient in its effect than the ascendant and ubiquitous cognitive framework, or even the humanistic framework, which underlies so much of the employee-involvement and participative-management thrusts in contemporary I-O. Yet the founders and prime movers of behaviorism did not ignore the workplace and the prospective application of their work to that setting. Skinner (e.g., 1948a, 1953, 1969) occasionally makes reference to the workplace to illustrate the applicability of EAB principles to the practical control of behavior. Even Watson (1919) did at times propose that behaviorism clearly and obviously had application to human affairs in the workplace. And I will suggest that early Watsonian/methodological behaviorism, to the extent it is simply the fundamental application of the scientific method to psychology, always has been visible, is clearly visible still, and will continue to be visible in much of the theory and practice of I-O psychology. I will further suggest that even in the more radical Skinnerian EAB-sense, several important areas of I-O research and practice are overtly behavioristic, and unabashedly acknowledge their debt to Skinner.

The Past: Watson and Skinner and the World of Work

John B. Watson, the so-called father of behaviorism, was interested not just in basic research, but also in applying the principles of the new science to the practical control of behavior in the real world, including the world of work. His introductory textbook of psychology (Watson 1919), written before his unceremonious exit from academia and entry into the practical world of work, includes a fascinating chapter titled "The Organism at Work," which confidently states as a "law" that "the higher the incentive and the more uniform the incentive the more rapid and steady will be the improvement" (1919, p. 390). Watson goes on to say that "the industries recognize the law and even during the earliest apprenticeship period the attempt is made to give extra monetary reward, promises of future position, advancement and the like to increase the speed of acquisition" (p. 390). It is interesting to me that Watson, who preferred Pavlov's approach over Thorndike's as the basic platform for learning in the behaviorism he championed, nonetheless speaks comfortably of "rewards" and "incentives" as critical to generating and maintaining productivity in the workplace. Presumably the Law of Effect is okay at work, if not in the laboratory. No foolish consistency here! So, without fitting such speculative work tightly into the rigorous scientific methodology of behaviorism, Watson clearly saw the need for psychology to deal with the issues addressed by the early I-O psychologists, and in ways at least broadly consistent with the scientific method.

Skinner also saw his work in the animal laboratory as revealing general principles that applied even to the most complex issues of human behavior. Indeed he is at times praised and at times castigated for going well beyond his data to speculate on the practical effectiveness of the control of behavior by reinforcement in the world outside the box, and on the philosophical (not to say moral and ethical) implications of such an approach for concepts such as "personal freedom." The particulars of this broad philosophical debate are well known, certainly to readers of this volume, and require no further elaboration here.

In *Science and Human Behavior* (1953), Skinner addresses organizations in the real world in an instructive chapter titled "Economic Control." Conceptually, some controlling authority identifies desirable, functional behaviors, then arranges contingencies of positive reinforcement (aided and abetted by appropriate discriminative stimulus conditions, appropriate initial shaping, etc.) to strengthen and sustain high rates of those behaviors. By the same token (no pun), inappropriate, dysfunctional behaviors are explicitly disconnected from positive reinforcement opportunities (time out from positive reinforcement), and are thus extinguished.

The obvious universal positive reinforcer in the EAB equation as applied to the workplace is pay. In addressing the issue of pay as reinforcement directly, Skinner (1953) draws parallels between various "wage schedules" and schedules of reinforcement, acknowledging at the same time that most wage schedules are not pure examples of reinforcement schedules, and that the optimal-in-the-lab variable schedules may be largely impractical in the world of work. Even so, Skinner generally appears to support the parallel, noting that "In general the performance of an employee, like that of a laboratory animal, adjusts quite accurately to the exact contingencies of reinforcement" (Skinner 1953, p. 389). Despite some analogical rough edges, pay is the pellet.

In general terms, then, Skinner saw behavior in the workplace as no different than operant behavior in any other setting, and further asserted that organizations necessarily set up contingencies of reinforcement in their effort to strengthen and maintain high levels of appropriate work behaviors. End of story.

The Recent Past and the Present: Uses of Skinnerian and Methodological Behaviorism

While the effects of the "cognitive revolution" in psychology, indeed inspired in part by reactions against Skinner, are more widespread in I-O than are the effects of Skinner's work, the EAB approach is hardly of mere historical interest. And, the influence of methodological behaviorism is more pervasive still in recent and current research and practice in I-O.

I-O Psychology's Direct Applications of Skinnerian Behaviorism

While essentially all of Skinner's "work" on organizational behavior as operant behavior was speculative and not empirical, as early as the 1960s and the 1970s others began boldly applying their understanding of EAB to organizational problems in the real world, with acknowledgment to Skinner as the inspiration. One of the earliest and best-known examples was a behavioral intervention at the Emery Air Freight Corporation.

Emery Air Freight An Emery vice president named Edward J. Feeney, impressed by Skinner's work, implemented a series of applied EAB interventions aimed at increasing sales, improving call-response time by customer service representatives, and, in the best-known of the interventions, improving utilization of large bulk-pack shipping containers (Whyte 1972; *Business Week* 1972). In the latter case, the defining example of Skinnerian behaviorism's early forays into the world of work, managers were instructed to set a goal of "90 percent utilization" of bulk containers, and to have employees track their own performance against those goals with a shift-by-shift checklist. Further, managers were encouraged to use "positive reinforcement," by which they meant rewarding satisfactory performance with praise and expressions of appreciation, and where performance was below expectation, praising employees' honest record keeping and encouraging improvement instead of punishing substandard results. Once these steps were taken (indeed once the "program" was announced), almost instantly performance met and exceeded the 90 percent goal, saving the company an estimated $3 million (in 1960s–1970s dollars) over a three-year period (Schultz and Schultz 2002). The Emery Air Freight example is often cited in general as a defining example of early operant interventions in the workplace, and sometimes more specifically as an example of the effectiveness of "self-feedback" as a kind of reinforcement.

Even setting aside the concept of "self-feedback as reinforcement," there is some legitimate question as to whether the Emery Air Freight intervention is in fact anything like a "pure" Skinnerian application. Nonetheless it was widely taken as such (there were no glowing paeans to Thorndike or Bandura, much less to cognitive psychology, in the recounting of the Emery story). It may be considered the opening chapter in what has become known as Organization Behavior Management (OBM), the most direct application of Skinner's approach to the workplace, to which we will return shortly.

Hawthorne Revisited by Skinnerian Behaviorism Around the time the Emery Air Freight story and a handful of other early applications of Skinner's approach to the workplace were being widely publicized, reanalyses of the original data from the classic "Hawthorne studies" conducted some 50 years earlier strongly challenged the prevalent "human relations" interpretation of the data (e.g., Mayo 1933; Roethlisberger and Dickson 1939). While Mayo et al. claimed to find (and secondary sources widely endorse that claim) that humane treatment of employees caused them to perform well and enjoy their work regardless of the physical working conditions to which they were exposed (the "Hawthorne Effect"), latter-day reanalyses suggested strongly that the productivity and job-satisfaction improvements were mainly attributable to performance-contingent pay/incentive systems, coupled with ongoing performance feedback. Things being equal (difficult to assess, as so many variables were changed concurrently in the Hawthorne studies), workers were more productive to the extent that their pay was tied contingently to their performance, and to the extent they had access to frequent ongoing performance feedback so they could know how they were doing at any point in time in terms of achieving their bonuses (e.g., Parsons 1974, 1992; Peach and Wren 1992; Rice 1982). Indeed, interviews with the Hawthorne workers had indicated that the workers not only "enjoyed the working conditions," but also that they "enjoyed the opportunity to make more money" (e.g., Peach and Wren 1992). If the lead researcher had been the young Harvard psychologist B. F. Skinner instead of the Harvard Business School professors Fritz Roethlisberger and Elton Mayo, how very different the Hawthorne conclusions might have been!

The Organization Behavior Management (OBM) Approach As much as Skinnerian behaviorism has been and is still controversial, and as much as it has diminished in impact on the field of psychology as a whole, there are several topic areas in I-O psychology which have imported Skinner's EAB methodology and philosophy rather directly, with credit given explicitly to Skinner. The form of "Applied Behavior Analysis" that uses operant methodology in the work setting, known sometimes in its early evolutions as "organizational behavior modification" or "O.B. Mod" (e.g., Kreitner and Luthans 1991), more commonly in recent years has gone by the name "Organization Behavior Management" or OBM. Examples of the basic OBM approach are sometimes labeled "A-B-C" models (e.g., Kreitner and Luthans 1991). In such terms, the C variable is the Consequence for behavior, ideally the positive reinforcer. The B variable is the target Behavior, on the basis of which the reinforcer is presented contingently. The A variable, heretofore not emphasized, is the "Antecedent" condition, or sometimes the "Activator," i.e., a cue which specifies the contingency, or sets the occasion for the response being reinforced. The A variable, then, "signals" the availability of reinforcement. In Skinnerian terms, A-variables are the equivalent of discriminative stimuli.

A foundational OBM model, developed by Komaki, Coombs, and Schepman (1991) and still widely cited, is typical of the general OBM approach. (See also Riggio 2000.) Komaki et al. suggest four steps, identified in a specific workplace safety intervention, as defining the OBM approach:

1. Specify desired behavior
2. Measure desired performance
3. Provide frequent, contingent positive consequences
4. Evaluate effectiveness on the job

Note that while the reinforcement in OBM studies commonly includes financial consequences (i.e., pay as the positive reinforcer), this is not inevitably true. According to Komaki et al. (1991), the reinforcing consequence may take any of several forms, including "organizational" (pay raise, promotion), "generalized" (cash incentive, gift certificate), "activity" (opportunity to engage in preferred activity contingent upon completing a less preferred activity), "social" (praise, recognition), and "informational" (performance feedback).

The OBM approach has been applied over the last 30 years or so to a wide array of organizational behaviors, including attendance/punctuality behaviors, sales/customer-service behaviors, and perhaps most prominently, safe work behaviors. The work of Scott Geller and his students and colleagues at Virginia Tech (e.g., Geller et al. 1986) represents some of the best work on "behavior-based safety." (For another early example of the use of a "token economy" to promote safe acts, see Fox, Hopkins, and Anger 1987.) The central thesis of the behavior-based approach to safety is that the problem is unsafe acts (rather than, say, negative attitudes, "accident proneness," or other underlying problems), and that the solution is simply to replace the unsafe behavior patterns with safe acts. The methodology for doing so is simply the positive reinforcement of targeted safe behaviors, and the prompting of them with effective antecedents to increase their likelihood of occurrence.

Where OBM strategies are applied to the workplace, there has always been a legitimate question as to the behavioristic "purity" of the interventions, going back at least as far as the Emery Air Freight example. As a practical matter, such reinforcement programs commonly supplement (in many cases heavily) the core A-B-C process with "explanation." That is to say, one does not simply one day start up an incentive program, and leave it to the employee/participants to gradually behave in ways consistent with the prevailing contingencies of reinforcement. Rather, meetings are commonly held in which the issues are identified and discussed, in some cases "commitment strategies" are used, and in general people are encouraged to think and make a public decision to participate, etc. (e.g., Kello, Geller, Rice, and Bryant 1988). In fairness then, the typical behavior-based safety intervention in fact is often a blend of behavioral and cognitive strategies (at least), which would be quite congenial to those of a social learning theory persuasion. To me as a sometime practitioner tutored by some of the best, OBM in practice, for all its Skinnerian trappings and overtly acknowledged debt to Skinner, looks and sounds a lot like cognitive behaviorism or social learning theory. Indeed, Kreitner and Luthans (1991) extol social learning theory as the step beyond OBM, as including the core behavioral elements of OBM, but also incorporating, appropriately they note, cognitive variables. But in OBM the behaviorist common core is inevitably there, and "to eliminate the reinforcer is to eliminate the effectiveness of the program."

I-O Psychology's Quasi-Applications of Skinnerian Behaviorism

There are areas of research and practice in recent and current I-O for which Skinner is often given direct credit, whether deserved or not.

Motivation Theory Contemporary I-O psychology shows the strong influence of "operant theory" or "reinforcement theory" in the venerable area of work motivation. An informal survey of several popular contemporary texts in I-O psychology indicates that "operant," "behavioral," or "reinforcement" approaches to motivation, traced explicitly and directly to Skinner alone (only rarely including any acknowledgment of debt to Thorndike—e.g., Hamner 1991; Steers and Porter 1991), are almost always presented as a class of motivation model, on a par with so-called need or content theories such as Maslow's hierarchy and Alderfer's Existence, Relatedness and Growth (ERG) Theory, and cognitive or expectancy theories such as Vroom's General Expectancy Theory and Adams's Equity Model (Dipboye, Smith, and Howell 1994; Jewell 1998; Landy 1989; Muchinsky 2000).

Within I-O psychology, some have noted the awkwardness attendant upon the notion of a Skinnerian "theory," or an operant focus on a hypothetical construct, at all (e.g., Landy 1989; Steers and Porter 1991). Yet philosophical consistency to the contrary, operant or behaviorist or reinforcement theory remains a centerpiece of motivation theory in contemporary I-O psychology.

Just how Skinnerian is the "operant theory" of motivation? To be sure, operant theory asserts that the essential key to building and sustaining work effort and performance, and hence ultimate worker productivity, is the contingency between the desired behavior and positive reinforcement. But while sometimes viewed as a distinguishing feature of the operant approach (e.g., Komaki, Coombs, and Schepman 1991) this core idea is obviously not proprietary to Skinner. The contingency-criticality assumption, clearly visible in Thorndike's Law of Effect, and with a history in philosophy pre-dating Thorndike by many, many years, is also central to several alternative theoretical approaches to motivation which are primarily identified as "cognitive" theories, and which otherwise are not in even any remote sense, Skinnerian. Indeed they are commonly somewhat *juxtaposed* to the "operant theory" of motivation. Thus, for example, Victor Vroom's (1964) influential cognitive, general expectancy, or VIE theory, as much as it depends on the internal workings of the worker's hypothesized mental calculus, also depends crucially on there being a relationship between performance and "valued outcomes" (as explained in the model, presumably an equivalent concept to "reinforcers"). Similarly, the influential Adams Equity Model of motivation (e.g., Adams 1963) centers on how people increase or decrease the amount and quality of their work as a function of their appraisal of their reward in comparison with the reward of others. While there is clearly much cognitive machination going on here, a central feature of Adams's theory is the assumed universal necessity of reward or reinforcement in any consideration of motivation. Reward (and its presumed contingent relationship with performance) is the ultimate anchor point of the equity assessment. The primary "inputs" that are gauged in the calculus of the cognitive models are considerations of performance-contingent reward, usually pay.

Additionally, as there is no generally agreed upon overarching motivation theory in I-O, many texts include in their stock chapter on Motivation (sometimes titled "Motivation and Job Satisfaction") a section on "integrative" or "synthetic" models, or at least list as practical guidelines an eclectic set of principles which attempt to combine the best features of the existing theories into a comprehensive and usable motivation framework for research and for practice (e.g., Jewell 1998). Virtually without exception a few core elements of the operant model are highlighted in such eclectic, integrative/synthetic approaches, including prominently that desired behaviors must be identified in very specific terms and that rewards must be contingent on those desired behaviors. Typically there is a grab bag of collateral assumptions, but the integrative models of motivation (e.g., Green and Hayes 1993; Katzell and Thompson 1990; Porter and Lawler 1968) universally incorporate a requisite performance/reinforcer contingency.

The operant approach to motivation largely reduces to the principle that response-contingent reward strengthens behavior. Little of the other apparatus of EAB is to be found there. "Reinforcement theory" of motivation may be Skinnerian only in the very loose sense that Skinner gets so much credit for popularizing the notion. The central issue may be whether the law of effect, empirical or otherwise, is considered proprietary to the EAB approach; if a theoretical approach to motivation asserts that performance-contingent financial incentives "work," is that approach *ipso facto* an operant theory?

Pay Systems? In Skinner's broad equation of pay systems with schedules of reinforcement, the most obvious reinforcer for functional work behaviors is pay. Monetary reward is certainly one of the most potent reinforcers or outcomes that make the various motivation models "work." The whole area of compensation systems would seem to be a natural point of contact between Skinner's behaviorism and motivation theory in I-O psychology. Thus one might well expect an extensive literature harmonizing pay systems with what is known about schedules of reinforcement, and giving practical Skinnerian guidelines for the design and implementation of more effective systems. There is indeed some literature on pay systems as schedules-of-reinforcement, though remarkably little given the prominence of operant motivation theory. By and large, actual hourly or salary pay systems are classical, traditional ones, developed and implemented independent of operant principles. Even newer pay systems such as "pay-for-knowledge" and "pay-for-skill," which are visible in some team-based organizations (Orsburn, Moran, Musselwhite, and Zenger 1990), and incentive-compensation systems such as "gainsharing," which are to some extent performance-based, are not drawn from the EAB well. In short, there is almost no intersection of actual pay systems with Skinner's principles. While one might speculate at length as to why this is so, one obvious reason is that despite Skinner's apparent comfort with the general pay-system/reinforcement schedule analogy, a weekly or monthly paycheck does not represent an FI schedule in any simple sense, and no one has figured out how to effectively pay on a VR or VI schedule (presumably in an effort to sustain high rates of appropriate target behaviors).

In sum, I argue that contemporary I-O psychology shows direct influence of the EAB approach, as reflected in the popularity of OBM interventions, especially in workplace safety; that contemporary I-O shows a more indirect influence of EAB in motivation theory, in that the "operant" or "reinforcement" theory, attributed to Skinner, continues to be prominently emphasized; and that there is some assumed parallel between pay systems and schedules of reinforcement, though that theme is much less prominent in I-O than the other two.

I will further assert that contemporary I-O psychology shows a strong influence of methodological behaviorism, in the original Watsonian sense of focusing attention on observable behavior, and in general applying the scientific method to the study of behavior.

I-O Psychology's Applications of Methodological Behaviorism: A Sampler

Independent of any direct tie to EAB methodology and language, much of contemporary I-O psychology takes a broadly methodological-behaviorist tack of focusing on observable behavior rather than on unobservable hypothetical constructs such as attitude and disposition when working a wide variety of specific I-O applications. Consider as just a modest sampling the following few diverse areas of I-O research and application which in my judgment clearly bear the strong stamp of methodological behaviorism. Again, my examples are selected to illustrate the breadth of application of methodological behaviorist thinking in the field, and are by no means exhaustive.

Performance Appraisal Systems A classical focus of I-O research has been, and continues to be, performance appraisal systems. Commonly, annual reviews of performance determine, at least in part, raises, promotion opportunities, and other rewards. In general there has been a historical progression from "trait-based" approaches to more outcomes-based and behavior-based approaches (e.g., Jewell 1998; Landy and Farr 1980).

The focus on employee behavior, which became prominent in research on performance appraisal systems starting in the 1960s (Jewell 1998; Smith and Kendall 1963), resulted in the development of several types of behavior-based instruments such as the prototype Behaviorally Anchored Rating Scale (BARS), and the derivative Behavioral Observation Scale (BOS) and Mixed Standard Scale (MSS). In each case the central point is to shift performance review away from the traditional/classical "trait-based" approach (which "measured" such personal characteristics as cooperativeness, dependability, and teamwork) and away from the outcomes-based approach (focusing for example on overall reduced cost, improved customer-satisfaction ratings, or increased volume of sales) to direct behavior-assessment approaches (e.g., number of sales calls made per week, or mean time to answer phone inquiries). Despite some criticism, and general waning of interest in finding the "ideal" performance appraisal instrument (e.g., Arvey and Murphy 1998; Dipboye, Smith, and Howell 1994; Landy and Farr 1980), the behavioral approach to performance appraisal continues to be quite visible in contemporary I-O psychology.

While some (e.g., Kreitner and Luthans 1991) have connected the behavioral approach to performance appraisal rather directly to OBM through the mere fact of the emphasis of such appraisal systems on observable behavior, the behavioral focus in performance appraisal is not usually linked conceptually to Skinnerian behaviorism at all.

CRM Methodology Another important and perhaps unlikely application of methodological behaviorism is in the area of "cockpit resource management" or "crew resource management" programs (e.g., Wiener, Kanki, and Helmreich 1993). These programs were first begun in commercial aviation (hence the "cockpit" designation), but subsequently applied to a wide variety of settings in which team-coordination under potentially stressful conditions is critical, such as the medical operating room, the nuclear control room, and the military-team setting (obviously of crucial and increasing importance in these uncertain times). These programs, at first, look a lot more like applied social psychology/group dynamics than they do behaviorism in any form. Admittedly, several of the prime movers in this area, including prominently Bob Helmreich and his colleagues and students at the University of Texas, are social psychologists by training and by persuasion. And, core elements of typical CRM training programs, whether aimed at airline pilots, medical OR teams, military combat teams, or nuclear control-room crews, do include questionnaire-based attitude measures. Indeed the earliest and most longstanding measures of the effectiveness of CRM programs have been "attitude change" measures (e.g., the Cockpit Management Attitudes Questionnaire (Helmreich 1984)). Historically, programs have been considered successful to the extent they were associated with a shift in the measured attitudes of participants toward more receptivity to the content of the program.

Yet some of the best "second-generation" work in CRM has focused not only or even mainly on group dynamics, climate, or attitude change *per se*, as important as those may be. Rather, it has focused on identifying the "behavioral markers" of effective crew performance (e.g., Helmreich, Kello, Chidester, Wilhelm, and Gregorich 1990), both to give pilots a clear sense of what good resource management looks and sounds like in very concrete and specific behavioral terms and to give their instructors similarly clear guidelines for evaluation of pilot performance. Simply put, how will a crew, or an evaluating flight instructor/check pilot, know when the crew is communicating and coordinating effectively? What is "good communication and coordination"—that is, how will we operationally define it in terms of observable behavior? The behavioral markers developed in each of these areas are now widely used in initial CRM training, and in post-training "checking" of pilots, to provide guidelines for check pilots to use in assessing the effectiveness of a cockpit crew and its individual members

(Helmreich, Wilhelm, Kello, Taggart, and Butler 1991). To the extent that I have personally contributed anything to this important applied area, it is the focus on behaviorally anchoring the competency areas or skill sets we are attempting to improve through CRM training.

Assessment Centers In the 1940s, in support of the war effort, the US Office of Strategic Services, with the help of I-O psychologists, developed a tool which has become known as the "assessment center" (Riggio 2000; Thornton and Byham 1982). Based on earlier seminal work by Henry Murray at Harvard University in the 1930s (Bray 1982), the OSS application involved putting candidates for highly sensitive military intelligence jobs through simulations of the types of stressful situations they might face in the field.

In the mid 1950s, the assessment center methodology as developed for the OSS was reportedly first applied to management development and selection at AT&T (e.g., Bray 1982; Muchinsky 2000; Thornton and Byham 1982). Since then, assessment centers have been used by many companies in the identification, selection, promotion, and development of talent for a variety of positions, most commonly managerial/leadership positions. While there are today many variations on the theme, there are some meaningful common denominators that apply to most iterations of the methodology. Thus, in a management assessment center, individual "candidates" might have to address problems (e.g., technical, personnel, safety) of the sort that incumbent managers in the organization would have to address. The tasks commonly come to them via an "in basket," i.e., memos and other communications which might come across the desk of an incumbent manager (these days, "in-basket" activities may include e-mail and voice mail, to the extent that these are appropriate to the role being assessed). As candidates work their way through the simulation (typically a multi-day process), the assessors observe and "score" them on a variety of performance dimensions that are central to the role for which they are being assessed.

One of the most critical elements in the contemporary assessment center is the "competencies set," which identifies the skills and abilities on which the participants are to be evaluated (e.g., Spychalski, Quinones, Gaugler, and Pohley 1997; International Task Force on Assessment Center Guidelines 2000). In the assessment center work I have done, the competencies list is abetted by a listing of "behavioral markers," which are observable manifestations of the competency in question. Much as with the work on CRM, the approach I have taken with the assessment center methodology is to take a general methodological behavioral orientation, to ground the work entirely in observable behaviors rather than global clinical impressions of "leadership."

The High Performance Organization Model In terms of macro organizational theory in I-O psychology, much contemporary thinking centers on the High Performance Organization (HPO) model (e.g., Gephardt and van Buren 1996; Neusch and Siebenaler 1998). The model derives from sociotechnical systems/whole-system theory, which took shape in the 1940s and the 1950s (e.g., Pasmore 1988; Weisbord 1992). The argument is that the early exemplars of mass manufacturing, often using an assembly-line-type production process, spawned a macro organizational model (today commonly referred to as the "traditional organization") that was basically a mechanistic, clockwork model. The organization was conceptualized as a big machine. In terms of this model, derived from the Scientific Management approach developed and popularized by Frederick W. Taylor around the turn of the century (see e.g. Taylor 1911), if the organizational production and support systems were designed well and every element played its part properly, a high volume of finished goods would roll off the end of the line and all would be well. Indeed, this mechanistic model of the organization predominated in American industry into the 1960s and the 1970s, and spread to a whole range of non-industrial organizations as well. It came to represent "how business was done."

In contrast to this model, the HPO model is an organic model, based on a qualitatively different view of the organization as an animate thing, a living biological system which exchanges inputs and outputs with an environment, and must adapt successfully to, and to some extent manage, that environment for its survival. Indeed, one of the seminal influences in the development of the HPO model was Ludwig von Bertalanffy's 1950 paper on open-systems theory in biology and physics. In HPO terms, then, the organization is better conceived as an organism or a superorganism (perhaps a colony or an ecosystem) than it is a big machine. Important components of this model in action include the use of teams rather than individuals as the primary working unit, multi-skilling of individuals into more flexible workers with broadened responsibilities, and developing supervisors into facilitators and coaches rather than workers and work-controllers (e.g., Gephardt and van Buren 1996).

One of the most important elements, often overlooked in our excitement about job enrichment, workplace democracy, participative management, etc., is the focus on behavior and the role of pay and other financial incentives in the HPO model. Thus, HPO models strongly encourage the use of any of a variety of forms of performance-based pay, i.e., establishing a clear contingency between performance (typically behaviors and results—which must be operationalized, stated to employees in specific terms, and measured) and pay. Beyond simple performance-based pay, the HPO approach also promotes "pay-for-knowledge" or "pay-for-skill" compensation plans. Simply put, these pay systems reward an employee for broadening his or her knowledge and skill base in ways which can be observed and measured. When an individual on such a system learns an expanded set of skills and is able to be more flexible, working any of a number of jobs, he or she is paid at a higher base level (whether the pay is hourly or monthly). Clearly, such a pay system supports the goal of a multi-skilled workforce (Orsburn et al. 1990).

The teams focus in the HPO is commonly linked with the concept of self-direction or self-management. It is expected that the team will be developed to the point that it can regulate itself and function as a semi-autonomous unit, in alignment with the rest of the organization. Part of the multi-skilling commonly includes not just learning more jobs ("horizontal loading") but learning to plan, coordinate, and manage jobs more autonomously ("vertical loading"). Admittedly, the literature on work teams rarely links explicitly with the literature of behaviorism. But, the self-management concept central to self-directed teams is addressed in the OBM literature (e.g., Komaki et al. 1991) as well as in cognitive-behavioral approaches such as social learning theory (e.g., Kreitner and Luthans 1991). While this link has not been well developed in the literature, at least on the surface there is some connection between the HPO concept of self-direction and the OBM concept of self-control. Here the behaviorist influence may be potentially even stronger than the general methodological behaviorist influence that pervades the HPO approach.

In sum, as far removed from behaviorism as the world of the HPO may seem at first glance, once again the focus on observable behavior is central, and "it is difficult to overestimate the pervasiveness of the idea of reinforcement contingency in human social thought" (Staddon 2001b, p. 112), even in I-O macro-organizational theory.

Whither Behaviorism in the Workplace?

I-O psychology seems to be a very self-conscious part of the discipline of psychology as a whole. There is a fair amount of interest in identifying where we have come from, where we have been, and where we are now. And there seems to be a great deal of interest in speculating about where we may be going next. On the latter topic, there are a number of thoughtful papers (e.g., Cascio 1995) and text chapters (e.g., Dipboye, Smith, and Howell 1994) which paint a common picture of the future of I-O psychology. The cognitive framework predominates. Behaviorism in any form is not seen as a major thrust in the field going forward (Dipboye, Smith, and Howell 1994; Jewell 1998). But as long as employee motivation, pay/reward systems, safety, absenteeism, and turnover continue to be important elements of the field of I-O, the impact of Skinnerian behaviorism will likely continue to be seen rather directly. As I have argued, methodological behaviorism is everywhere.

To take but one example, the relatively new I-O subfield of Organization Development (OD) is among the fastest-growing and highest-impact areas of the field (e.g., Jewell 1998), and will likely represent an increasingly salient trend in the future of I-O. Rooted in the work of Kurt Lewin, OD's founding and informing assumptions are those of experimental social psychology, the Hawthorne-inspired human relations movement (Roethlisberger and Dickson 1939), and humanistic psychology. Its more or less standard tools include team building, process consultation, and laboratory/sensitivity training, among other similar interactive problem-solving and relationship-building techniques (e.g., Cummings and Worley 1997). On the surface, and even at a bit of depth, there appears to be little intersection between OD and behaviorism. Yet I would argue that effective OD practitioners draw heavily on behaviorism in the daily practice of their craft. Consider the following case study drawn from my files.

Organization Development Case Study

A large division of a major industrial company was experiencing internal friction and strife between its Sales and Production groups. The problem was not new, but had escalated over recent months to the point that it was beginning to wear on the organization. Top leaders wanted the two warring factions to get along and work together for the benefit of the whole—now! So, they sat them down and told them so. Their exhortations to that effect mainly resulted in flurries of intensified finger pointing and blame assignment between Sales and Production, and no improvement in the working climate. Leaders then engaged me as an external third-party helper.

Management's first response was a "solution," namely that "the consultant do some teambuilding" and maybe reiterate management's "you oughtta wanna" speech, and that, perhaps combined with some so-called trust activities, would take care of it.

It would have been easy simply to accept the client's diagnosis and solution, and just do some generic teambuilding to help Sales and Production "make nice" because they oughtta wanna. But, in my experience, when there is perceived conflict and lack of cooperation, the causes are not automatically "personality clashes" or "blockers" with bad attitudes, as much as those prospective "causes" are commonly volunteered by the client, and as much as they may at times in fact play a substantial role. Rather, I would look first at the reward system. It is an excellent, highly serviceable heuristic in the OD business that lack of cooperation is often driven by incompatible rewards between groups or individuals. We can preach altruism until we are blue in the face, but the more effective strategy is to ensure that reward systems are aligned such that behaviors that are functional to the whole system are rewarded at the local level.

In this particular case, I first gathered my own independent view of the problem in behavioral terms, to determine who was doing what that was creating the perceived problem. I found that the Sales and Production groups had been traditionally "siloed," and from their perspective each saw the other as unhelpful. The expressed attitudes could be paraphrased thus: "We just don't get along, because they don't understand us (and won't try to), and we can't get through to them." Not surprisingly, my initial data gathering indicated that there was indeed significant misalignment of reward, though no one I interviewed or observed drew this conclusion. Indeed, a little poking around revealed that the reward systems were not just misaligned—they were actively at odds! The Sales organization was rewarded for a high-dollar sale, plain and simple. Sometimes customers asked Sales for products which were hard to make in Production, and in some cases relatively unprofitable to make, from a plant-budget perspective. Some of these products were nearly interchangeable with other products which Production had in abundance in existing inventory. No matter. That was not Sales's concern. As long as they "got the order," they were rewarded, they lived in their functional silo, and life was good.

Further, Sales set a forecast at the beginning of the year, which both established their sales goals, and separately strongly influenced Production budgets that were set at the plant level. If a sales representative beat his or her quota, he or she was rewarded additionally on a sales-incentive plan. Production, in sharp contrast, was rewarded for running their volume of product efficiently, and controlling costs in the plants, thus staying within their budgets. One of their high costs, a real drag on their budgets, was inventory. When Sales "dropped a big order on them" for an item not in inventory, and which they might lose money to produce, their budgets were wrecked for the month at least, and sometimes for the year. Compounding the problem, last-minute orders often required additional crewing and/or additional overtime scheduling, further torpedoing plant budgets.

The crux of this OD intervention was not teambuilding. It was a structural realignment of the reward system. Sales and Production were put on a common bonus plan which was anchored to the volume of profitable business sold, produced, and delivered. Sales made money when they sold a high-margin product and/or pushed inventory. Production made money essentially the same way, when they kept Sales informed about operating status and inventory, and thereby helped Sales move the heavily inventoried and/or cheap-to-produce products. The new reward system put a premium on joint planning and scheduling between Sales and Production, and naturally spawned regular joint Sales/Production meetings, which in and of themselves greatly improved the working relationship between the two groups. Such meetings would have been almost unthinkable under the former reward system.

Having thus helped to properly realign the reward system, I must now confess that as a second wave of this intervention we did indeed follow up with some teambuilding activities, targeted closely to the needs of the previously warring factions, to help them begin to learn more adaptive ways of working together in the new system. In the spirit of full disclosure, I will further acknowledge that some of this follow-up work approached what the client initially had in mind when they first represented the "problem" as "They need teambuilding." The former inter-departmental antagonists were given the venerable Myers-Briggs Type Indicator, and in later evolutions of the project, the more contemporary NEO PI-R tests based on the wildly popular Five Factor Model of personality (e.g., Costa and McCrae 1985), to identify personality profile variances among the Sales and Production groups. Such work went well beyond merely identifying dispositional differences between the Sales and Production folks ("You are High-E and she is Low-E—isn't that interesting?") to focus on so-called workaround behaviors and behavioral contracting, in an effort to improve their ability to get along and work collaboratively with different behavioral styles.

We did this group work in part because I think it is genuinely helpful to the players involved to reach a higher level of self-understanding and other-understanding (especially in usable behavioral terms), and partly because the client REALLY wanted it. But, to do so as the first or only strategy would, in my judgment, be tip-toeing around a rather large lump in the carpet, viz., the patently obvious mismatch in the reward structure for the two groups. Unless and until we created alignment and commonality in the reward systems for the two groups, no teambuilding of any sort would stand much of a chance of yielding durable positive change. Appeal as we might to their better instincts and the need for teamwork, enlighten them as we might about the inherent potential for conflict between "Judgers" and Perceivers," they would, not unlike the employees at the Hawthorne works some 75 years before, nonetheless continue to perform in accordance with the prevailing reward contingencies. Such is my passionate belief, based on abundant experience.

In general I think that it is common for effective OD consultants to bring the basic framework of methodological behaviorism to bear on organizational problems, which are usually client-identified in everyday commonsense terms of attitude, work ethic, teamwork, personality conflicts, and the like, and rarely specified as behavioral or reward-system problems. This is all reasonable enough from the layperson's perspective, and frankly I don't doubt that such problems as work ethic at times do exist. But I think most folks slide comfortably into what social psychologists call the Fundamental Attribution Error and assume that such problems are at their base dispositional ("that's just the way those guys are") and stop looking further even when the problems are in fact at their base situational/behavioral, as in my experience they very often are.

In sum, I must reemphasize that I think the behavioral approach to OD that I have illustrated here is by no means idiosyncratic to me. I think it is fair to say that the effective OD consultants I know of, that is, those whose work makes a tangible and durable difference in whatever ways that might be measured, necessarily use something like the same general approach. They use the client's "diagnosis" only as a starting point. They identify the problematic behaviors that are at issue, and look at effective ways of changing them. They definitely look at the reward system that is supporting those maladaptive behaviors. Their interventions commonly aim at aligning reward systems so that when individuals behave so as to get what they want, they thereby automatically contribute to the team, department, division, and company achieving their goals.

Concluding Thoughts

My central thesis is that behaviorism has contributed much to the field of I-O psychology throughout the short history of the discipline, although that contribution is usually explicitly acknowledged only in certain delimited areas of the field. Though the conventional wisdom has it that behaviorism is on the wane (or is dead, and has been so for some time now), behaviorism in many of its forms continues to influence I-O psychology, and strongly, as I hope I have illustrated in this essay. As much as we may trumpet the reassertion of cognitivism in psychology as a whole and in I-O as a part, the impact of behaviorism on I-O, whether acknowledged by that name or not, is likely to continue to be felt, even in such relatively "soft" areas of the field as OD. Indeed, for the advancement of I-O as a discipline it will continue to be critically important to focus on observable behavior, and on the techniques that actually work to promote constructive behavior change.

I owe a tremendous debt of gratitude to several mentors who have helped to shape my thinking about the issues addressed in this essay and have guided me in applying these ideas as a practitioner. While I have been privileged to learn from some of the very best, none of my mentors has done more to influence my thinking than the extraordinary scientist who is honored in this volume. My understanding of behaviorism and my conviction that a behavioral approach is a necessity for a science and practice of psychology were developed during my early apprenticeship under John Staddon. I have never sufficiently thanked him (nor could I), but I hope that this modest chapter in his honor will be accepted in the spirit of a very partial repayment of a very large debt.

IV Behaviorism and the Social Sciences

15 A New Paradigm for the Integration of the Social Sciences

Giulio Bolacchi

After more than a century of development, the social sciences, particularly economics, psychology, and sociology, face basic internal problems that each separately seems unable to solve.

The Need for Integration of the Social Sciences

Economics is the most developed social science on a syntactic level, since the consistency of its language is guaranteed by the use of mathematics and, in its more modern version, by axiomatization in algebraic and topological terms (formulated by Debreu (1959)). However, the *semantic interpretation*[1] (Carnap 1959, p. 202ff.) of economic language is not as certain, since there is still no experimental verification that makes this interpretation completely univocal, despite the many efforts have been and are still being made. Consequently, economic semantics usually falls back on common sense. Therefore only a normative value is commonly ascribed to economic theory in its present state (as well as to many social theories), since it is syntactically consistent[2] but it is lacking in experimental verification. This means, in behavioristic terms, that economics has to be learned in order to be implemented (even if economists generally are inclined not to agree with this conclusion).

Psychology is primarily divided into two approaches, which express themselves through two different languages: the cognitive language, which by definition considers mental states (thinking, mind, motivation) to be the causes of behavior (a position similar to that of sociology); and the behavioristic language, which is the only one founded on controlled experiment and whose semantic interpretation implies consequently a strictly scientific perspective (although it has not yet arrived at a univocally determinate and syntactically consistent theoretical paradigm).

Sociology and cognitive psychology at best use statistical (especially multivariate) analysis. Despite this, the semantic interpretation of their variables is devoid of any experimental context. Therefore they also rely on common sense, which results in a multiplicity of theoretical hypotheses that are often inconsistent with one another.

But an even more serious problem lies in the current *disjointness*[3] among the social sciences. Even though they all have as subject matter the study of man and society, they have no common ground; i.e., they do not attempt to make their own languages compatible with a consistent system of primary assumptions to which all the expressions of the different specific languages might be logically brought back.

This situation brings about an anomalous separation, involving both research and profession, among the different social sciences. It follows that the (more or less abstract) *domains of application* (Carnap 1959, pp. 52, 240) of the different languages fix limits to the single disciplines, ruling out any hypothesis of relations among the different language sets.

As a matter of fact, this situation should make us reflect on the adequacy of the languages related to the three fields of knowledge (each of which is subdivided into a more or less large number of specific languages) to explicate a set of phenomena that, in point of fact, are strictly related to each other (Bolacchi 2004, p. 475ff.).

If the phenomena concerning man and society are strictly related to each other, it appears difficult to justify the disjointness among economics, psychology and sociology. This disjointness, besides preventing the construction of a unitary theoretical reference paradigm, supports within the different disciplines such extensive "degrees of freedom" in research methods, theoretical schemata, and language tools that their languages often are not in accordance with the criteria for scientific (experimental) explanation (*explication*). In short, the partition[4] expresses disjoint equivalence classes founded on generic (indeterminate) experiential-type[5] properties,[6] lacking in experimental verification, and therefore cannot be held as a solid scientific basis of reference. This is confirmed by the common-sense arguments advanced within each separate social science that serve to emphasize the presumed differences and peculiarities that each one claims.

The Language of Science

Its Syntactic and Semantic Standards

Each science is a linguistic construction, quantitative in principle: (1) whose logical syntax is characterized, in the most abstract sense, by that specific subset of the Cartesian product $(A \times B)$,[7] where to each first element of any ordered pair there corresponds one and only one second element (function)[8]; (2) whose semantic interpretation is susceptible of different levels of abstraction, which correspond to the order[9] deriving from the (transitive) relation of inclusion[10] among subsets defined by specific properties (two-place or predicates).

These levels of abstraction can be made explicit or not in accordance with the state of progress of the research. They take their stand in a range from the highest levels of abstraction (which are expressed by the sets defined by the basic relations of a given scientific language) to lower levels (which are characterized by sets defined by a progressively larger number of two-place predicates). In science, predicates must be of an exclusively experimental type and/or statistical type and by no means of an experiential type. But experiential-type predicates are often found in sociological and cognitive research, and in economic research too (in the presence or not of intersections[11] with statistical type predicates).

Functions belonging to the highest levels of abstraction are poorer in semantic interpretations. Functions belonging to those sets characterized by lower levels of abstraction specify the theoretical predicates, i.e. they enrich them with more analytic meanings denoting situations (environments) where the multiplicity of variables and parameters tends toward individualization.

The case of technology points this out. Technological predicates define sets that express not only theoretical invariants (basic functions), but a much larger number of (specific) functions as well. These latter functions, which define the concrete environment where basic functions can work, specify the domains of application of the abstract basic functions. In this sense, the technological environment is richer (in semantic interpretations) compared to the poorer environment where the abstract basic functions take their place.

The order of the abstraction levels, which expresses the relation of inclusion from the most abstract (basic) to the less abstract (technological) sets of functions, is a partial order,[12] since the (sub)sets of the same level are not comparable by the relation of inclusion. Each level of abstraction is defined by one or more proper subsets[13] of functions, i.e., by one or more partitions of pairwise-disjoint subsets of functions corresponding to the equivalence classes that comprise functions of the same type (i.e., equivalent as to their experimental semantic interpretation).

Since functions are relations between independent and dependent variables, given certain parameters (namely certain factors which are kept constant within the examined function), the abstraction level can be modified by changing one or more parameters into variables or by specifying new *changing values* of parameters. This means defining further subsets of the examined function, i.e., functions with a lower abstraction level, which incorporate a larger number of specific semantic interpretations.

The function denotes the *system* that delimits the field of knowledge (laboratory experiment) and/or the field of operations (technology), whereas parameters denote all those factors external to the system. This does not mean that relations (functions) between system and outside do not exist. It only means that these relations are not taken into consideration; i.e., they are assumed to be non-influential with reference to the given system. If the relations between system and outside (*external system*) are taken into consideration, they extend the boundaries of the system and define new partitions within the system (i.e., functions with a lower abstraction level compared to the basic functions).

The language of science must be logically consistent, in accordance with the more or less advanced processes of knowledge. When the language is totally or partly axiomatized, consistency is quite evident. Seeing that a scientific language necessarily implies a strict and univocal (experimental and/or statistical) semantic interpretation of its syntactic terms, consistency concerns, in the final analysis, semantic interpretation too, since the latter determines those properties to which the syntactic relations refer.

The syntax and the semantics of a specific (and formalized) scientific language express a paradigm of reference that identifies the domain of application of this language, i.e. the properties characterizing each set (namely, each element of any set) belonging to the given language. In this sense, each property designates a subset of this language, i.e. the subset of elements which have that property. Therefore both the *intensional* perspective of properties (expressing the operational fields to which science refers: the properties) and the *extensional* perspective of the quantitative concepts according to which the properties are explicated are equally important for the language of science.

The reference paradigm is a strong one when the scientific language is constructed using the Galilean method of controlled (laboratory) experiment. In this case, the *intersubjectiveness* of the scientific language is guaranteed, together with its *operativeness,* because the scientific language is susceptible to experimental verification.

It may be that the language of a given science is constructed using a knowledge method weaker than controlled (laboratory) experiment. This happens when it is not possible to explicate a phenomenon with reference to all its paired variables and its parameters, i.e., when it is not possible to formulate the explicative functions of the given phenomenon in an exhaustive and univocal way. If, in principle, one cannot postulate a strict correspondence between the meaning (designation) of the linguistic terms and their experimental denotation (Morris 1955, p. 17ff.; Carnap 1956, p. 96ff.), the terms cannot be founded on direct verification. Then, indirect (non-experimental) verification is needed, through a statistical method that guarantees at least a probabilistic consistency of the scientific language.

There can be intersections between the experimental method and the statistical method (i.e. sets of knowledge methods combining experimental verification and statistical analysis). In the same way, there can be intersections between a consistent set of abstract theoretical predicates, devoid of experimental verification though they may be, and a set of statistical-type predicates, as happens in economics.

The positions that do not conform directly to the experimental and/or statistical methods of science, i.e., that do not use the logical syntax and semantics of the scientific language, refer to some (manifest or latent) metaphysical presuppositions—"mental biases" (prejudices) that the persistent common-sense culture cannot give up—which still hinders the construction of a unitary theoretical system as a basis for the integration of the social sciences.

Time in Science

All social interactions and behaviors take time. On this ground, it is important to state that they can be explicated in different ways, according to whether a cyclic sequence that defines *repetition time* (clock time) or a cumulative sequence that defines *evolution time* (history time) is used as reference point. Repetition time just expresses a measure of intervals interpreted as length. In physics (and in everyday experience) it is realized by repeating identically a (cyclic) set of operations—such as the oscillation of a pendulum, of a balance wheel, of a quartz crystal—which is an index to which an invariant numerical value is related (Faggiani 1957, p. 7ff.). Repetition time as a rule is used in scientific language as an implicit independent variable in the context of *reversible* processes. Evolution time expresses a different concept, which applies not to a relation concerning length, but rather to a concentration process or to a dissipation process (e.g., in physics the concentration of lead and uranium in uranium-rocks or the estimation of entropy (Faggiani 1957, p. 233)), or to the more general process of past-history change concerning living organisms; these cases refer to *irreversible* processes.

The difference between reversibility and irreversibility (Faggiani 1957, pp. 49ff., 232ff.) depends itself on the repeatability of the set of operations which change the system from its initial state to a different state, and particularly on the fact that the *tracks* of changes are assumed not to alter the (functional) dynamics of the system or to alter it. In the first case, tracks are considered in principle outside the system, and there is *free repeatability* (reversibility); in the second one tracks have cumulative effects, they cannot be considered outside the system, and there is *forced repeatability* (irreversibility).

The analyses of the existence of equilibrium, within (axiomatized) economic language, do not include time as an implicit independent variable; axiomatization is *atemporal*. The *theory of interests* (which I will discuss later) can be expressed as an atemporal theory, although behavior has by definition a temporal dimension in terms of repetition time, since that theory does not consider the dynamics of behavior, unlike experimental analysis; i.e. it does not consider the functional relations among behaviors, but only the structural relations among interests.

It is otherwise in the case of comparative static analyses and analyses on the global stability of equilibrium relating to whether a set of competing behaviors based on the exchange succeeds in directing itself toward some final optimal allocation of resources. In these cases, the (dynamic) language implicitly includes time as a variable and uses the relation "$+t$ *and* $-t$"; that is, it takes repetition time (the clock time) as temporal reference point.

The same can be said about the dynamic equations of motion and of electromagnetism in physics and about the experimental analysis of behavior, that both consider time as an implicit independent variable.

Analyses of social and economic development consider time with a different meaning. If these processes of change were expressed using a mathematical language, as happens with the (differential) evolutionistic equations of physics, such a language should implicitly contain time as a variable, but it should not admit the substitution between $+t$ and $-t$ (Faggiani 1957, p. 229ff.), since the semantic interpretation of the functions does not allow it.[14] All economic, sociological and psychological cumulative processes refer to this specific meaning of time (evolution time or history time), which still has to be held distinctly separate from repetition time.

Behavioral evolution time, which characterizes the past history (cumulative learning) of the organism, at present cannot be taken into consideration as a variable in the functions explicating the structural dynamics of behavior, but it must be set as a parameter. Much the same can be said for economics; for example: capital accumulation, innovation, and needs (i.e. cultural) change cannot be inserted as variables into the explicative functions of market equilibrium.

The scientific method imposes a clear-cut distinction between repetition time and evolution time, respectively related to reversibility and irreversibility. Every natural (physical), biological or behavioral phenomenon is characterized by evolution time, but the latter has to be considered as a parameter if one wants to explain the phenomenon in strict reversibility terms. Of course, also, the phenomena characterized by evolution time can be explicated from a scientific point of view, as is shown in physics; in this case too, however, the two temporal perspectives cannot be confused. So, corresponding to reversibility and irreversibility, structural dynamics must be distinguished from evolutionary (cumulative) dynamics.[15]

An Exemplary Case: The Language of Economics

The Semantic Interpretation of Economic Syntax At present economics is undeniably the most advanced social science. On the syntactic level, its language is characterized in mathematical terms by the structural dynamic function. Moreover, market economics has been partly axiomatized "with the standards of rigor of the contemporary formalist school of mathematics ... In the area under discussion it has been essentially a change from the calculus to convexity and topological properties, a transformation which has resulted in notable gains in the generality and in the simplicity of the theory." (Debreu 1959, p. viii)

In spite of this axiomatization (now a basic reference point for which all other social sciences should aim), within economics many problems referable to the uniqueness and global stability of equilibrium remain unsolved. But even more critical problems (perhaps including the first two) exist. They concern the semantic interpretation of the theory and are closely associated with the exclusion of the psychological and social variables by economic analysis.[16]

The ascription of a rigorous semantic interpretation to the mathematical syntax of economic language[17] has always been postulated *a priori* by economists, who have worked on the construction of a formalized scientific economics since the 1930s. Debreu explicitly points out that the axiomatized theory is absolutely autonomous from any possible interpretative hypothesis: "Allegiance to rigor dictates the axiomatic form of the analysis where the theory, in the strict sense, is logically entirely disconnected from its interpretations.... Such a dichotomy reveals all the assumptions and the logical structure of the analysis. It also makes possible immediate extensions of that analysis without modification of the theory by simple reinterpretations of concepts." (1959, p. viii)

Debreu closes chapter 2 (Commodities and Prices) of his 1959 book by systematizing those concepts drawn from what he calls "the language of the theory": "*The number l of commodities is a given positive integer. An action a of an agent is a point of R^l, the commodity space. A price system p is a point of R^l. The value of an action a, relative to a price system p, is the inner product $p \cdot a$.* All that precedes this statement is irrelevant for the logical development of the theory" (p. 35).

In chapter 4 (titled Consumers), Debreu states: "*Given the price system p and his wealth w_i, a real number, the* ith *consumer chooses his consumption x_i in his consumption set X_i so that his expenditure $p \cdot x_i$ satisfies the wealth constraint $p \cdot x_i \leqq w_i$. The point $w = (w_i)$ of R^m is called the wealth distribution. The point (p, w) of R^{l+m} is called the price-wealth pair.*" (p. 62, italics in original).

These are just two examples showing that Debreu does use a semantic interpretation, even though quite abstract, that allows him to let each term of the mathematical language (this latter, too, characterized from a more abstract syntax and semantics) correspond to an economic-type concept. Considering Debreu's sentences, the semantic interpretation of the syntactic expressions is given by concepts like: Commodity, Action/Agent, Price (System), Value (of an Action), Wealth (Constraint/Distribution), Consumer/Consumption, Expenditure.[18] Within axiomatization the semantic interpretation is assumed, but it is not taken into consideration explicitly, as the language is mainly formal (mathematical). If all the economic concepts (i.e., all the economic interpretations) were eliminated from Debreu's sentences, however, these sentences would become a pure mathematical language.

Economics and the Social System One of the basic problems for economics, and more generally for the social sciences, concerns the relations between variables and parameters that express the external system (i.e., the social environment) and variables and parameters that express the (theoretical) economic system.

Actually economics is characterized by a set of functions that define a system disjoined from the external system, which is expressed by a set of other social functions. In this case, to isolate a set of economic functions would mean to consider the variables of the external social system (such as population, technology, political and social institutions) as non-influential with reference to the economic system. It would mean, in short, to postulate that there is not, in principle, any (dynamic) function between the set of economic behaviors and the set of other social behaviors. If such a function was taken into consideration, it would express a change in the conditions under which economic variables are postulated to work.

It is for this reason that the rigorous construction of a scientific language, concerning solely economic behaviors first of all, has forced economists into defining the domain of application of their discipline, to make its semantic contents as univocal as possible. This can be done by assuming that a set of social operant behaviors (A^1) exists which is complementary (compared to a more abstract set S) to the set of economic operant behaviors (A), such that $A^1 = \{x | x \notin A\}$. In this sense, the two sets can be considered as disjoint, such that $A \cap A^1 = \varnothing$.

Such an ambiguous meaning has been ascribed to the disjointness, however, as to imply that all (operant) behaviors are necessarily economic behaviors. In this case, the set of other social behaviors would have no elements, or only pathological-type elements (behavior disorders). Therefore economics, on the one hand tends to include all behaviors and to explain them, in principle, as economic behaviors; on the other hand, it tends to consider those behaviors that it fails to deal with (those that don't fall within its explicative schemata) to be irrational (e.g., impulsive) behaviors.

As a matter of fact, the term "impulsive behavior" has been used by behaviorists to provide an explication for some experimental deviations from an explanatory model founded on a strictly rational concept of behavior in an economic sense. In particular, the postulate of transitivity that must characterize the (complete) preference preordering (in the language of Debreu: pp. 7–8, 54ff.) of a rational "agent" is often falsified with reference to human behavior and also by experimental verification on animal behaviors, as "the matching law predicts that as time passes the pigeon will change its preferences ('change its mind')" and that consequently "the matching law, which does predict reversals, posits value as a hyperbolic (an inverse), not exponential, function of delay. Behavior is often inconsistent in just this way, says the matching law." (Rachlin and Laibson 1997, p. 103)

On the topic of self-control, Rachlin and Laibson (1997) comment: "People who chose the larger-later are often said to be 'controlling themselves' (in the sense that they forgo a smaller but still positively valued alternative). By the same token, if they choose the smaller-sooner alternative they are said to be 'impulsive.'" (p. 101) In the same way Herrnstein (1997) states that "behavior is impulsive if it sacrifices long-range considerations for short-range gains; it is self-controlling if the reverse is the case" (p. 121). However this concept of impulsiveness does not make sense within economic language, since as Rachlin and Laibson (1997) note: "For an economist, rationality lies not in which alternative you choose but whether you choose that alternative *consistently* over time.... Therefore the only (economically) consistent account of the effect of delay on choice is by a discount function that predicts no reversals of preferences with time." (pp. 102–103)

All these experiments suggest that the instability of the transitivity of preferences, i.e., the assignment of *value* by a subject to his own behaviors over time, derives from the processes of learning (reinforcement). Therefore, it should be social variables that determine preference ordering and its reversal, with special reference to the transitivity of the "is not preferred to" relation. In this sense, it can be said that the consistency among two or more sets of behaviors realized by, or that could be realized by, a subject or by a group, as far as they result from a learning process, implies that such learning occurs within a consistent context of external stimuli.

The axiomatic analysis of economic equilibrium asserts the theoretical existence of a set of consistent exchange behaviors characterized by Pareto optimality (the problem of the existence of equilibrium). Usually it happens that economic equilibrium (and more generally economic behavior) loses its purity in the factual contexts in which it takes place, since it is not easy to distinguish other social variables from economic variables on a common-sense basis. The difficulty of operating such a kind of distinction at the factual (or broad economic-language-interpretation) level and the lack of a clear relation between the two sets (economic system and external social system) give rise to much ambiguity on both the theoretical and the operative level. Within economic language some of these difficulties are generally included in the concept of market failure, which expresses the market's inability to achieve an optimal employment of resources, i.e., a pure-competition equilibrium. In this sense, market failures prevent the achievement of economic efficiency and/or Pareto optimality.

Although economists tend to undervalue the set of other social behaviors that lie outside the language of economics, it is plain that if the assumption that all behaviors are in principle economic behaviors is rejected, then it is necessary to conclude that the set of factors distorting economic equilibrium is by definition exogenous to the economic system. It therefore becomes necessary to analyze the specific relations between the two sets and to define the functions between economic and other social operant-behaviors sets, so as to enlarge the economic system by inserting specific variables external to the system without them losing their primary characterization (i.e., without making them endogenous according to the schemata currently used by economists).

This situation will remain muddled until the relations between economic variables (which are endogenous to the system) and other social variables (which are exogenous, since they belong to the external system) are exactly specified. This is pointed out in the *theory of interest*, which shows that relations products between subsets of social behavior can exist; so specific functions can have both economic variables and variables belonging to the power and/or cooperation subsets.

The Verification of Economics in a Human Context If it is supposed that economics has the same characteristics as the natural sciences and thence expresses *behavioral invariants*, semantic interpretations of economics should be founded in principle on the controlled experiment. But it is hard to suppose that economic postulates can be verified in a complete way through experiments that use animal behavior, especially with reference to economic behavior related to the market. It is also hard to verify them using the behavior of human subjects, since in this case experiments cannot demonstrate whether the economic behavior shown by the subjects was learned during the socialization process or not; i.e., whether it was learned before the experiment or during the experiment.

For these reasons, current cognitive experimental research on economic behavior is affected by an error made by those who claim to study phenomena according to the Aristotelian method as they appear to common sense in everyday life. In the Aristotelian schema,

> "the behavior of any single object was regarded as determined by its relation to the rest of the cosmos, by the necessary role it must play in the whole drama. It was difficult, therefore, to think of events in isolation, for example, to concentrate attention on the behavior of a single object in a particular region rather than on events occurring in the universe as a whole.
>
> From the early 17th century on, scientific thinking tended more and more toward a narrow limitation of attention in a given experimental situation, concentrating upon those few factors that seemed most relevant and decisive. The great success of this approach became evident in Galileo's work on mechanics. To investigate the behavior of a body freed "from its weight," he asked us to consider a ball placed upon a frictionless horizontal plane . . . In Newton's first law of motion the conception of the isolated system is most evident, for the postulate allows us to think about the behavior of a totally isolated object, one which in thought is removed altogether from the influence of other objects." (Holton and Roller 1965, pp. 267–268)

I. P. Pavlov and B. F. Skinner operated on the experimental level by totally isolating the system from the outside. However, this fact did not obstruct the finding of the basic laws of behavior; on the contrary, it helped. Nevertheless modern Aristotelians seem not to follow the lesson of science. They persist in doing experiments that contradict the scientific method, and do not keep under control the stimuli that conditioned the past history (learning as irreversible process) and that condition the current behaviors (learning as reversible process) of the experimental subjects. Only "frictions" can emerge from these experiments, i.e., the behaviors clashing with the laws that should be verified. Those who claim to verify on humans economic laws of behavior, and social laws generally, behave in the same way as a physicist who claims to verify Newton's first law of motion (the principle of inertia) in a system full of frictions. In both cases, the law will fail.

Therefore, a "frictionless" experimental context would be necessary to verify the market equilibrium system, i.e., a context where all (learned) behaviors which are non-compatible with the principles of pure economic equilibrium are kept under control (like parameters) with reference to learned behavior. But such a context does not seem possible, neither with human subjects, nor (because of different reasons) with animals.

The behavioral interpretations ascribed to game-theory experiments point out this fact. In these experiments the convergence toward equilibrium (when it occurs) is usually based on the repetition of behaviors that give rise to a trial-and-error learning process. Such a process is driven both by the specific reinforcement contingencies and by the repetitive-trials procedure. Therefore, it is wrong to consider these arrangements as experimental verifications of economic dynamic functions formulated as equilibrium hypotheses inherent in the subjects' behaviors (or brain). And it is also wrong to consider game experiments of this type, currently popular among economists, to be suitable for founding a new theoretical model for economics or, in general, for social sciences (especially in terms of trust and fairness). Whether people are selfish or altruist is a matter of learning; subjects learn cooperation and conflict too (as in the zero-sum games, where players tend to the optimality[19] of their conflicting strategies) during experiments. In short, when game-theory experiments, and in general all (cognitive) experiments of different type, are interpreted according to the behavioral (not behavioristic) perspective, they express assertions on the experimental subjects' (current or past) behaviors, but these assertions cannot be generalized to all subjects as "natural laws".

From a behavioristic stand point all these types of experiments prove only that subjects do learn if their operant behaviors are reinforced; i.e., the experiments verify the hypothesis that learning is the reinforcement process and is either hindered or facilitated by different types of events, such as the repetition of the operative sequences, the subject's past history, and the specific social interactions that are the (external) behavioral stimuli reinforcing the subject's operant behavior.

The Verification of Economics with Animal Experiments The organism's past history and the control of the experimental context are not a real problem in animal experimentation. Other factors exist, however, that make these experiments unreliable in principle; particularly the fact that they refer to predicates and functions characterizing an abstract set of human operant behaviors. Moreover, the term "choice" is often used with an ambiguous meaning, that could make one think that animal organisms have some internal capabilities of this kind.

The results so far achieved by the experimental analysis of (animal) behavior can be synthesized by the *law of effect*: behaviors are reinforced by their effects and this relation takes place within a learning process, whose variables can be brought back to three quantitative dimensions characterizing reinforcement contingencies: rate of reinforcement, amount of reinforcer, delay of reinforcement. The *matching law* expresses these primary variables of the reinforcement process. Only the existence of these *invariants* of learning allows the experimenter to obtain specific behaviors from the organisms by manipulating the experimental reinforcement contingencies.

If an organism's behavior is the result of the experimental context, then (1) no autonomous "maximizing" principle can be attributed to the organism and (2) economic behavior, in case it is realized, depends solely on the experimental contingencies being compatible with the maximization, given the specific learning processes that can be realized by the organism. In this sense, the experimental results not conforming to the contingencies of reinforcement can express either an experimenter's "error" (a non-appropriate definition of reinforcement contingencies of maximization) or the existence of factors that lie outside the experimenter's control.

The same can be said for human subjects, who are able to realize operant behaviors in response to much more complicated reinforcement contingencies, such as those expressed by economic analysis. Therefore, also man must be enabled to learn these contingencies, that are typical not of his "nature," but rather of the multiplicity of factors and relations (functions) that can characterize all the aspects of human behavior. As a matter of fact, it so happens that man behaves *uneconomically* or even refuses an economic behavior. In this case too, uneconomic behavior must be necessarily learned (i.e., reinforced).

The hypothesis advanced in this chapter—that economic and social behaviors are learned behaviors—explains the non-conformity with theory of the results so far achieved by experimental economics. The general acceptance that these experiments still receive can be imputed to the error deriving from a misunderstanding of the distinction between scientific knowledge and common sense knowledge.

In the perspective of science, we can suppose that behavioral laws "exist", but these latter are only learning laws and must not be confused with the environmental contingencies (i.e., the "contents" of reinforcement schedules) on which also economic behavior depends. At present, economics is constructed as a theoretical system, but without the experimental analysis of behavior it is not possible to understand the limits and the real significance of economics and to use properly (and not blindly, as currently tried) this system. The *theory of interests* attempts to realize this connection, paving the way for theoretical systematisation and controlled experimental analysis of behavior.

The Problem of Inner States in Psychology and Sociology

With reference to sociology and cognitive psychology, as with economics, the experimental method cannot guarantee, at present, intersubjective results. The exact definition of the research field, which allows behaviorism to build on experimental bases an intersubjective and syntactically consistent explicative language founded on a set of relations (functions) between terms with univocal meanings (unlike common-language terms, that have vague domains of application), is considered by many social researchers to be an excessive simplification rather than an important achievement in knowledge.

The factors taken into consideration by sociologists and cognitive psychologists are all internal ones; i.e., they are cognitive states or, in a more general sense, states of consciousness that pertain in a strict sense to the experience of the individual subject.

Perceiving states of consciousness as prime causes of behavior brings about a radical distortion of the knowledge man has about himself, since it leads to concentrating attention solely upon internal processes (that cannot be submitted to an intersubjective, quantitative and experimental scientific analysis) and to building up a cultural context and a pseudo-explicative language in conformity with this representation.

Undoubtedly states of consciousness do exist for individual subjects, but outside the boundaries of subjectivity they can be known only through non-verbal or verbal behaviors. Non-verbal behaviors are by definition ignored, so as not to lapse into behaviorism, which is excluded as a rule by sociologists and cognitive psychologists. But verbal behaviors are considered to be reliable statements on which pseudo-experimental analyses are founded. In this case a typical methodological inconsistency occurs, since it claims to found the experimental method (which is by definition intersubjective) on the introspective method (which is by definition subjective).

This methodological inconsistency in some way hinders the development of an experimental science of behavior, too. So, the experiments carried out using cognitive-type predicates (i.e., ascribing cognitive meanings to variables and parameters) don't use an intersubjective abstract theoretical paradigm as their point of reference. This lack of a unified theoretical paradigm of reference is due not to the "complexity of phenomena," as it is superficially supposed, but to the fact that phenomena are analyzed using inadequate and generic research methods, that lead to an endless proliferation of theories which are often mutually incompatible and lacking real explicative power. Moreover, boundaries between the biological sciences on the one hand and psychology and sociology on the other hand are not exactly defined. This situation brings about an anomalous intersection among different languages (biological and psychological) that, on the contrary, denote disjoint sets; if these languages were formalized or axiomatized, the hypothesis of some equivalence relation or some isomorphism among them could be formulated (Bolacchi 2004, pp. 447–448).

The Theory of Interests

A Theoretical Hypothesis for the Study of Social Phenomena Founded on the Experimental Analysis of Behavior

The explication of behavior is based upon the definition of the organism (*subject*) as a set of responses to a set of environmental stimuli that can also be behaviors of other organisms. The role of reinforcement within the social interaction is explicated in its *structural invariants* (applied, by definition, to all living organisms, included man) through a very simple but significant experiment by Herrnstein (1964). The experiment is carried out with two pigeons, A and B, placed in a controlled environment and kept apart by a transparent wall. Pigeon A is previously trained to peck at a disk on the transparent wall and is reinforced with food (primary reinforcer).

The experiment is designed in order to let pigeon A receive food whenever it pecks at the disk, but only if pigeon B stands in the left corner of the experimental box with respect to A. If this situation (discriminative stimulus/secondary reinforcer) occurs, then B receives food too; but, if A pecks when B is anywhere else, then only B gets food. Since A's pecking is reinforced only when B stands in the left corner, A learns to peck only when B stands in that specific position. On the other hand, B is progressively reinforced only when it stands in the left corner of the experimental box, since in that position both pigeons receive food. Therefore B, instead of moving, learns to maintain the most favorable position for the other pigeon and, consequently, for itself too.

In this situation a new set of (social) stimuli joins with the (natural) stimuli of the physical environment. It follows that the discriminative stimulus S^D for A is not only the presence of the disk on the transparent wall (natural secondary reinforcer, S^{Dn}), but also B's instrumental behavior (response) when standing in the left corner (Rs^B, where s stands for 'instrumental'). In this case, actually, the second set of (social) stimuli does not remove the set of natural stimuli, but it does limit its range of control on behavior. B's position in the box is a social secondary reinforcer (S^{Ds}) with regard to A's behavior (Rs^A) instrumental to the food acquisition (Rc^A, where c stands for 'consummatory').

In the same way, the discriminative stimulus S^D for B is not only access to the left corner (natural secondary reinforcer, S^{Dn}), but also A's instrumental behavior (response) when pecking at the disk (Rs^A). As a matter of fact, B's standing in the left corner is reinforced only when A is in the pecking position. These relationships for subjects A and B are outlined in figure 15.1.

Therefore, the social context puts further constraints on the execution of the instrumental sequences of the subjects: it is necessary that the instrumental behavior, Rs, is compatible not only with the natural (physical) environment (S^{Dn}), but also with the social environment (S^{Ds}) in order for the subjects to realize their consummatory behavior Rc. This relation between the two reinforcement contexts is outlined in figure 15.1.

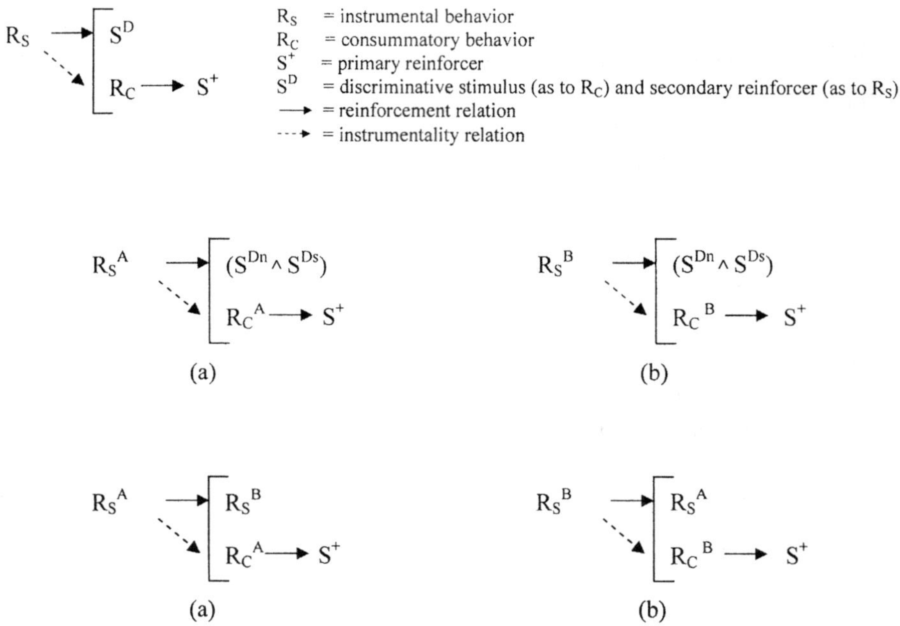

Figure 15.1
Representation of the relationships for subjects in the Herrnstein (1964) experiment.

For the purpose of analysis of the social interaction, only the relation (function) between the behavior of the subject and the social stimuli is examined. The natural environment is considered a parameter, taking for granted the presence of natural discriminative stimuli or secondary reinforcers. As a matter of fact, it is possible to suppose that an instrumental sequence takes place in a context which is characterized solely by physical-type variables and parameters (constraints) in the absence of any social variable and parameter, but it is by no means possible to suppose that an instrumental sequence takes place in the absence of physical-type variables and parameters.

All possible types of social interaction have to be explicated in terms of reinforcement, because the reinforcing stimuli for one subject's social behavior sequences are, by definition, the behaviors of other subjects. As stated above, the set of social stimuli (the social environment) does not replace or remove the set of natural stimuli, but it widens the extent of control on behavior, determining a further constraint on the execution of instrumental sequences: in order that the subject can complete his sequence with the consummatory behavior, it is necessary that the instrumental behavior is compatible not only with the physical environment, but also with the social environment. In short, these are the basic reference points for the experimental analysis of social behavior.

At the level of abstract language, there is a correspondence between the experimental language of behavior analysis and the *theory of interests* (which is concisely outlined in this chapter[20]); the latter fits more easily in dealing with the difficulties inherent in the explication of social phenomena. The relation between experimental language and abstract language (theory of interests) is based on the correspondence between the predicate "operant behavior" (*minimal unit of analysis*) and the (primitive) predicate "interest." In this way, the concept of interest loses the motivational connotations that the common language ascribes to it and designates only instrumental sequences of operant behaviors. Therefore, saying that an interest is satisfied or not satisfied (sacrificed) is equivalent to saying that a behavior is realized or is not realized.

Within the abstract language of the theory of interests, each subject is defined as a set of *instrumental* and *final* interests (*field of interests*), which is characterized by two relations which refer to the instrumental interests (Is, where s stands for 'instrumental') and the final interests (IF, where F stands for 'final'), respectively:

(a) an *order relation* between interests according to their *instrumentality degree*, which is given by the position of each interest in an ordered set that has on one side the final interests and on the other side the instrumental interests. The "is instrumental to" relation implies that (1) each interest can be satisfied (i.e., each sequence of operant behaviors can take place) only if the preceding interest in the order relation (i.e., the interest having higher instrumentality degree) has been satisfied (i.e., the preceding sequence of operant behaviors has taken place); (2) each interest can be regarded as an instrumental interest with respect to the interests that follow it and as a final interest with respect to the interests that precede it;

(b) an *order relation* between interests according to their *intensity level*, which is given by the position of each interest in a set of preferences. The "is not preferred to" relation implies that (1) when confronted with the satisfaction of one interest or another interest, the subject satisfies that interest with the highest intensity level; (2) two final interests can be disjunctively satisfied.[21]

The structure of the field of interests is formed by orderly pairs of interests, which express the instrumentality and the preference respectively. In the first case (*instrumentality*): (1) the pair is composed of an instrumental interest and a final interest which define the instrumental sequence of interests $\{Is \rightarrow I_F\}$[22]; (2) the measure of instrumentality is expressed by the instrumentality degree. In the second case (*preference*): (1) the pair is composed of two final interests; (2) the measure of preference is expressed by the intensity level (ι). The sequence of instrumental interests and the sequence of final interests are subsets of the field of interests.

The structure of the social interaction is formed by pairs belonging to different fields of interests (subjects A's and B's fields), which express the (*positive* or *negative*) *involvement* between final interests and the (*conjunct* or *disjunct*) *interrelation* between instrumental interests.

Given two instrumental sequences of interests $\{Is^{A.1} \rightarrow I_F^{A.1}\}$ and $\{Is^{B.1} \rightarrow I_F^{B.1}\}$ belonging to subject A's field of interests and to subject B's field of interests respectively, the possible basic relations among interests (social interactions) are the following:

(a) a relation between the two final interests $I_F^{A.1}$ and $I_F^{B.1}$ exists, such that the satisfaction of A's interest $I_F^{A.1}$ can occur only if B's interest $I_F^{B.1}$ is contextually satisfied, and vice versa. Consequently there is also a relation between the two interests $Is^{A.1}$ and $Is^{B.1}$ such that A's interest $Is^{A.1}$ (instrumental one with respect to $I_F^{A.1}$) cannot be satisfied if B's interest $Is^{B.1}$ is not satisfied, and B's interest $Is^{B.1}$ (instrumental one with respect to $I_F^{B.1}$) cannot be satisfied if A's interest $Is^{A.1}$ is not satisfied;

(b) a relation between the two final interests $I_F^{A.1}$ and $I_F^{B.1}$ exists, such that the satisfaction of A's interest $I_F^{A.1}$ can occur only if B's interest $I_F^{B.1}$ is contextually not satisfied, and vice versa. Consequently there is also a relation between the two interests $Is^{A.1}$ and $Is^{B.1}$ such that A's interest $Is^{A.1}$ (instrumental one with respect to $I_F^{A.1}$) cannot be satisfied if B's interest $Is^{B.1}$ is satisfied and B's interest $Is^{B.1}$ (instrumental one with respect to $I_F^{B.1}$) cannot be satisfied if A's interest $Is^{A.1}$ is satisfied.

These relations between subject A's field of interests and subject B's field of interests can be represented by figure 15.2, where (1) in the oriented segments *ab* and *cd* the final interests are plotted, for subject A and subject B respectively, ordered according to their intensity level (increasing from left to right); (2) in the oblique segments the instrumental interests are plotted

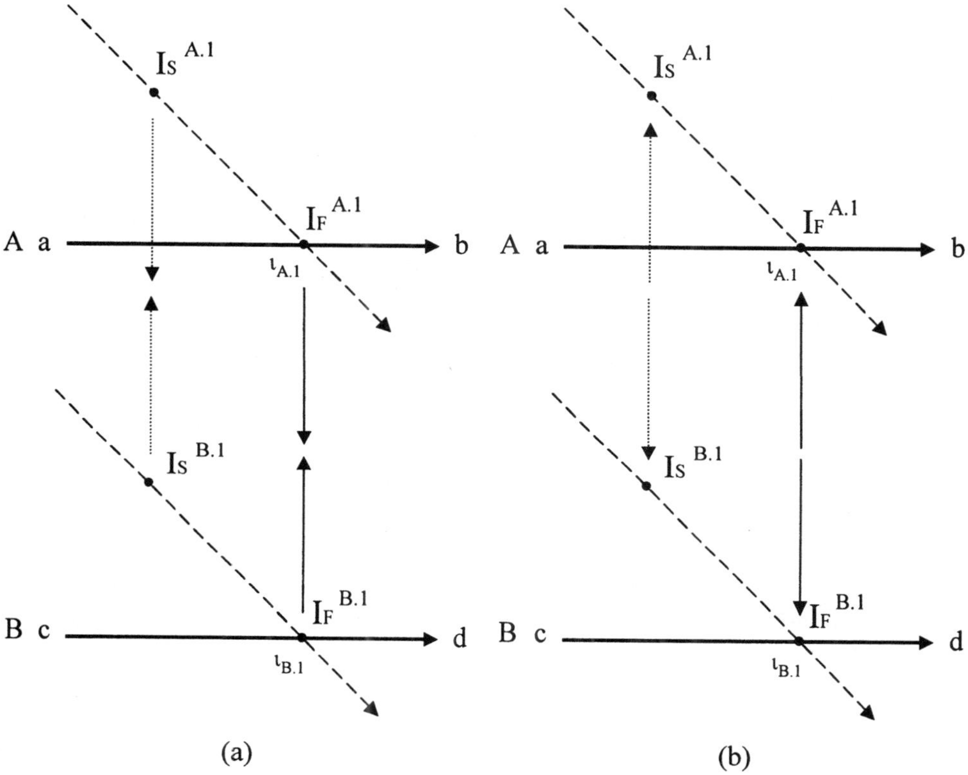

Figure 15.2
Diagrams for the basic typologies of social interactions: (a) positive involvement and conjunct interrelation, and (b) negative involvement and disjunct interrelation.

for each final interest (identified by the point of intersection with the horizontal oriented segment), ordered according to their instrumentality degree (decreasing from the top to the bottom).

For clarity of explication, the abstract schemata of the theory of interests—and the corresponding experimental analysis—take the simplest and most basic case into consideration, in which each instrumental sequence is composed of only one instrumental interest (namely, only one instrumental behavior). So diagrams represent only pairs of interests.

In case a in figure 15.2, it is necessary that the two subjects contextually satisfy their two final interests and carry out, in principle, two distinct but complementary instrumental sequences. In this case, the two final interests $I_F^{A.1}$ and $I_F^{B.1}$ are *positively involved* (PI) and the two instrumental interests

$Is^{A.1}$ and $Is^{B.1}$ are *conjunctly interrelated* ("related" for the notation) (CR): $[IF^{A.1}]$ PI $[IF^{B.1}]$ and $[Is^{A.1}]$ CR $[Is^{B.1}]$. The PI (positive involvement) relation is represented by the convergent solid-line arrows; the CR (conjunct interrelation) relation is represented by the convergent dotted-line arrows. The two-pigeon experiment by Herrnstein (discussed above) designates this type of relation between interests.

In case (b) in figure 15.2, only one of the two subjects can satisfy his own final interest, since the realization of an instrumental sequence by one of the subjects precludes the other from realizing the instrumental sequence aimed at satisfying his own final interest. In this case, the two final interests $IF^{A.1}$ and $IF^{B.1}$ are *negatively involved* (NI) and the two instrumental interests $Is^{A.1}$ and $Is^{B.1}$ are *disjunctly interrelated* ("related" for the notation) (DR): $[IF^{A.1}]$ NI $[IF^{B.1}]$ and $[Is^{A.1}]$ DR $[Is^{B.1}]$. The NI (negative involvement) relation is represented by the divergent solid-line arrows; the DR (disjunct interrelation) relation is represented by the divergent dotted-line arrows.

The positive involvement (with the consequent conjunct interrelation) and the negative involvement (with the consequent disjunct interrelation) define the two basic typologies of social interaction.[23] In the structural theory of interests, they are two primitive dyadic predicates (primitive ordered pairs), corresponding to the relation (function) of social reinforcement within the experimental dynamics of operant behavior.

It is possible to change from the abstract analysis of the theory of interests to the experimental (dynamic) analysis of behavior (founded on functions) by establishing a correspondence between the terms denoting interests and the terms denoting operant behaviors, in their different specifications given by the instrumental behavior (Rs) and consummatory behavior (Rc):

$$Is^{A.1} \leftrightarrow Rs^{A.1},$$

$$Is^{B.1} \leftrightarrow Rs^{B.1},$$

$$IF^{A.1} \leftrightarrow Rc^{A.1},$$

$$IF^{B.1} \leftrightarrow Rc^{B.1}.$$

In the case of *conjunct interrelation* there are the following social reinforcement relations (figure 15.3):

(a) for subject A, $Rs^{A.1}$ is the behavior (corresponding to the interest $Is^{A.1}$) reinforced by the behavior $Rs^{B.1}$ (corresponding to the interest $Is^{B.1}$) of

Figure 15.3
Representation of the conjunct interrelation in terms of social reinforcement.

subject B. The latter behavior is a discriminative stimulus in the presence of which A realizes the consummatory behavior $\text{Rc}^{A.1}$, which is reinforced by S^+ (i.e., he satisfies his interest $\text{IF}^{A.1}$);

(b) for subject B, $\text{Rs}^{B.1}$ is the behavior (corresponding to the interest $\text{Is}^{B.1}$) reinforced by the behavior $\text{Rs}^{A.1}$ (corresponding to the interest $\text{Is}^{A.1}$) of subject A. The latter behavior is a discriminative stimulus in the presence of which B realizes the consummatory behavior $\text{Rc}^{B.1}$, which is reinforced by S^+ (i.e., he satisfies his interest $\text{IF}^{B.1}$). It is worth noting that both $\text{Rc}^{A.1}$ and $\text{Rc}^{B.1}$ are reinforced by the same reinforcer S^+, since the interests $\text{IF}^{A.1}$ and $\text{IF}^{B.1}$ are positively involved.

On that account, the *reciprocal complementarity* of the two subsets of instrumental interests belonging to different fields of interests, which characterizes positive involvement, is specified on the experimental level by the *reciprocal positive reinforcement* of the corresponding sequences of operant behaviors.

The concept of reciprocal complementarity is different from the concept of instrumental order of operant sequences. The basic factor of positive involvement is not the instrumental order of operant sequences, and hence of instrumental interests (although the order is in any case presupposed), but rather the reciprocal positive reinforcement as is made evident by the experimental analysis of behavior; even if common sense cannot discover it, as it perceives only the instrumental order of behaviors. As a matter of fact, there can be sets of instrumentally ordered behaviors of two (or more) subjects, but if the behavioral sequences do not positively reinforce each others, they on their own don't bring about positive involvement.

In the case of *disjunct interrelation* there are the following social reinforcement relations, as shown in figure 15.4:

(a) for subject A, $\text{Rs}^{A.1}$ is the behavior (corresponding to the interest $\text{Is}^{A.1}$) reinforced by the absence of behavior $\text{Rs}^{B.1}$ (corresponding to the interest $\text{Is}^{B.1}$) of subject B. The absence of $\text{Rs}^{B.1}$ is a discriminative stimulus in the

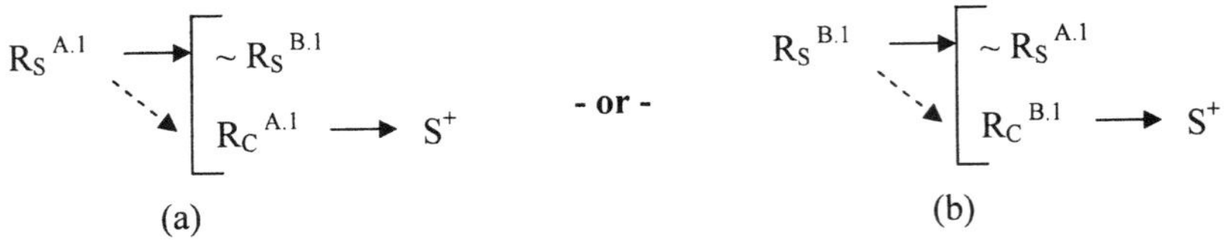

Figure 15.4
Representation of the disjunct interrelation in terms of social reinforcement.

presence of which A realizes the consummatory behavior $Rc^{A.1}$, which is reinforced by S^{+} (i.e., he satisfies his interest $I_F^{A.1}$);

(b) for subject B, $Rs^{B.1}$ is the behavior (corresponding to the interest $Is^{B.1}$) reinforced by the absence of behavior $Rs^{A.1}$ (corresponding to the interest $Is^{A.1}$) of subject A. The absence of $Rs^{A.1}$ is a discriminative stimulus in the presence of which B realizes the consummatory behavior $Rc^{B.1}$, which is reinforced by S^{+} (i.e., he satisfies his interest $I_F^{B.1}$).

In the case of disjunct interrelation only one of the two subjects can realize an instrumental behavior and thence a consummatory behavior, i.e., only one of the two subjects can satisfy his own interest. In fact, interests $I_F^{A.1}$ and $I_F^{B.1}$ are negatively involved. This implies that only one of the two interests can be satisfied and therefore only the behavioral sequence corresponding to the interest which is satisfied can be realized.

Explication of Three Fundamental Concepts for the Integration of the Social Sciences: Power, Exchange, Organization

I conclude from the basic explicative relations of social interaction formulated within the theory of interests that positive involvement and negative involvement are the more basic relations of the scientific analysis of social behavior. Positive involvement explicates the pre-scientific concept of cooperation and negative involvement explicates the pre-scientific concept of conflict.

One of the most important problems in the field of social studies is how to overcome *conflict* (negative involvement of interests). In fact, negative involvement expresses a situation of perfect *social inertia*, since neither of the two subjects is able to carry out autonomously his own operant sequence as the other subject, bringing into action the opposite operant sequence, blocks him (bars the reinforcement of the other subject's instrumental sequence). Both operant sequences exclude each other, since it is impossible, by definition, that one subject can share the sequence that the other subject can carry out, and vice versa.

Leaving aside a resort to physical force, which is not taken into consideration within social science, there are only three modalities by which to overcome the inherent inertia of negative involvement. The first one concerns the change of one or both subjects' field of interests, which occurs in the context of evolutionary dynamics (history time). By definition, it is not taken into consideration within the theory of interests and the experimental analysis of behavior founded on functions that include only repetition time as an implicit independent variable. The second and the third modalities concern power (typical of *institutions*) and exchange (typical of the *market*).

The explication of power and exchange is obtained starting from the two more basic relations (i.e., positive and negative involvement), and by inserting in the context further relations that define more specific social-interaction situations.

Power, in its more abstract definition, occurs when a majority group (with greater *social strength*) opposes a (deviant) subject or a minority group (deviant too) that has one of his interests conflicting (negatively involved) with the interest (positively involved) that establishes the majority group. The *relation of power* can be described by figure 15.5, which shows:

the relation $[\mathrm{IF}^{A.1}]$ **PI** $[\mathrm{IF}^{B.1}]$, which defines the social strength of the majority group (in this case composed of A and B)

the relation $[\mathrm{IF}^{B.1}]$ **NI** $[\mathrm{IF}^{C.1}]$, which defines the situation of conflict between the majority group and the subject C (deviant)

and

the relation $[\mathrm{IF}^{B.1}]$ **PI** $[\mathrm{IF}^{C.2}]$, which defines the condition that makes possible for the majority group to impose on subject C an exclusive disjunction between two interests with different intensity level: the interest $\mathrm{IF}^{C.1}$ (lower in intensity) and the interest $\mathrm{IF}^{C.2}$ (higher in intensity: $\iota_{C.2} > \iota_{C.1}$). The majority group settles (on the grounds of social strength) a new positive-involvement relation between $\mathrm{IF}^{B.1}$ and $\mathrm{IF}^{C.2}$. In fact, if subject C satisfies $\mathrm{IF}^{C.2}$, then he necessarily *sacrifices* $\mathrm{IF}^{C.1}$ and the majority group's interest $\mathrm{IF}^{B.1}$ (together with the positively involved interest $\mathrm{IF}^{A.1}$) is necessarily satisfied—in accordance with the negative involvement between $\mathrm{IF}^{B.1}$ and $\mathrm{IF}^{C.1}$.

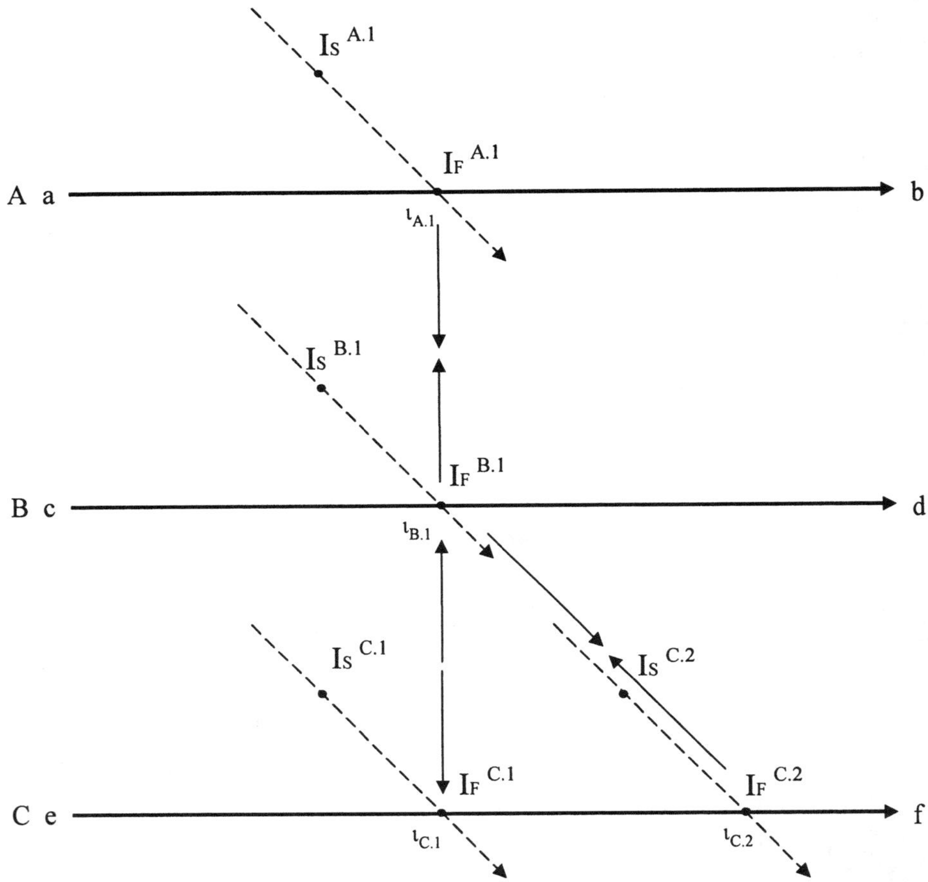

Figure 15.5
Diagram for the relation of power between the majority group (composed by A and B) and the deviant subject (C).

In this case a *mediate* (*indirect*) positive involvement (acting by power) is established between the majority group's interest $I_F^{B.1}$ and the deviant's interest $I_F^{C.2}$, and the latter subject becomes a *potential deviant*. On the contrary, subject C becomes an *actual deviant* if he satisfies his own interest $I_F^{C.1}$, which is negatively involved with the interest $I_F^{B.1}$, that represents the positive involvement of interests of the majority group. This occurs when the deviant's interest $I_F^{C.1}$ holds the highest intensity level and, therefore, there is not any interest in the deviant subject's field that makes it possible for the group with larger social strength to establish a relation of power (i.e., to impose an effective exclusive disjunction between the sacrifice of one interest and the satisfaction of another one).

Therefore, social strength is a necessary, but not sufficient, condition for power.[24] A further condition is needed: that at least one interest with a higher intensity level than the interest in conflict (i.e., the interest which is negatively involved with the majority group's interest) exists in the deviant's field. This condition is related to the problem of effectiveness of punishment in preventing violations from the rules (where punishment is the sacrifice of $\text{IF}^{C.2}$ when $\text{IF}^{C.1}$ is satisfied and $\text{IF}^{B.1}$ is consequently sacrificed—in accordance with the mediate positive involvement). It is worth noting that effectiveness of punishment implies only that the deviant subject does not become an actual deviant, whereas the negatively involved interest remains in his field of interests, as the subject is a potential deviant. To *obey* the rules (mediate positive involvement) does not mean to *agree* with the rules (immediate positive involvement).

Another modality to overcome the negative involvement, totally different from power, concerns two subjects, each of whom has two interests negatively involved with as many corresponding interests of the other subject; with the further condition that the two negative-involvement relations take place only between subjects' interests with a transposed intensity-level order (i.e., with the exclusion of the case in which the two subjects' interests that are negatively involved are the ones with higher intensity level or the ones with lower intensity level). Under this modality, the subjects establish a *relation of exchange,* that can be described by figure 15.6, which shows

the relations $[\text{IF}^{A.1}]$ NI $[\text{IF}^{B.2}]$ and $[\text{IF}^{A.2}]$ NI $[\text{IF}^{B.1}]$, which define the specific *crossed* negative involvements among interests under which neither subject can satisfy both interests of his own field (since, by definition, the social strength is excluded in this situation), but each one of them can satisfy only one of the two interests negatively involved with as many interests of the other subject and sacrifice the other one—in accordance with the transposed intensity-level order

and

the relation $[\text{IF}^{A.2}]$ PI $[\text{IF}^{B.2}]$, which defines the *mediate* (*indirect*) positive involvement (acting by exchange) requiring that both subjects satisfy their interest with the higher intensity level and contextually sacrifice their

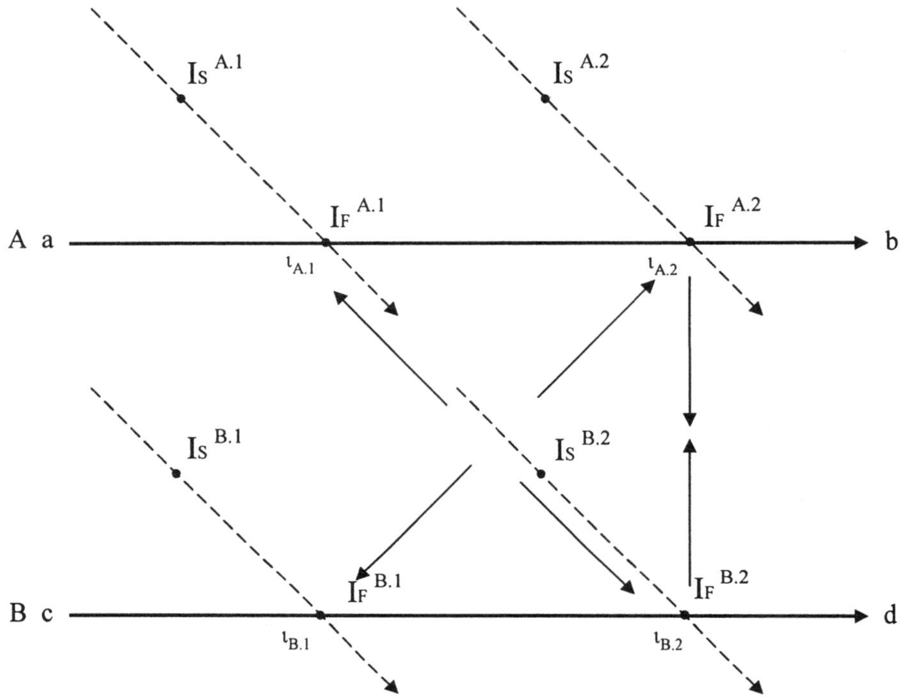

Figure 15.6
Diagram for the relation of exchange.

interest with the lower intensity level. It takes place, as to A, with the satisfaction of the interest $I_F^{A.2}$ (higher in intensity) and the contextual sacrifice of the interest $I_F^{A.1}$ (lower in intensity: $\iota_{A.1} < \iota_{A.2}$) and, as to B, with the satisfaction of the interest $I_F^{B.2}$ (higher in intensity) and the contextual sacrifice of the interest $I_F^{B.1}$ (lower in intensity: $\iota_{B.1} < \iota_{B.2}$).

The explication of exchange[25] within the theory of interests proves that the "is not preferred to" relation, which is the only one economists take into consideration, is coupled with the "is instrumental to" relation. As stated above, both the "is instrumental to" and the "is not preferred to" relations derive from the experimental analysis of behavior. Within the theory of interests, they are expressed by the instrumentality degree and the intensity level, respectively. Therefore it can be confirmed that economic behavior is a subset of social behavior.

With reference to exchange, the "is not preferred to" relation has to be supposed between a behavior that is realized (preferred) and a (non-preferred) behavior whose non-realization is made instrumental to the behavior that is realized. Therefore, it is not sufficient that one behavior is preferred to another. A further condition is required, which is expressed by the theory of interests: the non-preferred interest has to be sacrificed (not satisfied) and its sacrifice has to be made *instrumental* to the satisfaction of the preferred interest.

This specific compatibility between a subset of interests ordered by the "is not preferred to" relation and a corresponding subset of interests ordered by the "is instrumental to" relation defines the concept of *choice*. The assumptions characterizing the consumption sets on the economic analysis level (Debreu 1959, p. 52ff.) apply to it. In this particular case, the position of a subject achieving the exchange can be expressed by saying that the marginal rate of substitution (MRS) between the interest ($\text{IF}^{A.2}$ for subject A and $\text{IF}^{B.2}$ for subject B) with higher intensity level ($\iota_{A.2}$ and $\iota_{B.2}$ respectively) and the interest ($\text{IF}^{A.1}$ for subject A and $\text{IF}^{B.1}$ for subject B) with lower intensity level ($\iota_{A.1}$ and $\iota_{B.1}$ respectively) concerns the degree of satisfaction of the interest $\text{IF}^{A.1}$ or $\text{IF}^{B.1}$, which the subject who exchanges renounces in order to obtain an increase in the degree of satisfaction for the interest $\text{IF}^{A.2}$ or $\text{IF}^{B.2}$. Moving downward along the indifference curve for the two interests $\text{IF}^{A.1}$ and $\text{IF}^{A.2}$ (for subject A) or $\text{IF}^{B.1}$ and $\text{IF}^{B.2}$ (for subject B), the subject who exchanges determines a decrease of the $\text{MRS}(\text{IF}^{A.1}, \text{IF}^{A.2})$ or $\text{MRS}(\text{IF}^{B.1}, \text{IF}^{B.2})$.

Simplifying the notation with reference to marginal utility (MU), it can be said that MRSxy = MUx/MUy. The exchange is mutually profitable when given a subject A with MRSxy and a subject B with MRSx′y′ the condition MRSxy ≠ MRSx′y′ (and the corresponding MUx/MUy ≠ MUx′/MUy′) occurs.

In economic language, the quantities Qx, Qy of the two goods x and y (namely, the interests $\text{IF}^{A.1}$ and $\text{IF}^{A.2}$—or $\text{IF}^{B.1}$ and $\text{IF}^{B.2}$—or rather the two given consumption sets) establish a curve which is usually interpreted as an equivalence class with respect to the indifference relation "$x_i^1 \underset{i}{\lesssim} y_i^2$ and $y_i^2 \underset{i}{\lesssim} x_i^1$" which is denoted "$x_i^1 \underset{i}{\sim} y_i^2$." In this sense the equivalence class is named an indifference class (Debreu 1959, p. 54).

The theory of interests proves that the equivalence class—with respect to the indifference relation between $\{\text{IF}_i^{A.1}$ and $\text{IF}_i^{A.2}\}$ or $\{\text{IF}_i^{B.1}$ and $\text{IF}_i^{B.2}\}$—can be interpreted as an equivalence class in terms of instrumentality involving the sacrifice of one interest and the corresponding satisfaction of another interest, i.e., an equivalence class with respect to the instrumentality relation between $\{\sim IF_i^{A.1} \rightarrow IF_i^{A.2}\}$ or $\{\sim IF_i^{B.1} \rightarrow IF_i^{B.2}\}$.

In this sense, equivalence classes are not indifference classes, but rather instrumentality classes of one interest, which is sacrificed, with respect to another interest, which is satisfied. That is, they are equivalence classes with respect to the instrumentality relation between two sets in terms of sacrifice-satisfaction (choice). On that account, these equivalence classes assume that the two interests are ordered primarily according to their intensity level, which determines which of the two interests has to be satisfied and which one has to be instrumentally sacrificed. Therefore, the order of intensity is a premise for the order of instrumentality in terms of sacrifice-satisfaction.

This interpretation can be used to explicate the concepts of *preference* and *utility* within the more general behavioristic language. Preference expresses the order of intensity levels, whereas utility, in a general sense, does not express a property of one interest, but rather an instrumentality relation between two interests, one of which is sacrificed in order to gain the satisfaction of the other one. The utility of one interest is determined by the instrumentality of the sacrifice of another interest.

In economic language, utility is defined by the order of indifference classes, i.e., by the partitions of the consumption set obtained using the equivalence classes with respect to the *indifference relation*. On this subject Debreu (1959) states: "Is it possible to associate with each class a real number in such a way that, if a class is preferred to another, the number of the first is greater than the number of the second? In other words, given a set completely preordered by preferences, does there exist an increasing ... real-valued function on that set? Such a function is called a *utility function*" (pp. 55–56).

In the same way, the concept of utility can be applied to the order of equivalence classes with respect to the *instrumentality relation*. The two definitions of utility, the one based on instrumentality classes and the other based on indifference classes (to which economists refer), are consistent with the theory of interests and with the economic theory.

There is also another important side for the characterization of exchange: *competition*. Exchange refers to the activity of those subjects who transfer services and obtain other services, so that in the subset of economic behavior the individual utility functions are in principle maximized. Competition refers to the activity of producers, each of whom acts with reference to the behavior of the other producers in the subset of exchange behavior. Competitive activity also can be analyzed in terms of interests.

Given two producers, A and C, there is a negative involvement between their interests, since each of them has an interest in removing the consumers from the other. But it is different from the negative involvement that takes place between the subjects that engage in exchange. Unlike exchange, it is not possible that both subjects benefit in the case of competition, since the advantage of one necessarily leads to the disadvantage of the other. Moreover, unlike power, the conflict between producers cannot be resolved through a social interaction in which A's actions are aimed to change C's behavior, or vice versa. As a matter of fact, the possibility that the conflict between two competitors can be resolved through social strength has to be ruled out. Subject A can resolve the conflict to his favor with subject C in only one way: by offering to consumers a greater advantage than the one they would obtain if they exchanged with C. This situation can be described by figure 15.7, which shows

the relations $[\text{IF}^{B.1}]$ NI $[\text{IF}^{A.2}]$ and $[\text{IF}^{B.2}]$ NI $[\text{IF}^{A.1}]$, which define the exchange conditions between B (consumer) and A (producer),

the relations $[\text{IF}^{B.1'}]$ NI $[\text{IF}^{C.2}]$ and $[\text{IF}^{B.2}]$ NI $[\text{IF}^{C.1}]$, which define the exchange conditions between B (consumer) and C (the producer competing with A who is left out of the exchange with B),

and

the relation $[\text{IF}^{B.2}]$ PI $[\text{IF}^{A.2}]$, which defines the exchange interaction between B (consumer) and A (producer) (see explication of figure 15.6).

The exclusion of C is due to the fact that B (consumer) has a lower advantage in realizing the exchange behavior with him, since such behavior would imply that B sacrifices interest $\text{IF}^{B.1'}$, with an intensity level higher than the intensity level of interest $\text{IF}^{B.1}$ $(\imath_{B.1'} > \imath_{B.1})$ which is sacrificed when he exchanges with A. Consequently B must exchange (i.e., is conditioned to exchange, in conformity with the explicative postulates of behavior) with A instead of C. In this case exchange is more profitable for B also in the economic perspective.

The social interaction between the two producers A and C, which is implicit in figure 15.7, can be clarified by reversing the positions of A's and B's fields of interests. Figure 15.8 shows

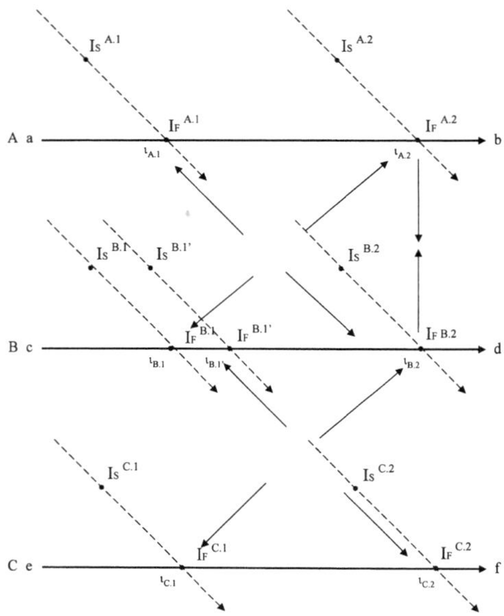

Figure 15.7
Diagram for the situation of competition, which points out the exchange between the consumer B and producer A, resulting from the different exchange conditions fixed by the two producers A and C, as represented by the different intensity levels of the interest to be sacrificed by the consumer B.

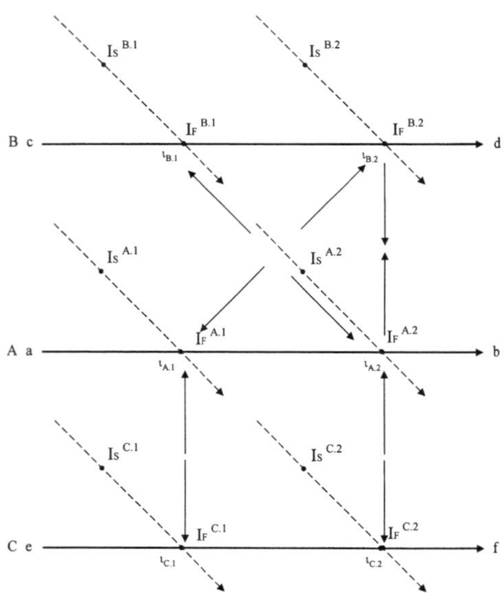

Figure 15.8
Diagram for the situation of competition, which points out the "conflict" (negative involvement) between the interests of producer A and producer C. Note that this diagram is a transformation of figure 15.7 obtained by reversing the position of A's and B's fields of interests.

the relations $[IF^{A.1}]$ NI $[IF^{B.2}]$, $[IF^{A.2}]$ NI $[IF^{B.1}]$ and $[IF^{A.2}]$ PI $[IF^{B.2}]$, which define the exchange interaction between A (producer) and B (consumer) (see explication of figure 15.6)

and

the relations $[IF^{A.1}]$ NI $[IF^{C.1}]$ and $[IF^{A.2}]$ NI $[IF^{C.2}]$, which define the competition between the two producers A and C.

From the above relations it follows that the satisfaction of A's interest $IF^{A.2}$, with an intensity level higher than $IF^{A.1}$, corresponds to the non-satisfaction of C's interest $IF^{C.2}$; and, vice versa, the sacrifice of A's interest $IF^{A.1}$ corresponds to the satisfaction of C's interest $IF^{C.1}$, which holds however an intensity level lower than $IF^{C.2}$, namely the interest that C would had satisfied if he was not left out of the exchange.

In competition, therefore, conflict can be resolved by one of the competitors when he offers to consumers an advantage greater than the one they could obtain if they exchanged with the other competitor. Such advantage takes place when, given the same intensity level of the satisfied interest, the intensity level of the sacrificed interest is lower; or when, given the same intensity level of the sacrificed interest, the intensity level of the satisfied interest is higher.

Summing up, the theory of interests identifies one type of negative involvement and two types of positive involvement: (1) the *immediate (direct) positive involvement,* which occurs when the positively involved interests are stabilized in each subject's field of interests, apart from any exchange or power relation; (2) the *mediate* (*indirect*) *positive involvement* obtained through exchange or power, which are the two specific social interactions that make it possible to overcome situations of conflict (negative involvement of interests).

On the logical level, both typologies of positive involvement are characterized by two necessary conditions: *mutual implication of final interests* and *reciprocal complementarity of instrumental interests*. The difference between the two forms of positive involvement is given by a further condition, that must be necessarily fulfilled only in the case of mediate (indirect) positive involvement: at least one of the two subjects (as stated above, the subject having less social strength in the case of power, both subjects in the case of exchange) not only must realize the instrumental sequence related to the positively involved (in the mediate way) interest, which is complementary to the other subject's sequence, but must also instrumentally sacrifice the interest with an intensity level lower than the one positively involved (in the mediate way). That is, at least one of the two subjects must realize a *sacrifice-satisfaction instrumentality relation* (choice).

In the case where one subject is in a position to realize autonomously (also without the other subject's consent) the entire sequence of instrumental behaviors related to the consummatory behavior corresponding to the satisfaction of one of his own final interests, there is not any positive involvement (neither an immediate nor a mediate one), even when the satisfaction of his final interest implies the satisfaction of another subject's interest. This is what happens with reference to the *"altruistic behavior."* In this case the essential conditions for a positive involvement between the two interests do not exist, since the satisfaction of the second subject's interest is not necessary for the first subject's interest to be satisfied, because the satisfaction of the second subject's interest is a mere consequence of the first subject's interest satisfaction.[26]

Organization is explicated in scientific terms by the positive involvement, with specific reference to the essential condition of the reciprocal complementarity of the two distinct instrumental interests sequences carried out by each subject. This reciprocal complementarity among instrumental interests belonging to different fields of interests implies that the set of all conjointly interrelated instrumental interests is such that, in principle, each instrumental interest defines an organizational role and each role, thus differentiated, is assigned to either subject whose interests are positively involved.

That being said, given that at the most abstract level the founding element of an organization is immediate (direct) positive involvement of interests, it may be that access to organizational roles (defined by sequences of complementary instrumental behaviors) is realized through exchange. In this specific case, exchange works as a tool to acquire or to assign organizational roles, but it does not qualify these roles, whose only reference point is immediate (direct) positive involvement of interests of those subjects who have their interests in organization not mediated by exchange. Therefore, organization must not be confused either with exchange or with power—even if both exchange and power can be utilized to integrate (but not found) an organization on the basis of mediate (indirect) positive involvement.[27]

Conclusion

I have proposed a concise outline of a model for integration among economics, psychology and sociology using basic concepts of behaviorism, together with other primitive theoretical concepts. My aim has been to construct an abstract language (the theory of interests) which is strictly consistent with both the behavioristic language (related to experimental analysis) and the formalized and axiomatized economic language (related to market equilibrium), as well as the sociological language; that is, with all the languages of the social sciences.

This model, which I cannot work out here more analytically, points out how difficult is the way to a real integration among the social sciences and how many logical and methodological obstacles still have to be overcome before behavior can be explained with a unitary perspective. The model also points out that many of the problems and questions, that are still the subject of tenacious debate within each narrow specialty, turn out to be false problems when considered from the wider point of view of the real social science.

I did not meet John Staddon in a university lecture hall, but I knew him from the pages of journals and books. The article "The 'superstition' experiment: A re-examination of its implications for the principles of adaptive behavior" (by Staddon and Simmelhag) and Staddon's books *Limits to Action* (1980) and *Adaptive Behavior and Learning* (1983) corroborated my opinion that he was a scholar who did not consider experiments *per se*, but as a basis to try to construct a theoretical perspective that was missing in behaviorism.

Thus, in the 1990s, when I was appointed to design and manage the International Graduate Program in Science of Organization by AILUN, I invited John to participate, since the program had the object of integrating social sciences under a behavioristic point of view. But I feared that such a rash enterprise, in addition to its location in an inner area of Sardinia (Nuoro), would arouse questions and reservations. On the contrary, I found enthusiastic acceptance, and every year since then John has participated in the program. The serene profundity of his thought, together with his distinguished humor and his human kindness rich in emotional contents, even if hidden by very controlled (but always sincere, refined, and spontaneous) operant behaviors, made our relationship more and more friendly and hearty.

Notes

1. The attribution of properties to the domain and the range of every function (in general to every set of functions) to make it possible for the logical-mathematical language, in its formal configuration, to fit the specific fields of scientific knowledge.

2. Generally, a set of postulates is consistent if it does not imply contradictory statements.

3. $A \cap B = \varnothing$: two sets are disjoint if their intersection is the null set.

4. $A \neq 0$, $B \neq 0$; $A \cap B = \varnothing$; $A \cup B = S$: S is partitioned into two (or more) subsets. The partition of S originates an equivalence relation in S of the type "from the same subset as" (in extensional terms) or "has the same property as" (in intensional terms concerning the property that defines the subset). The equivalence relation is between all pairs of elements in the same subset; so every subset of the partition is an equivalence class.

5. Experiential as the opposite of experimental (i.e., common sense versus scientific sense).

6. A distinctive character or attribute typical of all the elements belonging to a set, which defines the set.

7. $A \times B$: the set of ordered pairs, with a as first element and b as second element, such that $a \in A$ and $b \in B$.

8. Function: if $(a_1\, b_1) \in f$ and $(a_2\, b_2) \in f$ and $a_1 = a_2$, then $b_1 = b_2$. More simply: if $(a_1\, b_1) \in f$ and $(a_1\, b_2) \in f$, then $b_1 = b_2$.

9. In a general sense an order relation is transitive: if $(A, B) \in R$ and $(B, C) \in R$, then $(A, C) \in R$.

10. $A \subseteq B$: A is a subset of B. The relation "is a subset of" is reflexive: $(A \subseteq A)$, and antisymmetric: $(A, B) \in R$ and $(B, A) \in R$ imply $A = B$.

11. $A \cap B$: the set of elements belonging to both A and B.

12. A partially ordered set (poset): for any pair of elements in S, R is reflexive, antisymmetric, transitive, and not all pairs of elements in S are comparable by R.

13. $A \subset B$ and $A \neq B$: A is a proper subset of B. The relation "is a proper subset of" is asymmetric: $(A, B) \in R$ implies $(B, A) \notin R$.

14. In this case, only the relation "$+t$ or $-t$" is significant, where 'or' stands for an exclusive disjunction.

15. On this subject, Staddon writes: "The central fact about behavior is that it is a *process*, a series of events that occur in time. It is *dynamic*. So my main emphasis is on the way behavior changes in time" (p. xi). But this fact does not prevent him from acknowledging that "the specific reason is my belief that the within-subject method is essential if our aim is to understand learning at the most fundamental level. But it must be accompanied, as in the past it has not been, by theoretical exploration" (2001a, p. 8).

16. When social variables are made endogenous (i.e., transformed into economic variables), they lose their distinctive connotation.

17. Mathematical language becomes economic language by its interpretation. The interpretation consists essentially of the rules of designation (Carnap 1959, p. 24ff.) that (together with the other semantic rules) lay down conventions (in a metalanguage) concerning the domain of application of a given object language.

18. This interpretation could be improved if it were brought back to the strict logic of behavior and to the theory of interests.

19. With reference to the optimality approach to operant behavior, Staddon states that "no optimality model works in every situation. Animals are rarely, if ever, 'literal optimizers'; they don't remember the average payoff associated with a given pattern of responding, compare it with the payoffs for the other patterns (from a well-defined set of possibilities), and then pick the best pattern—as some views of optimal responding seem to imply. Under most conditions, people don't behave in this way either." (2001a, p. 76)

20. The basic outline of the theory of interests was first published in Bolacchi 1963a,b and Bolacchi 1964. The technical analysis was further developed in Bolacchi 1974 and subsequent publications.

21. This is the case of exclusive disjunction (truth table: 0110).

22. The instrumental sequence of interests corresponds, in the behavioral perspective, to the basic experimental set "instrumental operant and consummatory operant": $\{\mathrm{Rs} \rightarrow \mathrm{Rc}\}$.

23. In logical terms, the *positive involvement* can be expressed by the formula: $\{([\mathrm{IF}^{A.1}] \supset [\mathrm{IF}^{B.1}]) \wedge ([\mathrm{IF}^{B.1}] \supset [\mathrm{IF}^{A.1}])\}$, which is equivalent to: $[\mathrm{IF}^{A.1}] \equiv [\mathrm{IF}^{B.1}]$. The *negative involvement* can be expressed by the formula: $\{([\mathrm{IF}^{A.1}] \supset [\sim\mathrm{IF}^{B.1}]) \wedge ([\sim\mathrm{IF}^{A.1}] \supset [\mathrm{IF}^{B.1}])\}$, which is equivalent to $\{([\mathrm{IF}^{B.1}] \supset [\sim\mathrm{IF}^{A.1}]) \wedge ([\sim\mathrm{IF}^{B.1}] \supset [\mathrm{IF}^{A.1}])\}$. Each formula of negative involvement is equivalent to: $\sim([\mathrm{IF}^{A.1}] \equiv [\mathrm{IF}^{B.1}])$.

24. In logical terms, *power* can be expressed by the conjunction of the formulas concerning the negative involvement (conflict) and the mediate positive involvement (related to social strength): $\{\sim([\mathrm{IF}^{B.1}] \equiv [\mathrm{IF}^{C.1}]) \wedge ([\mathrm{IF}^{B.1}] \equiv [\mathrm{IF}^{C.2}])\}$; from these formulas it can be derived the exclusive disjunction: $\{([\mathrm{IF}^{C.1}] \vee [\mathrm{IF}^{C.2}]) \wedge \sim([\mathrm{IF}^{C.1}] \wedge [\mathrm{IF}^{C.2}])\}$. It follows that if $[\mathrm{IF}^{C.2}]$ (given $\iota_{C.2} > \iota_{C.1}$), then $([\sim\mathrm{IF}^{C.1}] \wedge [\mathrm{IF}^{B.1}])$.

25. In logical terms, *exchange* can be expressed by the conjunction of the formulas concerning the crossed negative involvements: $\{\sim([\mathrm{IF}^{A.1}] \equiv [\mathrm{IF}^{B.2}]) \wedge \sim([\mathrm{IF}^{A.2}] \equiv [\mathrm{IF}^{B.1}])\}$; from these formulas it can be derived two exclusive disjunctions: $\{([\mathrm{IF}^{A.1}] \vee [\mathrm{IF}^{A.2}]) \wedge \sim([\mathrm{IF}^{A.1}] \wedge [\mathrm{IF}^{A.2}])\}$ and $\{([\mathrm{IF}^{B.1}] \vee [\mathrm{IF}^{B.2}]) \wedge \sim([\mathrm{IF}^{B.1}] \wedge [\mathrm{IF}^{B.2}])\}$ that express the mediate positive involvement $([\mathrm{IF}^{A.2}] \equiv [\mathrm{IF}^{B.2}])$. It follows that if $([\mathrm{IF}^{A.2}] \wedge [\mathrm{IF}^{B.2}])$ (given $\iota_{A.2} > \iota_{A.1}$ and $\iota_{B.2} > \iota_{B.1}$), then $([\sim\mathrm{IF}^{A.1}] \wedge [\sim\mathrm{IF}^{B.1}])$.

26. This case might be the one economists refer to when they talk about *externalities* of production and consumption. Furthermore, this case also allows us to analyze the problem of *free riding*, which is usually examined with reference to public goods. The free rider's behavior can be generalized in a more abstract perspective within the theory of interests, as an element of the more general set of behaviors realized by the subjects who profit (without any positive involvement) by positive involvement among other subjects' interests. With reference to the free rider, no cooperation can exist in the sense of immediate (direct) positive involvement. Only a mediate (indirect) positive involvement based upon a power relation established by a majority group of subjects can exist, expressing an immediate (direct) positive involvement in an interest in supporting the cost of financing the public good. This interest is negatively involved with the free rider's interest in not contributing to financing of the public good.

27. This points out shows that it is not possible to define cooperation by using the reference schema of the exchange, as a branch of economic analysis claims to do (Buchanan 1964). Under this logic, cooperation would arise when the expected benefits related to the achievement of a given social object (that cannot be attained directly by the single subjects through the market, owing to the lack of sufficient incentives) are higher than the costs inherent in some "adaptation" to a "voluntary cooperation" among several subjects. Thus "voluntary cooperation" is regarded as a type of social interaction (in which the *firm*, as an *organization*, can also be included) aimed at satisfying those interests that get no incentive from the market, through a multiplicity of exchanges (among subjects cooperating in satisfying what should be a common interest), so that an equilibrium situation takes place, optimizing the cooperation positions of the single subjects. The theory of interests points out the inconsistency of Buchanan's argumentations. He confuses cooperation with exchange when he states that, on the one hand, cooperation aims at satisfying those (common) interests that get no incentive from the market and that, from the other hand, this satisfaction should take place through a multiplicity of exchanges among cooperating subjects. It is true that those interests which are satisfied through cooperation get no incentive from the market; this is explicated in the theory of interests by the positive involvement. However, it is contradictory to state that cooperation should always take place through a multiplicity of exchanges, because cooperation and exchange are two different types of social behavior (belonging to two disjoint sets). Buchanan and several other economists, such as R. H. Coase, M. Olson, K. J. Arrow, H. A. Simon, who have turned their attention to this problem, did not notice

that the definition of cooperation (and of organization) by means of exchange can be referred only to the mediate (indirect) positive involvement and not to the immediate (direct) positive involvement.

Since exchange entails a mediate positive involvement, and it can concern any type of interest (or, in economic terms, and type of service), it is possible that the interest in not bearing the costs of cooperation could be sacrificed, to satisfy the interest in gaining the (expected) benefits of cooperation. This is exactly the case of an interest (lower in intensity) sacrificed to satisfy another interest (higher in intensity), as occurs in the exchange (as well as in the power). Therefore cooperation cannot be explained by exchange, even though it can be derived from exchange as mediate (indirect) positive involvement. Really the difference between these concepts is founded on the primitive relations of immediate (direct) positive involvement and of negative involvement. These primitive relations, which are considered basic preliminary assumptions (postulates), have a logical (syntactic) meaning (which points out their *disjunctness*) and a semantic interpretation founded on experimental analysis of behavior (when the behavior of a subject A is dynamically related to a social stimulus, that is a behavior of a subject B presenting or removing a positive "pleasant" reinforcer, according to whether A's behavior is socially admitted or not admitted—as illustrated in this chapter). Starting from these basic assumptions every social behavior can be explicated (scientifically explained); but, accordingly, we cannot assume only one of the two postulates to explain all social behaviors. But economists do it.

References

Adams, J. S. 1963. Toward an understanding of equity. *Journal of Abnormal and Social Psychology* 67: 422–436.

Adret, P. 1993. Vocal learning induced with operant techniques: An overview. *Netherlands Journal of Zoology* 43: 125–142.

Allan, L. G. 1992. The internal clock revisited. In *Time, Action, and Cognition: Towards Bridging the Gap*, ed. F. Macar, V. Pouthas, and W. Friedman. Kluwer.

Antonitis, J. J. 1951. Response variability in the white rat during conditioning, extinction, and reconditioning. *Journal of Experimental Psychology* 42: 273–281.

Arvey, R. D., and Murphy, K. R. 1998. Performance evaluation in work settings. *Annual Review of Psychology* 49: 141–168.

Bachelard, G. 1968. *The Philosophy of No: A Philosophy of the New Scientific Mind*. Orion. Original work published 1940.

Baddeley, A. D., and Hitch, G. 1974. Working memory. In *The Psychology of Learning and Motivation*, volume 8, ed. G. Bower. Academic Press.

Bailey, D. W., Rittenhouse, L. R., Hart, R. H., and Richards, R. W. 1989. Characteristics of spatial memory in cattle. *Applied Animal Behavior Science* 23: 331–340.

Bailey, J. T., and Mazur, J. E. 1990. Choice behavior in transition: Development of preference for the higher probability of reinforcement. *Journal of the Experimental Analysis of Behavior* 53: 409–422.

Baptista, L. F., and Petrinovich, L. 1986. Song development in the white-crowned sparrow: Social factors and sex differences. *Animal Behaviour* 34: 1359–1371.

Baum, W. M. 1973. The correlation-based law of effect. *Journal of the Experimental Analysis of Behavior* 20: 137–153.

Baum, W. M. 1974. On two types of deviation from the matching law: Bias and undermatching. *Journal of the Experimental Analysis of Behavior* 22: 231–242.

Baum, W. M. 1979. Matching, undermatching, and overmatching in studies of choice. *Journal of the Experimental Analysis of Behavior* 32: 269–281.

Baum, W. M. 1993. Performance on ratio and interval schedules of reinforcement: Data and theory. *Journal of the Experimental Analysis of Behavior* 59: 245–264.

Baum, W. M. 2002. From molecular to molar: A paradigm shift in behavior analysis. *Journal of the Experimental Analysis of Behavior* 78: 95–116.

Baum, W. M., and Rachlin, H. C. 1969. Choice as time allocation. *Journal of the Experimental Analysis of Behavior* 12: 861–874.

Belke, T. W. 1992. Stimulus preference and the transitivity of preference. *Animal Learning and Behavior* 20: 401–406.

Bem, D. J. 1967. Self perception: An alternative interpretation of cognitive dissonance phenomena. *Psychological Review* 74: 183–200.

Bertalanffy, L. von. 1950. The theory of open systems in physics and biology. *Science* 111: 23–29.

Best, J. B. 1995. *Cognitive Psychology*, fourth edition. West.

Bizo, L. A., and White, K. G. 1994. Pacemaker rate in the behavioral theory of timing. *Journal of Experimental Psychology: Animal Behavior Processes* 20: 308–321.

Bolacchi, G. 1963a. *Teoria delle classi sociali*. Edizioni Ricerche.

Bolacchi, G. 1963b. *Metodologia delle scienze sociali*. Edizioni Ricerche.

Bolacchi, G. 1974. Concorrenza, collettivismo e pianificazione. *Studi di economia* 5: 3–49.

Bolacchi, G. 2006. On "social sciences" and science. *Behavior and Philosophy* 32: 465–478.

Boyd, R. 1984. The current status of scientific realism. In *Scientific Realism*, ed. J. Leplin. University of California Press.

Bray, D. W. 1982. The assessment center and the study of lives. *American Psychologist* 37: 180–189.

Breland, K., and Breland, M. 1961. The misbehavior of organisms. *American Psychologist* 16: 681–684.

Bronowski, J. 1974. *The Ascent of Man*. Little, Brown.

Brown, B. L., Hemmes, N. S., and Cabeza de Vaca, S. 1992. Effects of intratrial stimulus change on fixed-interval performance: The roles of clock and memory processes. *Animal Learning and Behavior* 20: 83–93.

Brown, M. F. 1992. Does a cognitive map guide choices in the radial-arm maze? *Journal of Experimental Psychology: Animal Behavior Processes* 18: 56–66.

Brown, M. F., and Demas, G. E. 1994. Evidence for spatial working memory in honeybees (*Apis mellifera*). *Journal of Comparative Psychology* 108: 344–352.

Brunner, D., Kacelnik, A., and Gibbon, J. 1992. Optimal foraging and timing processes in the starling, *Sturnus vulgaris*: Effect of inter-capture interval. *Animal Behaviour* 44: 597–613.

Buhusi, C. V., and Meck, W. H. 2000. Timing for the absence of a stimulus: The gap paradigm reversed. *Journal of Experimental Psychology: Animal Behavior Processes* 26: 305–322.

Bush, R. R., and Mosteller, F. 1955. *Stochastic Models for Learning*. Wiley.

Business Week. 1972. Where Skinner's theories work. December 2: 64–65.

Cabeza de Vaca, S., Brown, B. L., and Hemmes, N. S. 1994. Internal clock and memory processes in animal timing. *Journal of Experimental Psychology: Animal Behavior Processes* 20: 184–198.

Campbell, D. T. 1960. Blind variation and selective retention in creative thought as in other knowledge processes. *Psychological Review* 67: 380–400.

Caraco, T., Martindale, S., and Whitham, T. S. 1980. An empirical demonstration of risk sensitive foraging preferences. *Animal Behaviour* 28: 820–830.

Carnap, R. 1959. *Introduction to Semantics*. Harvard University Press.

Cascio, W. F. 1995. Whither industrial and organizational psychology in a changing world of work? *American Psychologist* 50: 928–939.

Catania, A. C. 1963. Concurrent performances: A baseline for the study of reinforcement magnitude. *Journal of the Experimental Analysis of Behavior* 6: 299–300.

Catania, A. C. 1970. Reinforcement schedules and psychophysical judgments: A study of some temporal properties of behavior. In *The Theory of Reinforcement Schedules*, ed. W. Schoenfeld. Appleton-Century-Crofts.

Catania, A. C. 1971. Reinforcement schedules: The role of responses preceding the one that produces the reinforcer. *Journal of the Experimental Analysis of Behavior* 15: 271–287.

Catania, A. C., and Reynolds, G. S. 1968. A quantitative analysis of the responding maintained by interval schedules of reinforcement. *Journal of the Experimental Analysis of Behavior* 11: 327–383.

Catania, A. C., Sagvolden, T., and Keller, K. J. 1988. Reinforcement schedules: Retroactive and proactive effects of reinforcers inserted into fixed-interval performances. *Journal of the Experimental Analysis of Behavior* 49: 49–73.

Cerutti, D. T., and Staddon, J. E. R. 2003. Time and rate measures in choice transitions. *Journal of the Experimental Analysis of Behavior* 81: 135–154.

Chaiken, M., Böhner, J., and Marler, P. 1983. Song acquisition in the European Starling (*Sturnus vulgaris*): A comparison of the songs of live-tutored, untutored, and wild-caught males. *Animal Behaviour* 46: 1079–1090.

Cheng, K., and Roberts, W. A. 1989. Timing multimodal events in pigeons. *Journal of the Experimental Analysis of Behavior* 52: 363–376.

Cheng, K., Spetch, M. L., and Miceli, P. 1996. Averaging temporal duration and spatial position. *Journal of Experimental Psychology: Animal Behavior Processes* 22: 175–182.

Chomsky, N. 1959. A review of Skinner's "Verbal Behavior." *Language* 35: 26–58.

Christopher, R., and Neuringer, A. 2002. Reinforcement of variations and repetitions along three independent response dimensions. *Behavioural Processes* 57: 199–209.

Church, R. M. 1978. The internal clock. In *Cognitive Processes in Animal Behavior*, ed. S. Hulse, H. Fowler, and W. Honig. Erlbaum.

Church, R. M. 1984. Properties of an internal clock. In *Annals of the New York Academy of Sciences*, volume 423: *Timing and Time Perception*, ed. J. Gibbon and L. Allan.

Church, R. M. 1997. Timing and temporal search. In *Time and Behaviour: Psychological and Neurobehavioural Analyses*, ed. C. Bradshaw and E. Szabadi. Elsevier.

Church, R. M., and Broadbent, H. A. 1990. Alternative representations of time, number and rate. *Cognition* 37: 55–81.

Church, R. M., and Broadbent, H. A. 1991. A connectionist model of timing. In *Neural Network Models of Conditioning and Action*, ed. M. Commons, S. Grossberg, and J. Staddon. Erlbaum.

Church, R. M., Meck, W. H., and Gibbon, J. 1994. Application of scalar timing theory to individual trials. *Journal of Experimental Psychology: Animal Behavior Processes* 20: 135–155.

Clark, B. C. 1979. The evolution of genetic diversity. *Proceedings of the Royal Society of London Series B* 205: 453–479.

Clayton, N. S., Yu, K. S., and Dickinson, A. 2003. Interacting cache memories: Evidence for flexible memory use by Western Scrub-jays (*Aphelocoma californica*). *Journal of Experimental Psychology: Animal Behavior Processes* 29: 14–22.

Cleaveland, J. M. 1999. Interresponse-time sensitivity during discrete-trial and free-operant concurrent variable-interval schedules. *Journal of the Experimental Analysis of Behavior* 72: 317–339.

Cleaveland, J. M. 2002. Beyond trial-and-error in a selectionist psychology. *Behavior and Philosophy* 30: 73–99.

Cleaveland, J. M., Jäger, R., Rössner, P., and Delius, J. D. 2003. Ontogeny has a phylogeny: Background to adjunctive behaviors in budgerigars and pigeons. *Behavioral Processes* 61: 143–158.

Cohen, J. 1960. A coefficient of agreement for nominal scales. *Educational and Psychological Measurement* 20: 37–46.

Colbert, E. H., Morales, M., and Minkoff, E. C. 2001. *Colbert's Evolution of the Vertebrates*, fifth edition. Wiley-Hiss.

Collins, H. 1992. *Changing Order: Replication and Induction in Scientific Practice*. University of Chicago Press.

Conover, D. O., and Van Voorhees, D. A. 1990. Evolution of a balanced sex ratio by frequency-dependent selection in a fish. *Science* 250: 1556–1557.

Costa, P. T., Jr., and McCrae, R. 1985. *NEO Personality Inventory*. Psychological Assessment Resources.

Couvillon, P. A., and Bitterman, M. E. 1985. Analysis of choice in honeybees. *Animal Learning and Behavior* 13: 246–252.

Couvillon, P. A., and Bitterman, M. E. 1988. Compound-component and conditional discrimination of colors and odors by honeybees: Further tests of a continuity model. *Animal Learning and Behavior* 16: 67–74.

Cummings, T. G., and Worley, C. G. 1997. *Organization Development and Change*, sixth edition. South-Western.

Dale, R. H. I. 1982. Parallel-arm maze performance of sighted and blind rats: Spatial memory and maze structure. *Behaviour Analysis Letters* 2: 127–139.

Dale, R. H. I. 1987. Similarities between human and animal spatial memory: Item and order information. *Animal Learning and Behavior* 15: 293–300.

Dale, R. H. I., and Bedard, M. 1984. Limitations on spatial memory in mice. *The Southern Psychologist* 2: 23–26.

Dale, R. H. I., and Innis, N. K. 1986. Interactions between response stereotypy and memory strategies on the eight-arm radial maze. *Behavioural Brain Research* 19: 17–25.

Dale, R. H. I., Peterson, J. R., and Shyan, M. R. 1995. Too much of a good thing: African elephants get confused when given three memory tests in a row. Paper presented at Elephant Managers Workshop, Tacoma.

Dale, R. H. I., Shyan, M. R., and Hagan, D. A. 1994a. Preliminary studies of the spatial memory abilities of captive African elephants (*Loxodonta africana*). In Proceedings of 13th Annual International Elephant Workshop, Atlanta, 1992.

Dale, R. H. I., Shyan, M. R., and Hagan, D. A. 1994b. Long-term retention of a short-term retention task by five female African elephants (*Loxodonta africana*). In Proceedings of 14th Annual Elephant Managers Conference, Vallejo, California, 1993.

Daly, H. B., and Daly, J. T. 1982. A mathematical model of reward and aversive non-reward: Its application in over 30 appetitive learning situations. *Journal of Experimental Psychology: General* 111: 441–480.

Darwin, C. 1896. *The Variation of Animals and Plants Under Domestication*. Appleton.

Davies, N. B., and Houston, A. I. 1981. Owners and satellites: The economics of territory defence in the pied wagtail, *Motacilla alba*. *Journal of Animal Ecology* 50: 157–180.

Davis, D. G. S., and Staddon, J. E. R. 1990. Memory for reward in probabilistic choice: Markovian and non-Markovian properties. *Behaviour* 114: 37–64.

Davis, D. G. S., Staddon, J. E. R., Machado, A., and Palmer, R. G. 1993. The process of recurrent choice. *Psychological Review* 100: 320–341.

Davison, M., and Baum, W. 2000. Choice in a variable environment: Every reinforcer counts. *Journal of the Experimental Analysis of Behavior* 74: 1–24.

Dawkins, R. 1978. *The Selfish Gene*. Oxford University Press.

Debreu, G. 1959. *Theory of Value: An Axiomatic Analysis of Economic Equilibrium*. Yale University Press.

Dember, W. N., and Fowler, H. 1958. Spontaneous alternation behavior. *Psychological Bulletin* 55: 412–428.

Dews, P. B. 1962. The effect of multiple S^{Δ} periods on responding on a fixed-interval schedule. *Journal of the Experimental Analysis of Behavior* 5: 369–374.

Dews, P. B. 1965. The effect of multiple S^{Δ} periods on responding on a fixed-interval schedule: III. Effect of changes in pattern of interruptions, parameters and stimuli. *Journal of the Experimental Analysis of Behavior* 8: 427–435.

Dews, P. B. 1966. The effect of multiple S^{Δ} periods on responding on a fixed-interval schedule: IV. Effect of continuous S^{Δ} with only short S^{D} probes. *Journal of the Experimental Analysis of Behavior* 9: 147–151.

Dews, P. B. 1970. The theory of fixed-interval responding. In *The Theory of Reinforcement Schedules*, ed. W. Schoenfeld. Appleton-Century-Crofts.

Dipboye, R. L., Smith, C. S., and Howell, W. C. 1994. *Understanding Industrial and Organizational Psychology: An Integrated Approach*. Harcourt Brace.

Donahoe, J. W., and Burgos, J. E. 1999. Timing without a timer. *Journal of the Experimental Analysis of Behavior* 71: 257–263.

Douglas, R. J., Mitchell, D., and Del Valle, R. 1974. Angle between choice alleys as a critical factor in spontaneous alternation. *Animal Learning and Behavior* 2: 218–220.

Dragoi, V. 1997. A dynamic theory of acquisition and extinction in operant learning. *Neural Networks* 10: 201–229.

Dragoi, V., and Staddon, J. E. R. 1999. The dynamics of operant conditioning. *Psychological Review* 106: 20–61.

Dragoi, V., Staddon, J. E. R., Palmer, R. G, and Buhusi, C. V. 2003. Interval timing as an emergent learning property. *Psychological Review* 110: 126–144.

Dreyfus, L. R. 1991. Local shifts in relative reinforcement rate and time allocation on concurrent schedules. *Journal of Experimental Psychology: Animal Behavior Processes* 17: 486–502.

Ebbinghaus, H. 1964. *Memory: A Contribution to Experimental Psychology*. Dover. Original work published 1885.

Epstein, R., Kirshnit, C. E., Lanza, R. P., and Rubin, L. C. 1984. "Insight" in the pigeon: Antecedents and determinants of an intelligent performance. *Nature* 308: 61–62.

Estes, W. K. 1979. *Experimental Psychology: An Overview*. Erlbaum.

Faggiani, D. 1957. *La struttura logica della fisica*. Edizioni Scientifiche Einaudi.

Fantino, E. 1969. Choice and rate of reinforcement. *Journal of the Experimental Analysis of Behavior* 12: 723–730.

Fantino, E. 1981. Contiguity, response strength, and the delay-reduction hypothesis. In *Advances in Analysis of Behavior*, volume 2: *Predictability, Correlation, and Contiguity*, ed. P. Harzem and M. Zeiler. Wiley.

Fantino, E., and Davison, M. 1983. Choice: Some quantitative relations. *Journal of the Experimental Analysis of Behavior* 40: 1–13.

Fantino, E., and Logan, C. A. 1979. *The Experimental Analysis of Behavior: A Biological Perspective*. Freeman.

Fantino, E., Preston, R. A., and Dunn, R. 1993. Delay reduction: Current status. *Journal of the Experimental Analysis of Behavior* 60: 159–169.

Farabaugh, S. M., Linzenbold, A., and Dooling, R. J. 1994. Vocal plasticity in budgerigars (*Melopsittacus undultus*): Evidence for social factors in the learning of contact calls. *Journal of Comparative Psychology* 108: 1–11.

Farmer, J., and Schoenfeld, W. N. 1966. Varying temporal placement of an added stimulus in a fixed-interval schedule. *Journal of the Experimental Analysis of Behavior* 9: 369–375.

Ferster, C. B., and Skinner, B. F. 1957. *Schedules of Reinforcement.* Appleton-Century-Crofts.

Fetterman, J. G., and Killeen, P. R. 1991. Adjusting the pacemaker. *Learning and Motivation* 22: 226–252.

Fetterman, J. G., and Killeen, P. R. 1992. Time discrimination in *Columba livia* and *Homo sapiens. Journal of Experimental Psychology: Animal Behavior Processes* 18: 80–94.

Fetterman, J. G., Killeen, P. R., and Hall, S. 1998. Watching the clock. *Behavioural Processes* 44: 211–224.

Fetterman, J. G., and Stubbs, D. A. 1982. Matching, maximizing, and the behavioral unit: Concurrent reinforcement of response sequences. *Journal of the Experimental Analysis of Behavior* 37: 97–114.

Findley, J. D. 1958. Preference and switching under concurrent scheduling. *Journal of the Experimental Analysis of Behavior* 1: 123–144.

Fisher, R. A. 1930. *The Genetical Theory of Natural Selection.* Oxford University Press.

Flanagan, O. J. 1991. *The Science of the Mind.* MIT Press.

Fleshler, M., and Hoffman, H. S. 1962. A progression for generating variable-interval schedules. *Journal of the Experimental Analysis of Behavior* 5: 529–530.

Fox, M. L., Hopkins, B. L., and Anger, W. K. 1987. The long-term effects of a token economy on safety performance in open-pit mining. *Journal of Applied Behavior Analysis* 20: 215–224.

Freeman, J. S., Cody, F. W. J., O'Boyle, D. J., Crauford, D., Neary, D., and Snowden, J. S. 1996. Abnormalities of motor timing in Huntington's disease. *Parkinsonism Related Disorders* 2: 81–93.

Freeman, J. S., Cody, F. W. J., and Scahdy, W. 1993. The influence of external timing cues upon the rhythm of voluntary movements in Parkinson's disease. *Journal of Neurology, Neurosurgery and Psychiatry* 56: 1078–1084.

Friman, P. C., Hayes, S. C., and Wilson, K. G. 1998. Why behavior analysts should study emotion: The example of anxiety. *Journal of Applied Behavior Analysis* 31: 137–156.

Galbicka, G. 1997. Rate and the analysis of behavior: Time to move forward? In *Investigations in Behavioral Epistemology,* ed. L. Hayes and P. Ghezzi. Context.

Gallistel, C. R. 1999. Can a decay process explain the timing of conditioning responses? *Journal of the Experimental Analysis of Behavior* 71: 264–271.

Geller, E. S., Rudd, J. R., Streff, F. M., Berry, T. D., Kalsher, M. J., Lehman, G. R., and Kello, J. E. 1986. Power Lockout and Occupational Safety: Guidelines for a Comprehensive Program. Prepared for Motor Vehicle Manufacturers Association.

Gephardt, M. A., and van Buren, M. E. 1996. Building synergy: The power of high performance work systems. *Training and Development*, October: 21–26.

Gibbon, J. 1977. Scalar expectancy theory and Weber's law in animal timing. *Psychological Review* 84: 279–325.

Gibbon, J. 1991. Origins of scalar timing. *Learning and Motivation* 22: 3–38.

Gibbon, J. 1992. Ubiquity of scalar timing with a Poisson clock. *Journal of Mathematical Psychology* 36: 283–293.

Gibbon, J. 1995. Dynamics of time matching: Arousal makes better seem worse. *Psychonomic Bulletin and Review* 2: 208–215.

Gibbon, J., and Church, R. M. 1981. Linear versus logarithmic subjective time. *Journal of Experimental Psychology: Animal Behavior Processes* 7: 87–108.

Gibbon, J., and Church, R. M. 1984. Sources of variance in an information processing theory of timing. In *Animal Cognition*, ed. H. Roitblat, T. Bever, and H. Terrace. Erlbaum.

Gibbon, J., and Church, R. M. 1990. Representation of time. *Cognition* 37: 23–54.

Gibbon, J., Church, R. M., Fairhurst, S., and Kacelnik, A. 1988. Scalar expectancy theory and choice between delayed rewards. *Psychological Review* 95: 102–114.

Gibbon, J., Church, R. M., and Meck, W. H. 1984. Scalar timing in memory. In *Annals of the New York Academy of Sciences*, volume 423: *Timing and Time Perception*, ed. J. Gibbon and L. Allan.

Gibbon, J., and Fairhurst, S. 1994. Ratio versus difference comparators in choice. *Journal of Experimental Analysis of Behavior* 62: 105–124.

Gibbon, J., Malapani, C., Dale, C. L., and Gallistel, C. R. 1997. Toward a neurobiology of temporal cognition: Advances and challenges. *Current Opinion in Neurobiology* 7: 170–184.

Gibson, J. J. 1966. *The Senses Considered as Perceptual Systems*. Houghton Mifflin.

Gibson, J. J. 1979. *The Ecological Approach to Visual Perception*. Houghton Mifflin.

Glanz, J. 1998. Magnetic brain imaging traces a stairway to memory. *Science* 280: 37.

Glymour, C., ed. 1997. Déjà vu all over again. In *Proceedings of the 1994 Carnegie Symposium*, ed. J. Cohen. Erlbaum.

Goetz, E. M., and Bear, D. M. 1973. Social control of form diversity and emergence of new forms in children's blockbuilding. *Journal of Applied Behavior Analysis* 6: 209–217.

Goldstone, S., Lhamon, W. T., and Sechzer, J. 1979. Light-intensity and judged duration. *Bulletin of the Psychonomic Society* 12: 83–84.

Gomez, L. M., and Robertson, L. C. 1979. The filled-duration illusion: The function of temporal and nontemporal set. *Perception and Psychophysics* 25: 432–438.

Gould, S. J. 1980. *The Panda's Thumb*. Norton.

Gould, S. J. 2002. *The Structure of Evolutionary Theory*. Belknap.

Gould-Beierle, K. 2000. A comparison of four corvid species in a working memory and reference memory task using a radial maze. *Journal of Comparative Psychology* 114: 347–356.

Grace, R. C. 2002. Acquisition of preference in concurrent chains: Comparing linear-operator and memory representation models. *Journal of Experimental Psychology: Animal Behavior Processes* 28: 257–276.

Grau, J. W. 2002. Learning and memory without a brain. In *The Cognitive Animal: Empirical and Theoretical Perspectives On Animal Cognition*, ed. M. Bekoff, C. Allen, and G. Burghardt. MIT Press.

Green, T., and Hayes, M. A. 1993. *The Belief System: The Secret to Motivation and Improved Performance*. Beechwood.

Grondin, S. 2001. From physical time to the first and second moments of psychological time. *Psychological Bulletin* 127: 22–44.

Grossberg, S., and Schmajuk, N. A. 1989. Neural dynamics of adaptive timing and temporal discrimination during associative learning. *Neural Networks* 2: 79–102.

Grunow, A., and Neuringer, A. 2002. Learning to vary and varying to learn. *Psychonomic Bulletin and Review* 9: 250–258.

Grzimek, B. 1944. Gedaechtnisversuche mit elephanten. *Zeitschrift für Tierpsychologie* 6: 126–140.

Hacking, I. 1983. *Representing and Intervening*. Cambridge University Press.

Hamilton, W. D. 1972. Altruism and related phenomena, mainly in the social insects. *Annual Review of Ecology and Systematics* 3: 193–232.

Hamner, W. C. 1991. Reinforcement theory and contingency management in organizational settings. In *Motivation and Work Behavior*, ed. R. Steers and L. Porter. McGraw-Hill.

Hardy, G. H. 1908. Mendelian proportions in a mixed population. *Science* 28: 49–50.

Harrington, D. L., Haaland, K. Y., and Hermanowicz, N. 1998. Temporal processing in basal ganglia. *Neuropsychology* 12: 3–12.

Harzem, P. 1969. Temporal discrimination. In *Animal Discrimination Learning*, ed. R. Gilbert and N. Sutherland. Academic Press.

Haykin, S. 1999. *Neural Networks—A Comprehensive Foundation*. Prentice-Hall.

Hediger, H. 1955. *Studies of The Psychology and Behaviour of Captive Animals in Zoos and Circuses*. Butterworth.

Hefferline, R. F., and Keenan, B. 1963. Amplitude-induction gradient of a small scale (covert) operant. *Journal of the Experimental Analysis of Behavior* 6: 307–315.

Heisenberg, W. 1971. *Physics and Beyond; Encounters and Conversations*. Harper and Row.

Helmreich, R. L. 1984. Cockpit management attitudes. *Human Factors* 26: 583–589.

Helmreich, R. L., Kello, J. E., Chidester, T. R., Wilhelm, J. A., and Gregorich, S. 1990. Maximizing the impact of line oriented flight training (LOFT): Lessons from initial observations. NASA/UT Technical Report 90–1.

Helmreich, R. L., Wilhelm, J. A., Kello, J. E., Taggart, W. R., and Butler, R. E. 1991. Reinforcing and evaluating crew resource management: Evaluator/LOS instructor reference manual. NASA/UT Technical Manual 90–2, Revision 1.

Herrnstein, R. J. 1961. Relative and absolute strength of response as a function of frequency of reinforcement. *Journal of the Experimental Analysis of Behavior* 4: 267–272.

Herrnstein, R. J. 1964. Will. *Proceedings of the American Philosophical Society* 108: 455–458.

Herrnstein, R. J. 1970. On the law of effect. *Journal of the Experimental Analysis of Behavior* 13: 243–266.

Herrnstein, R. J. 1997. Self-control as response strength. In *The Matching Law: Papers in Psychology and Economics*, ed. H. Rachlin and D. Laibson. Harvard University Press.

Herrnstein, R. J. 1990. Rational choice theory: Necessary but not sufficient. *American Psychologist* 45: 356–367.

Herrnstein, R. J., and Hineline, P. N. 1966. Negative reinforcement as shock frequency reduction. *Journal of the Experimental Analysis of Behavior* 9: 421–430.

Herrnstein, R. J., and Loveland, D. H. 1975. Matching and maximizing on concurrent ratio schedules. *Journal of the Experimental Analysis of Behavior* 24: 107–116.

Herrnstein, R. J., and Vaughan, W. 1980. Melioration and behavioral allocation. In *Limits to Action: The Allocation of Individual Behavior*, ed. J. Staddon. Academic Press.

Heyman, G. M. 1979. A Markov model description of changeover probabilities on concurrent variable-interval schedules. *Journal of the Experimental Analysis of Behavior* 7: 133–140.

Heyman, G. M., and Luce, R. D. 1979. Operant matching is not a logical consequence of maximizing reinforcement rate. *Animal Learning and Behavior* 7: 133–140.

Heyman, G. M., and Tanz, L. 1995. How to teach a pigeon to maximize overall reinforcement rate. *Journal of the Experimental Analysis of Behavior* 64: 277–297.

Higa, J. J. 1996. The dynamics of time discrimination II: The effects of multiple impulses. *Journal of the Experimental Analysis of Behavior* 66: 117–134.

Higa, J. J., and Staddon, J. E. R. 1997. Dynamic models of rapid temporal control in animals. In *Time and Behavior: Psychological and Neurobehavioral Analysis*, ed. C. Bradshaw and E. Szabadi. Elsevier.

Higa, J. J., Thaw, J. M., and Staddon, J. E. R. 1993. Pigeons' wait time responses to transitions in interfood trial duration: Another look at cyclic schedule performance. *Journal of the Experimental Analysis of Behavior* 59: 529–541.

Higa, J. J., Wynne, C. D. L., and Staddon, J. E. R. 1991. Dynamics of time discrimination. *Journal of Experimental Psychology: Animal Behavior Processes* 17: 281–291.

Hilgard, E. R. 1987. *Psychology in America: A historical survey*. Harcourt Brace Jovanovich.

Hinson, J. M., and Staddon, J. E. R. 1978. Behavioral competition: A mechanism for schedule interactions. *Science* 202: 432–434.

Hinson, J. M., and Staddon, J. E. R. 1983a. Hill-Climbing by pigeons. *Journal of the Experimental Analysis of Behavior* 39: 25–47.

Hinson, J. M., and Staddon, J. E. R. 1983b. Matching, maximizing and hill-climbing. *Journal of the Experimental Analysis of Behavior* 40: 321–331.

Hobhouse, L. T. 1901. *Mind in Evolution*. Macmillan.

Holden, A. V. 1986. *Chaos*. Princeton University Press.

Holton, G., and Roller, D. D. 1965. *Foundation of Modern Physical Science*. Addison-Wesley.

Honig, W. K. 1978. Studies of working memory in the pigeon. In *Cognitive Processes in Animal Behavior*, ed. S. Hulse, H. Fowler, and W. Honig. Erlbaum.

Honig, W. K., and Staddon, J. E. R., eds. 1977. *Handbook of Operant Behavior*. Prentice-Hall.

Hopson, J. W. 1999. Gap timing and the spectral timing model. *Behavioural Processes* 45: 23–31.

Hori, M. 1993. Frequency-dependent natural selection in the handedness of scale-eating cichlid fish. *Science* 260: 216–219.

Horner, J. M. 2002. Information in the behavior stream. *Behavioural Processes* 58: 133–147.

Horner, J., and Staddon, J. E. R. 1987. Probabilistic choice: A simple invariance. *Behavioural Processes* 15: 59–92.

Horner, J. M., Staddon, J. E. R., and Lozano, K. K. 1997. Integration of reinforcement effects over time. *Animal Learning and Behavior* 25: 84–98.

Hosoi, E., Rittenhouse, L. R., Swift, D. M., and Richards, R. W. 1995. Foraging strategies of cattle in a Y-maze: influence of food availability. *Applied Animal Behaviour Science* 43: 189–196.

Hosoi, E., Swift, D. M., Rittenhouse, L. R., and Richards, R. W. 1995. Comparative foraging strategies of sheep and goats in a T-maze apparatus. *Applied Animal Behaviour Science* 44: 37–45.

Houk, C., Davis, J. L., and Beiser, D. G., eds. 1998. *Models of Information Processing in Basal Ganglia*. MIT Press.

Houston, A. 1986. The matching law applies to wagtails' foraging in the wild. *Journal of the Experimental Analysis of Behavior* 45: 15–18.

Hughes, R. N., and Blight, C. M. 1999. Algorithmic behavior and spatial memory are used by two intertidal fish species to solve the radial maze. *Animal Behaviour* 58: 601–613.

Hull, C. L. 1943. *Principles of Behavior*. Appleton-Century-Crofts.

Hume, D., Norton, D. F., and Norton, M. J. 2000. *A Treatise of Human Nature*. Oxford University Press.

Innis, N. K. 1981. Reinforcement as input: Temporal tracking on cyclic interval schedules. In *Quantitative Analysis of Behavior: Discriminative Properties of Reinforcement Schedules*, ed. M. Commons and J. Nevin. Pergamon.

Innis, N. K., Mitchell, S. K, and Staddon, J. E. R. 1993. Temporal control on interval schedules: What determines the postreinforcement pause? *Journal of the Experimental Analysis of Behavior* 60: 293–311.

Innis, N. K., and Staddon, J. E. R. 1971. Temporal tracking on cyclic-interval reinforcement schedules. *Journal of the Experimental Analysis of Behavior* 16: 411–423.

International Task Force on Assesment Center Guidelines. 2000. *Public Personnel Management* 29: 315–331.

Ivry, R. B. 1996. The representation of temporal information in perception and motor control. *Current Opinion in Neurobiology* 6: 851–857.

Iwata, B. 1994. Toward a functional analysis of self injury. *Journal of Applied Behavior Analysis* 27: 197–209.

James, W. 1904. Does consciousness exist? *Journal of Philosophy* 1: 477–491.

James, W. 1971/1879. The sentiment of rationality. In *William James: The Essential Writings*, ed. B. Wilshire. Harper and Row.

Jenkins, J. J. 1974. Remember that old theory of memory? Well forget it! *American Psychologist* 29: 785–795.

Jenkins, J. J. 1981. Can we have a fruitful cognitive psychology? In *Nebraska Symposium On Motivation*, volume 28, ed. J. Flowers. University of Nebraska Press.

Jewell, L. N. 1998. *Contemporary Industrial/Organizational Psychology*, third edition. Brooks Cole.

Jog, M. S., Connolly, C. I., Kubota, Y., Iyengar, L., Garrido, L., Harlan, R., and Graybiel, A. M. 2002. Tetrode technology: advances in implantable hardware, neuroimaging, and data analysis techniques. *Journal of Neuroscience Methods* 117: 141–152.

Jog, M. S., Kubota, Y., Connolly, C. I., Hillegart, V., and Graybiel, A. M. 1999. Building neural representations of habits. *Science* 286: 1745–1749.

Kacelnik, A. 1984. Central place foraging in Starlings (*Sturnus vulgaris*). I. Patch residence time. *Journal of Animal Ecology* 53: 283–299.

Kacelnik, A., Krebs, J. R., and Ens, B. 1987. Foraging in a changing environment: An experiment with starlings (*sturnus vulgaris*). In *Quantitative Analyses of Behavior VI: Foraging*, ed. M. Commons, A. Kacelnik, and S. Shettleworth. Erlbaum.

Katzell, R. A., and Thompson, D. 1990. An integrative model of work attitudes, motivation, and performance. *Human Performance* 3: 63–85.

Kelleher, R. T., Fry, W., and Cook, L. 1959. Interresponse time distribution as a function of differential reinforcement of temporally spaced responses. *Journal of the Experimental Analysis of Behavior* 2: 91–106.

Kello, J. E., Geller, E. S., Rice, J. C., and Bryant, S. L. 1988. Motivating auto safety belt wearing in industrial settings: From awareness to behavior change. *Journal of Organizational Behavior Management* 9: 7–21.

Killeen, P. 1968. On the measure of reinforcement frequency in the study of preference. *Journal of the Experimental Analysis of Behavior* 11: 263–269.

Killeen, P. R. 1991. The behavior's time. In *The Psychology of Learning and Motivation*, volume 27, ed. G. Bower. Academic Press.

Killeen, P. R., and Fetterman, J. G. 1988. A behavioral theory of timing. *Psychological Review* 95: 274–285.

Killeen, P., Hanson, S. J., and Osborne, S. R. 1978. Arousal: its genesis and manifestation as response rate. *Psychological Review* 85: 571–581.

King, A. P., and West, M. J. 1989. Presence of female cowbirds (*Molothrus ater ater*) affects vocal improvisation in males. *Journal of Comparative Psychology* 103: 39–44.

Klopf, A. H. 1988. A neuronal model of classical conditioning. *Psychobiology* 16: 85–125.

Komaki, J. L., Coombs, T., and Schepman, S. 1991. Motivational implications of reinforcement theory. In *Motivation and Work Behavior,* ed. R. Steers and L. Porter. McGraw-Hill.

Kraemer, P. J., Brown, R. W., and Randall, C. K. 1995. Signal intensity and duration estimation in rats. *Behavioural Processes* 344: 265–268.

Kraemer, P. J., Randall, C. K., and Brown, R. W. 1997. The influence of stimulus attributes on duration matching-to-sample in pigeons. *Animal Learning and Behavior* 25: 148–157.

Kreitner, R., and Luthans, F. 1991. A social learning approach to behavioral management; Radical behaviorists "mellowing out." In *Motivation and Work Behavior,* ed. R. Steers and L. Porter. McGraw-Hill.

Kuhn, T. S. 1970. *The Structure of Scientific Revolutions,* second edition. University of Chicago Press.

Lamal, P. A. 1998. Advancing backwards. *Journal of Applied Behavior Analysis* 31: 705–706.

Landy, F. J. 1989. *Psychology of Work Behavior,* fourth edition. Brooks-Cole.

Landy, F. J., and Farr, J. L. 1980. Performance rating. *Psychological Bulletin* 87: 72–107.

Lea, S. E., and Dow, S. M. 1984. The integration of reinforcement effects over time. In *Annals of the New York Academy of Sciences,* volume 423: *Timing and Time Perception,* ed. J. Gibbon and L. Allan.

Leahey, T. H. 1992. *A History of Psychology: Main Currents in Psychological Thought,* third edition. Prentice-Hall.

Leak, T. M., and Gibbon, J. 1995. Simultaneous timing of multiple intervals: Implications of the scalar property. *Journal of Experimental Psychology: Animal Behavior Processes* 21: 3–19.

Leigland, S., ed. 1997. *Systems and Theories in Behavior Analytic Science: An Overview of Alternatives*. Context.

Lejeune, H. 1998. Switching or gating? The attentional challenge in cognitive models of psychological time. *Behavioural Processes* 44: 127–145.

Lejeune, H., Macar, F., and Zakay, D. 1999. Attention and timing; Dual-task performance in pigeons. *Behavioural Processes* 45: 141–157.

Lejeune, H., and Wearden, J. H. 1991. The comparative psychology of fixed-interval responding: Some quantitative analyses. *Learning and Motivation* 22: 84–111.

Lima, S. L., Valone, T. J., and Caraco, T. 1985. Foraging efficiency-predation risk trade-off in the grey squirrel. *Animal Behaviour* 33: 155–165.

Lloyd, G. E. R., ed. 1978. *Hippocratic Writings*. Penguin.

Lowe, C. F., and Harzem, P. 1977. Species differences in temporal control of behavior. *Journal of the Experimental Analysis of Behavior* 28: 189–201.

MacDonald, S. E. 1994. Gorillas' (*Gorilla gorilla gorilla*) spatial memory in a foraging task. *Journal of Comparative Psychology* 108: 107–113.

MacDonald, S. E., and Wilkie, D. M. 1990. Spatial memory in yellow-nosed monkeys (*Cercopithecus ascanius whitesidei*) in a simulated foraging environment. *Journal of Comparative Psychology* 104: 382–387.

Machado, A. 1989. Operant conditioning of behavioral variability using a percentile reinforcement schedule. *Journal of the Experimental Analysis of Behavior* 52: 155–166.

Machado, A. 1992. Behavioral variability and frequency-dependent selection. *Journal of the Experimental Analysis of Behavior* 58: 241–263.

Machado, A. 1993. Learning variable and stereotypical sequences of responses: Some data and a new model. *Behavioural Processes* 30: 103–130.

Machado, A. 1997a. Increasing the variability of response sequences in pigeons by adjusting the frequency of switching between two keys. *Journal of the Experimental Analysis of Behavior* 68: 1–25.

Machado, A. 1997b. Learning the temporal dynamics of behavior. *Psychological Review* 104: 241–265.

Machado, A., and Keen, R. 1999. The learning of response patterns in choice situations. *Animal Learning and Behavior* 27: 251–271.

Mackintosh, N. J. 1974. *The Psychology of Animal Learning*. Academic Press.

Malapani, C., Rakitin, B., Levy, R., Meck, W. H., Deweer, B., Dubois, B., and Gibbon, J. 1998. Coupled temporal memories in Parkinson's disease: A dopamine-related dysfunction. *Journal of Cognitive Neuroscience* 10: 316–31.

Malone, J. C., Jr. 1975. William James and B. F. Skinner: Behaviorism, reinforcement, and interest. *Behaviorism* 3: 140–151.

Malone, J. C., Jr. 1987. Skinner, the behavioral unit, and current psychology. In *B. F. Skinner: Consensus and Controversy*, ed. S. Modgill and C. Modgill. Falmer.

Malone, J. C., Jr. 1991. *Theories of Learning: A Historical Approach*. Wadsworth.

Mammen, D. L., and Nowicki, S. 1981. Individual differences and within-flock convergence in chickadee calls. *Behavioral Ecology and Sociobiology* 9: 179–186.

Manabe, K. 1990. Determinants of pigeon's waiting time: Effect of interreinforcement interval and food delay. *Journal of the Experimental Analysis of Behavior* 53: 123–132.

Manabe, K. 1997. Vocal plasticity in budgerigars: Various modifications of vocalization by operant conditioning. *Biomedical Research* 18, Supplement 1: 125–132.

Manabe, K., and Dooling, R. J. 1997. Control of vocal production in budgerigars (*Melopsittacus undulatus*). Selective reinforcement, call differentiation, and stimulus control. *Behavioural Processes* 41: 117–132.

Manabe, K., and Kawashima, T. 2001. Differential reinforcement of variability of pecking location in budgerigars. In Proceedings of 19th Convention of Japanese Association for Behavior Analysis.

Manabe, K., and Kawashima, T. 2002. Differential reinforcement of variability of pecking location in budgerigars: A comparison between two kinds of *N*-back procedures. In Proceedings of 20th Convention of Japanese Association for Behavior Analysis.

Manabe, K., and Kawashima, T. In preparation. Differential reinforcement of variability of pecking location in reinforcement-based N-back procedures in budgerigar.

Manabe, K., Kuwata, S. Kurashige, N., Chino, K., and Ogawa, T. Time allocation of various activities under multiple schedules in pigeons. *Behavioural Processes* 26: 113–123.

Manabe, K., Staddon, J. E. R., and Cleaveland, J. M. 1997. Control of vocal repertoire by reward in budgerigars (*Melopsittacus undulatus*). *Journal of Comparative Psychology* 111: 50–62.

Mantanus, H. 1981. Empty and filled interval discrimination by pigeons. *Behaviour Analysis Letters* 1: 217–224.

Margulies, S. 1961. Response duration in operant level, regular reinforcement, and extinction. *Journal of the Experimental Analysis of Behavior* 4: 317–321.

Maricq, A. V., Roberts, S., and Church, R. M. 1981. Methamphetamine and time estimation. *Journal of Experimental Psychology: Animal Behavior Processes* 7: 18–30.

Marinier, S. L., and Alexander, A. J. 1994. The use of a maze in testing learning and memory in horses. *Applied Animal Behaviour Science* 39: 177–182.

Mark, T. A., and Gallistel, C. R. 1994. Kinetics of matching. *Journal of Experimental Psychology: Animal Behavior Processes* 20: 79–95.

Markowitz, H. Schmidt, M., Nadal, L., and Squier, L. 1975. Do elephants ever forget? *Journal of Applied Behavior Analysis* 8: 333–335.

Marler, P. 1990. Song learning: The interface between behaviour and neuroethology. *Philosophical Transactions of the Royal Society (London)* 329: 109–114.

Marler, P. 1991. Song-learning behavior: the interface with neuroethology. *Trends in Neuroscience* 14: 199–206.

Mazur, J. E. 1992. Choice behavior in transition: Development of preference with ratio and interval schedules. *Journal of Experimental Psychology: Animal Behavior Processes* 18: 364–378.

Mazur, J. E. 1995. Development of preference and spontaneous recovery in choice behavior with concurrent variable-interval schedules. *Animal Learning and Behavior* 23: 93–103.

Mazur, J. E. 1998. *Learning and Behavior,* fourth edition. Prentice-Hall.

Mazur, J. E., and Ratti, T. A. 1991. Choice behavior in transition: Development of preference in a free-operant procedure. *Animal Learning and Behavior* 19: 241–248.

Mayo, E. 1933. *The Human Problems of an Industrial Civilization.* Macmillan.

McCullock, W. S., and Pitts, W. 1943. A logical calculus of the ideas immanent in nervous activity. *Bulletin of Mathematical Biophysics* 5: 115–133.

McElroy, E., and Neuringer, A. 1990. Effects of alcohol on reinforced repetitions and reinforced variations in rats. *Psychopharmacology* 102: 49–55.

Meck, W. H. 1983. Selective adjustment of the speed of internal clock and memory processes. *Journal of Experimental Psychology: Animal Behavior Processes* 9: 171–201.

Meck, W. H. 1996. Neuropharmacology of timing and time perception. *Cognitive Brain Research* 3: 227–242.

Meck, W. H., Church, R. M., and Olton, D. S. 1984. Hippocampus, time, and memory. *Behavioral Neurosciences* 98: 3–22.

Mendl, M., Laughlin, K., and Hitchcock, D. 1997. Pigs in space: Spatial memory and its susceptibility to interference. *Animal Behaviour* 54: 1491–1508.

Mettler, L. E., Gregg, T. G., and Schaffer, H. E. 1988. *Population Genetics and Evolution,* second edition. Prentice-Hall.

Michelson, A. A., and Morley, E. W. 1887. On the relative motion of the earth and the luminiferous ether. *American Journal of Science,* Third Series 34: 52.

Miller, G. A. 1962. *Psychology: The Science of Mental Life.* Harper and Row.

Miller, N. E. 1959. Liberalization of basic S-R concepts: Extensions to conflict behavior, motivation, and social learning. In *Psychology: A Study of a Science,* volume 2, ed. S. Koch. McGraw-Hill.

Minsky, M. L. 1967. *Computation: Finite and Infinite Machines*. Prentice-Hall.

Morgan, L., and Lee, K. 1996. Extinction-induced response variability in humans. *The Psychological Record* 46: 145–159.

Morgan, L., and Neuringer, A. 1990. Behavioral variability as a function of response topography and reinforcement contingency. *Animal Learning and Behavior* 18: 257–263.

Morris, C. J. 1989. The effects of lag value on the operant control of response variability under free-operant and discrete-response procedures. *Journal of the Experimental Analysis of Behavior* 39: 263–270.

Morrison, S. K., and Brown, M. F. 1990. The touch screen system in the pigeon laboratory: An initial evaluation of its utility. *Behavior Research methods, Instruments, and Computers* 22: 123–126.

Morse, D. H., and Stephens, E. G. 1996. The consequences of adult foraging success on the components of lifetime fitness in a semelparous, sit-and-wait predator. *Evolutionary Ecology* 10: 361–373.

Morse, W. H., and Kelleher, R. T. 1977. Determinants of reinforcement and punishment. In *Handbook of Operant Behavior*, ed. W. Honig and J. Staddon. Prentice-Hall.

Moss, C. J., and Poole, J. H. 1983. Relationships and social structure of African elephants. In *Primate Social Relationships: An Integrated Approach*, ed. R. Hinde. Sinauer.

Muchinsky, P. M. 2000. *Psychology Applied to Work: An Introduction to Industrial and Organizational Psychology*, sixth edition. Brooks-Cole.

Munro, H. H. 1904. *Reginald*. London: Methuen.

Myers, D. L., and Myers, L. E. 1977. Undermatching: A reappraisal of performance on concurrent variable-interval schedules of reinforcement. *Journal of the Experimental Analysis of Behavior* 27: 203–214.

Myerson, J., and Miezin, F. M. 1980. The kinetics of choice: An operant systems analysis. *Psychological Review* 87: 160–174.

Nakamura, R., Nagasaki, H., and Narabayashi, H. 1978. Disturbances of rhythm formation in patients with Parkinson's disease: Part 1. Characteristic of tapping response to the periodic signals. *Perceptual and Motor Skills* 46: 63–75.

Neisser, U. 1967. *Cognitive Psychology*. Appleton-Century-Crofts.

Neisser, U. 1976. *Cognition and Reality: Principles and Implications of Cognitive Psychology*. Freeman.

Neisser, U. 1978. Memory: What are the important questions? In *Practical Aspects of Memory*, ed. M. Gruneberg, P. Morris, and R. Sykes. Academic Press.

Neisser, U. 1982. *Memory Observed: Remembering in Natural Context.* Freeman.

Neuringer, A. J. 1967. Effects of reinforcement magnitude on choice and rate of responding. *Journal of the Experimental Analysis of Behavior* 10: 417–424.

Neuringer, A. 1990. Behavioral variability as a function of response topography and reinforcement contingency. *Animal Learning and Behavior* 18: 257–263.

Neuringer, A. 1991. Operant variability and repetition as functions of interresponse time. *Journal of Experimental Psychology: Animal Behavior Processes* 17: 3–12.

Neuringer, A. 1992. Choosing to vary and repeat. *Psychological Science* 3: 246–250.

Neuringer, A. J., and Chung, S. 1967. Quasi-reinforcement: Control of responding by a percentage reinforcement schedule. *Journal of the Experimental Analysis of Behavior* 10: 45–54.

Neuringer, A., Kornell, N., and Olufs, M. 2001. Stability and variability in extinction. *Journal of Experimental Psychology: Animal Behavior Processes* 27: 79–94.

Neusch, D. R., and Siebenaler, A. F. 1998. *The High Performance Enterprise: Reinventing The People Side of Your Business*, second edition. Wiley.

Nevin, J. A. 1969. Interval reinforcement of choice behavior in discrete trials. *Journal of the Experimental Analysis of Behavior* 12: 875–885.

Nevin, J. A. 1979. Overall matching versus momentary maximizing: Nevin (1969) revisited. *Journal of the Experimental Psychology: Animal Behavior Processes* 5: 300–306.

Nevin, J. A. 1988. Behavioral momentum and the partial reinforcement effect. *Psychological Bulletin* 103: 44–56.

Nevin, J. A., Mandell, C., and Yarenski, P. 1981. Response rate and resistance to change in chained schedules. *Journal of Experimental Psychology: Animal Behavior Processes* 7: 278–294.

Newell, A., Shaw, J. C., and Simon, H. A. 1958. Elements of a theory of human problem solving. *Psychological Review* 65: 151–166.

Nicolelis, M. A. L., ed. 1999. *Methods For Neural Ensemble Recordings.* CRC Press.

Nisbett, R., and Wilson, T. 1977. Telling more than we can know: Verbal reports on mental processes. *Psychological Review* 84: 231–259.

Nordeen, K., and Nordeen, E. 1992. Auditory feedback is necessary for the maintenance of stereotyped song. *Behavioral and Neural Biology* 334: 149–151.

Nottebohm, F. 1984. Bird song as a model in which to study brain processes related to learning. *The Condor* 86: 227–236.

Nottebohm, F., and Nottebohm, M. E. 1978. Relationship between song repertoire and age in the canary (*Serinus canaria*). *Zeitschrift für Tierpsychologie* 46: 298–305.

Nowicki, S. 1989. Vocal plasticity in captive Black-capped Chickadees: The acoustic basis and rate of call convergence. *Animal Behaviour* 37: 64–73.

O'Boyle, D., Freeman, J. S., and Cody, F. W. J. 1996. The accuracy and precision of timing of self-paced, repetitive movements in subjects with Parkinson's disease. *Brain* 119: 51–70.

Olton, D. S., Becker, J. T., and Handelmann, G. E. 1979. Hippocampus, space, and memory. *Behavioral and Brain Sciences* 2: 313–365.

Olton, D. S., and Samuelson, R. J. 1976. Remembrance of places passed: Spatial memory in rats. *Journal of Experimental Psychology: Animal Behavior Processes* 2: 97–116.

Olton, D. S., and Schlosberg, P. 1978. Food-searching strategies in young rats: Win-shift predominates over win-stay. *Journal of Comparative and Physiological Psychology* 92: 609–618.

Orsburn, J. D., Moran, L., Musselwhite, E., and Zenger, J. H. 1990. *Self-Directed Work Teams: The New American Challenge*. Business One Irwin.

Page, S., and Neuringer, A. 1985. Variability is an operant. *Journal of Experimental Psychology: Animal Behavior Processes* 11: 429–452.

Parsons, H. M. 1974. What happened at Hawthorne? *Science* 183: 922–932.

Parsons, H. M. 1992. Hawthorne: An early OBM experiment. *Journal of Organizational Behavior Management* 12: 27–34.

Pasmore, W. A. 1988. *Designing Effective Organizations: The Sociotechnical Systems Perspective*. Wiley.

Pastor, M. A., Jahanashi, M., Artieda, J., and Obeso, J. A. 1992a. Time estimation and reproduction is abnormal in Parkinson's disease. *Brain* 115: 211–225.

Pastor, M. A., Jahanashi, M., Artieda, J., and Obeso, J. A. 1992b. Performance of repetitive wrist movements in Parkinson's disease. *Brain* 115: 875–891.

Palya, W. L., Walter, D., Kessel, R., and Lucke, R. 1996. Investigating behavioral dynamics with a fixed-time extinction schedule and linear analysis. *Journal of the Experimental Analysis of Behavior* 66: 391–409.

Peach, E. B., and Wren, D. A. 1992. Pay for performance from antiquity to the 1950s. *Journal of Organizational Behavior Management* 12: 5–26.

Peirce, C. S. 1878/1955. How to make our ideas clear. In *Philosophical Writings of Peirce*, ed. J. Buchler. Dover.

Peirce, C. 1962. How to make our ideas clear. In *Philosophy in The Twentieth Century*, volume 1, ed. W. Barrett and H. Aiken. Random House.

Pepperberg, I. M. 1993. A review of the effects of social interaction on vocal learning in African Grey Parrots (*Psittacus erithacus*). *Netherlands Journal of Zoology* 43: 104–124.

Piaget, J. 2000. Piaget's theory. In *Childhood Cognitive Development: The Essential Readings*, ed. K. Lee. Blackwell.

Pisacreta, R. 1982. Some factors that influence the acquisition of complex, stereotyped response sequences in pigeons. *Journal of the Experimental Analysis of Behavior* 37: 359–369.

Plotkin, H. 1993. *Darwin Machines and the Nature of Knowledge*. Harvard University Press.

Popper, K. 1972. *Objective Knowledge: An Evolutionary Approach*. Oxford University Press.

Porter, L., and Lawler, E. E. 1968. *Managerial Attitudes and Performance*. Irwin-Dorsey.

Posner, R. A. 1990. *The Problems of Jurisprudence*. Harvard University Press.

Powell, R. A., Symbaluk, D. G., and Macdonald, S. E. 2002. *Introduction to Learning and Behavior*. Wadsworth.

Price, P. H. 1979. Developmental determinants of structure in zebra finch song. *Journal of Comparative and Physiological Psychology* 93: 260–277.

Pryor, K. W., Haag, R., and O'Reilly, J. 1969. The creative porpoise: Training for novel behavior. *Journal of the Experimental Analysis of Behavior* 12: 653–661.

Putnam, H. 1978. *Meaning and Moral Science*. Routledge and Kegan Paul.

Rachlin, H. 1987a. Rachlin replies to Lacey and Schwartz. 1987. In *B. F. Skinner: Consensus and Controversy*, ed. S. Modgil and C. Modgil. Falmer.

Rachlin, H. 1987b. The explantory power of Skinner's radical behaviorism. In *B. F. Skinner: Consensus and Controversy*, ed. S. Modgil and C. Modgil. Falmer.

Rachlin, H. 1994. *Behavior and Mind: The Roots of Modern Psychology*. Oxford University Press.

Rachlin, H. 1999. Teleological behaviorism. In *Handbook of Behaviorism*, ed. W. O'Donohue and R. Kitchener. Academic Press.

Rachlin, H., and Laibson, D. I., eds. 1997. *The Matching Law: Papers in Psychology and Economics*. Harvard University Press.

Rashotte, M. E., and Amsel, A. 1999. Hull's behaviorism. In *Handbook of Behaviorism*, ed. W. O'Donohue and R. Kitchener. Academic Press.

Rasmussen, L. E. L., and Krishnamurthy, V. 2000. How chemical signals integrate Asian elephant society: The known and the unknown. *Zoo Biology* 19: 405–423.

Reed, P., Schachtman, T. R., and Hall, G. 1991. Effect of signaled reinforcement on the formation of behavioral units. *Journal of Experimental Psychology: Animal Behavior Processes* 17: 475–485.

Reid, A. K. 1994. Learning new response sequences. *Behavioural Processes* 32: 147–162.

Reid, A. K., Chadwick, C. Z., Dunham, M., and Miller, A. 2001. The development of functional response units: The role of demarcating stimuli. *Journal of the Experimental Analysis of Behavior* 76: 303–320.

Reid, A. K., and Staddon, J. E. R. 1997. A reader for the cognitive map. *Information Sciences* 100: 217–228.

Reid, A. K., and Staddon, J. E. R. 1998. A dynamic route-finder for the cognitive map. *Psychological Review* 105: 385–601.

Rensch, B. 1957. The intelligence of elephants. *Scientific American* 196: 44–49.

Rescorla, R. A., and Wagner, A. R. 1972. A theory of Pavlovian conditioning: Variations in the effectiveness of reinforcement and nonreinforcement. In A. H. Black and W. F. Prokasy, eds. *Classical Conditioning II: Current Research and Theory*. Appleton-Century-Crofts.

Rice, B. 1982. The Hawthorne defect: Persistence of a flawed theory. *Psychology Today* 16, no. 2: 70–74.

Richelle, M., and Lejeune, H. 1980. *Time in Animal Behavior*. Pergamon.

Richman, C. L., Dember, W. N., and Kim, P. 1986. Spontaneous alternation behavior in animals: A review. *Current Psychological Research and Reviews* 5: 358–391.

Riggio, R. E. 2000. *Introduction to Industrial/Organizational Psychology*, third edition. Prentice-Hall.

Roberts, S. 1981. Isolation of an internal clock. *Journal of Experimental Psychology: Animal Behavior Processes* 7: 242–268.

Roberts, S., and Church, R. M. 1978. Control of an internal clock. *Journal of Experimental Psychology: Animal Behavior Processes* 4: 318–337.

Roberts, S., and Holder, M. D. 1984. What starts an internal clock? *Journal of Experimental Psychology: Animal Behavior Processes* 10: 273–296.

Roberts, W. A., Cheng, K., and Cohen, J. S. 1989. Timing light and tone signals in pigeons. *Journal of Experimental Psychology: Animal Behavior Processes* 15: 23–35.

Roberts, W. A., and Dale, R. H. I. 1981. Remembrance of places lasts: Proactive inhibition and patterns of choice in rat spatial memory. *Learning and Motivation* 12: 261–281.

Roethlisberger, F. L., and Dickson, W. J. 1939. *Management and the Worker*. Harvard University Press.

Roitblat, H. L., Tham, W., and Golub, L. 1982. Performance of *Betta splendens* in a radial arm maze. *Animal Learning and Behavior* 10: 108–114.

Roper, T. J. 1978. Diversity and substitutability of adjunctive activities under fixed-interval schedules of food reinforcement. *Journal of the Experimental Analysis of Behavior* 30: 83–96.

Rubin, D. C., Hinton, S., and Wenzel, A. 1999. The precise time course of retention. *Journal of Experimental Psychology: Learning, Memory, and Cognition* 25: 1161–1176.

Rubin, D. C., and Wenzel, A. E. 1996. One hundred years of forgetting: A quantitative description of retention. *Psychological Review* 103: 734–760.

Rumelhart, D. E., McClelland, J. L., and the PDP Research Group. 1986. *Parallel Distributed Processing: Explorations in the Microstructure of Cognition*, volumes 1 and 2. MIT Press.

Santayana, G. 1905. *Life of Reason*, volume 1. Scribner.

Schmid-Hempel, P., Kacelnik, A., and Houston, A. I. 1985. Honeybees maximise efficiency by not filling their crop. *Behavior Ecology and Sociobiology* 17: 61–66.

Schneider, B. A. 1969. A two-state analysis of fixed-interval responding in pigeons. *Journal of the Experimental Analysis of Behavior* 12: 667–687.

Schneider, S. M., and Morris, E. K. 1992. Sequences of spaced responses: Behavioral units and the role of contiguity. *Journal of the Experimental Analysis of Behavior* 58: 537–555.

Schultz, D., and Schultz, S. E. 2002. *Psychology and Work Today*, eighth edition. Prentice-Hall.

Schulz, W., Apicella, P., Romo. R., and Scarnati, E. 1998. Context-dependent activity in primate striatum refelecting past and future behavioral events. In *Models of Information Processing in the Basal Ganglia*, ed. C. Houk, J. Davis, and D. Beiser. MIT Press.

Schultz, W., Dayan, P., and Montague, P. R. 1997. A neural substrate of prediction and reward. *Science* 275: 1593–1599.

Schwartz, B. 1980. Development of complex, stereotyped behavior in pigeons. *Journal of the Experimental Analysis of Behavior* 11: 153–166.

Schwartz, B. 1981. Reinforcement creates behavioral units. *Behaviour Analysis Letters* 1: 33–41.

Schwartz, B. 1982a. Failure to produce response variability with reinforcement. *Journal of the Experimental Analysis of Behavior* 37: 171–181.

Schwartz, B. 1982b. Interval and ratio reinforcement of a complex, sequential operant in pigeons. *Journal of the Experimental Analysis of Behavior* 37: 349–357.

Schwartz, B. 1986. Allocation of complex, sequential operants on multiple and concurrent schedules of reinforcement. *Journal of the Experimental Analysis of Behavior* 45: 283–295.

Shaw, R. S. 1984. *The Dripping Faucet as a Model Chaotic System*. Aerial.

Shettleworth, S. 1972. Consraints on learning. In *Advances in the Study of Behavior*, volume 4, ed. D. Lehrman, R. Hinde, and E. Shaw. Academic Press.

Shimp, C. P. 1966. Probabilistically reinforced choice behavior in pigeons. *Journal of the Experimental Analysis of Behavior* 9: 443–455.

Shimp, C. P. 1969. Optimal behavior in free-operant experiments. *Psychological Review* 76: 97–112.

Shimp, C. P. 1981. The local organization of behavior: Discrimination of and memory for simple behavioral patterns. *Journal of the Experimental Analysis of Behavior* 36: 303–315.

Shimp, C. P. 1982. Choice and behavioral patterning. *Journal of the Experimental Analysis of Behavior* 37: 157–169.

Shimp, C. P., Fremouw, T., Ingebritsen, L. M., and Long, K. A. 1994. Molar function depends on molecular structure of behavior. *Journal of Experimental Psychology: Animal Behavior Processes* 20: 96–107.

Shoshani, J. 2000. *Elephants: Majestic Creatures of the Wild*, revised edition. Checkmark Books.

Shull, R. L. 1970a. A response-initiated fixed-interval schedule of reinforcement. *Journal of the Experimental Analysis of Behavior* 13: 13–15.

Shull, R. L. 1970b. The response-reinforcement dependency in fixed-interval schedules of reinforcement. *Journal of the Experimental Analysis of Behavior* 14: 55–60.

Shull, R. L., And Pliskoff, S. S. 1967. Changeover delay and concurrent schedules: some effects on relative performance measures. *Journal of the Experimental Analysis of Behavior* 10: 517–527.

Sikstrom, S. 2002. Forgetting curves: implications for connectionist models. *Cognitive Psychology* 45: 95–152.

Silberberg, A., Hamilton, B., Ziriax, J. M., and Casey, J. 1978. The structure of choice. *Journal of Experimental Psychology: Animal Behavior Processes* 4: 368–398.

Skinner, B. F. 1931. The concept of the reflex in the description of behavior. *Journal of General Psychology* 5: 427–458.

Skinner, B. F. 1935. The generic nature of the concepts of stimulus and response. *Journal of General Psychology* 12: 40–65.

Skinner, B. F. 1938. *The Behavior of Organisms*. Appleton-Century-Crofts.

Skinner, B. F. 1945. The operational analysis of psychological terms. *Psychological Review* 52: 270–277.

Skinner, B. F. 1948a. *Walden Two*. Macmillan.

Skinner, B. F. 1948b. "Superstition" in the pigeon. *Journal of Experimental Psychology* 38: 198–172.

Skinner, B. F. 1950. Are theories of learning really necessary? *Psychological Review* 57: 193–216.

Skinner, B. F. 1953. *Science and Human Behavior*. Macmillan.

Skinner, B. F. 1963. Behaviorism at fifty. *Science* 140: 951–958.

Skinner, B. F. 1966a. The phylogeny and ontogeny of behavior. *Science* 153: 1205–1213.

Skinner, B. F. 1966b. An operational analysis of problem solving. In *Problem Solving*, ed. B. Kleinmuntz. Wiley.

Skinner, B. F. 1969. *Contingencies of Reinforcement: A Theoretical Analysis*. Appleton-Century-Crofts.

Skinner, B. F. 1972. The generic nature of the concepts of stimulus and response. In *Cumulative Record*, third edition. Appleton-Century-Crofts.

Skinner, B. F. 1976. *About Behaviorism*. Vintage.

Skinner, B. F. 1981. Selection by consequences. *Science* 213: 501–504.

Skinner, B. F. 1983. Can the EAB rescue psychology? *The Behavior Analyst* 6: 9–17.

Skinner, B. F. 1987. *Upon Further Reflection*. Prentice-Hall.

Skinner, B. F. 1988. Methods of behavioral science: In *The Selection of Behavior: The Operant Behaviorism of B. F. Skinner*, ed. A. Catania and S. Harnad. Cambridge University Press.

Smith, P. C., and Kendall, L. M. 1963. Retranslation of expectations. An approach to the construction of unambiguous anchors for rating scales. *Journal of Applied Psychology* 47: 149–155.

Spetch, M. L., and Edwards, C. A. 1986. Spatial memory in pigeons (*Columba livia*) in an open-field feeding environment. *Journal of Comparative Psychology* 100: 266–278.

Spetch, M. L., and Wilkie, D. M. 1983. Subjective shortening: A model of pigeons' memory for event durations. *Journal of Experimental Psychology: Animal Behavior Processes* 9: 14–30.

Spychalski, A. C., Quinones, M. A., Gaugler, B. B., and Pohley, K. 1997. A survey of assessment center practices in the United States. *Personnel Psychology* 50: 71–90.

Staddon, J. E. R. 1963. The effect of knowledge of 'knowledge of results' on timing behavior in the pigeon. Doctoral dissertation, Harvard University.

Staddon, J. E. R. 1964. Reinforcement as input: Cyclic variable-interval schedule. *Science* 45: 410–412.

Staddon, J. E. R. 1965. Some properties of spaced responding in pigeons. *Journal of the Experimental Analysis of Behavior* 8: 19–27.

Staddon, J. E. R. 1968. Spaced responding and choice: A preliminary analysis. *Journal of the Experimental Analysis of Behavior* 11: 669–682.

Staddon, J. E. R. 1969a. The effect of informative feedback on temporal tracking in the pigeon. *Journal of the Experimental Analysis of Behavior* 12: 27–38.

Staddon, J. E. R. 1969b. Inhibition and the operant. *Journal of the Experimental Analysis of Behavior* 12: 481–487.

Staddon, J. E. R. 1974. Temporal control, attention and memory. *Psychological Review* 81: 375–391.

Staddon, J. E. R. 1977a. Schedule-induced behavior. In *Handbook of Operant Behavior,* ed. W. Honig and J. Staddon. Prentice-Hall.

Staddon, J. E. R. 1977b. Behavioral competition in conditioning situations: Notes toward a theory of generalization and inhibition. In *Operant-Pavlovian Interactions,* ed. H. Davis and H. Hurwitz. Erlbaum.

Staddon, J. E. R. 1979a. Conservation and consequences—theories of behavior under constraint: An overview. *Journal of Experimental Psychology: General* 108: 1–3.

Staddon, J. E. R. 1979b. Operant behavior as adaptation to constraint. *Journal of Experimental Psychology: General* 108: 48–67.

Staddon, J. E. R., ed. 1980a. *Limits to Action: The Allocation of Individual Behavior.* Academic Press.

Staddon, J. E. R. 1980b. Optimality analyses of operant behavior and their relation to optimal foraging. In *Limits to Action: The Allocation of Individual Behavior,* ed. J. Staddon. Academic Press.

Staddon, J. E. R. 1983. *Adaptive Behavior and Learning.* Cambridge University Press. Second edition (2003) available at http://psychweb.psych.duke.edu.

Staddon, J. E. R. 1984. Time and memory. *Annals of the New York Academy of Sciences* 423: 322–334.

Staddon, J. E. R. 1991. Scientific autobiography. Unpublished manuscript.

Staddon, J. E. R. 1992. Rationality, melioration, and law-of-effect models for choice. *Psychological Science* 3: 136–141.

Staddon, J. 1993a. *Behaviorism: Mind, Mechanism and Society*. Duckworth.

Staddon, J. E. R. 1993b. On rate-sensitive habituation. *Adaptive Behavior* 1: 421–436.

Staddon, J. E. R. 1997. Why behaviorism needs internal states. In *Investigations in Behavioral Epistemology*, ed. L. Hayes and P. Ghezzi. Context.

Staddon, J. E. R. 1999. Theoretical behaviorism. In *Handbook of Behaviorism*, ed. W. O'Donohue and R. Kitchener. Academic Press.

Staddon, J. E. R. 2001a. *Adaptive Dynamics: The Theoretical Analysis of Behavior*. MIT Press.

Staddon, J. 2001b. *The New Behaviorism: Mind, Mechanism and Society*. Psychology Press.

Staddon, J. E. R., and Bueno, J. L. O. 1991. On models, behaviorism, and the neural basis of learning. *Psychological Science* 2: 3–11.

Staddon, J. E. R., and Cerutti, d. T. 2003. Operant behavior. Annual review of Psychology 54: 115–144.

Staddon, J. E. R., Chelaru, I. M., and Higa, J. J. 2002a. A tuned-trace theory of interval-timing dynamics. *Journal of the Experimental Analysis of Behavior* 77: 105–124.

Staddon, J. E. R., Chelaru, I. M., and Higa, J. J. 2002b. Habituation, memory and the brain: The dynamics of interval timing. *Behavioural Processes* 57: 71–88.

Staddon, J. E. R., and Ettinger, R. H. 1989. *Learning: An Introduction to the Principles of Adaptive Behavior*. Harcourt Brace Jovanovich.

Staddon, J. E. R., and Higa, J. J. 1991. Temporal learning. In *The Psychology of Learning and Motivation*, volume 27, ed. G. Bower. Academic Press.

Staddon, J. E. R., and Higa, J. J. 1996. Multiple time scales in simple habituation. *Psychological Review* 103: 720–733.

Staddon, J. E. R., and Higa, J. J. 1999. Time and memory: Towards a pacemaker-free theory of interval timing. *Journal of the Experimental Analysis of Behavior* 71: 215–251.

Staddon, J. E. R., Higa, J. J., and Chelaru, I. M. 1999. Time, trace, memory. *Journal of the Experimental Analysis of Behavior* 71: 293–301.

Staddon, J. E. R., Hinson, J. M., and Kram, R. 1981. Optimal choice. *Journal of the Experimental Analysis of Behavior* 35: 397–412.

Staddon, J. E. R., and Horner, J. M. 1989. Stochastic choice models: A comparison between Bush-Mosteller and a source-independent reward-following model. *Journal of the Experimental Analysis of Behavior* 52: 57–64.

Staddon, J. E. R., and Innis, N. K. 1969. Reinforcement omission on fixed-interval schedules. *Journal of the Experimental Analysis of Behavior* 12: 689–700.

Staddon, J. E. R., and Simmelhag, V. 1971. The "superstition" experiment: A reexamination of its implications for the principles of adaptive behavior. *Psychological Review* 78: 3–43.

Staddon, J. E. R., Wynne, C. D. L., and Higa, J. J. 1991. The role of timing in reinforcement schedule performance. *Learning and Motivation* 22: 200–225.

Staddon, J. E. R., and Zhang, Y. 1991. On the assignment-of-credit problem in operant learning. In *Neural Networks of Conditioning and Action*, ed. M. Commons, S. Grossberg, and J. Staddon. Erlbaum.

Starr, B., and Staddon, J. E. R. 1974. Temporal control on fixed-interval schedules: Signal properties of reinforcement and blackout. *Journal of the Experimental Analysis of Behavior* 22: 535–545.

Steers, R., and Porter, L., eds. 1991. *Motivation and Work Behavior*. McGraw-Hill.

Stephens, D. W., and Krebs, J. R. 1986. *Foraging Theory*. Princeton University Press.

Straub, R. O., and Terrace, H. S. 1981. Generalization of serial learning in the pigeon. *Animal Learning and Behavior* 9: 454–468.

Stubbs, D. A., Dreyfus, L. R., Fetterman, J. G., Boynton, D. M., Locklin, N., and Smith, L. D. 1994. Duration comparison: Relative stimulus differences, stimulus age and stimulus predictiveness. *Journal of the Experimental Analysis of Behavior* 62: 15–32.

Stubbs, D. A., Fetterman, J. G., and Dreyfus, L. R. 1987. Concurrent reinforcement of response sequences. In *Quantitative Analyses of Behavior*, volume 5: *The Effect of Delay and of Intervening Events On Reinforcement Value*, ed. M. Commons, J. Mazur, J. Nevin, and H. Rachlin. Erlbaum.

Sutton, R. S., and Barto, A. G. 1981. Toward a modern theory of adaptive networks: expectation and prediction. *Psychological Review* 88: 135–170.

Suzuki, S., Augerinos, G., and Black, A. 1980. Stimulus control of spatial behavior on the eight-arm maze in rats. *Learning and Motivation* 11: 1–18.

Swartz, K. B., Chen, S., and Terrace, H. S. 1991. Serial learning by rhesus monkeys. I: Acquisition and retention of multiple four-item lists. *Journal of Experimental Psychology: Animal Behavior Processes* 17: 396–410.

Taylor, F. W. 1911. *The Principles of Scientific Management.* Harper and Row.

Taylor, R., and Davison, M. 1983. Sensitivity to reinforcement in concurrent arithmetic and exponential schedules. *Journal of the Experimental Analysis of Behavior* 39: 191–198.

Terman, M., Gibbon, J., Fairhurst, S., and Waring, A. 1984. Daily meal anticipation: Interaction of circadian and interval timing. In *Annals of the New York Academy of Sciences,* volume 423: *Timing and Time Perception,* ed. J. Gibbon and L. Allan.

Terrace, H. S. 1984. Simultaneous chaining: The problem it poses for traditional chaining theory. In *Quantitative Analyses of Behavior: Discrimination Processes,* ed. M. Commons, R. Herrnstein, and A. Wagner. Ballinger.

Thompson, D. 1973. Repeated acquisition as a behavioral base line for studying drug effects. *Journal of Pharmacology and Experimental Therapeutics* 185: 506–514.

Thompson, T., and Zeiler, M., eds. 1986. *Analysis and Integration of Behavioral Units.* Erlbaum.

Thornton, G. C., and Byham, W. C. 1982. *Assessment Centers and Managerial Performance.* Academic Press.

Tinbergen, N. 1963. On aims and methods of ethology. *Zeitschrift für Tierpsychologie* 20: 410–433.

Todorov, J. C., Souza, D. G., and Bori, C. M. 1993. Momentary maximizing in concurrent schedules with a minimum interchangeover interval. *Journal of the Experimental Analysis of Behavior* 60: 415–435.

Tolman, E. C. 1932. *Purposive Behavior in Animals and Men.* Appleton-Century-Crofts.

Tolman, E. C. 1948. Cognitive maps in rats and men. *Psychological Review* 55: 189–208.

Tolman, E. C. 1966. *Behavior and Psychological Man: Essays in Motivation and Learning.* University of California Press.

Treisman, M. 1963. Temporal discrimination and the indifference interval: Implications for a model of the "internal clock." *Psychological Monographs* 77: 1–31.

Trevett, A. J., Davison, M. C., and Williams, R. J. 1972. Performance in concurrent interval schedules. *Journal of the Experimental Analysis of Behavior* 17: 369–374.

Tufillaro, N. B., Abbott, T., and Reilly, J. 1992. *An Experimental Approach to Nonlinear Dynamics and Chaos.* Addison-Wesley.

Van Fraassen, B. 1989. *Laws and Symmetry.* Oxford University Press.

Vaughan, W. 1981. Melioration, matching, and maximization. *Journal of the Experimental Analysis of Behavior* 36: 141–149.

Vogel, R., and Annau, Z. 1973. An operant discrimination task allowing variability of reinforced response patterning. *Journal of the Experimental Analysis of Behavior* 20: 1–6.

Vroom, V. H. 1964. *Work and Motivation*. Wiley.

Waring, G. H. 2002. *Horse Behavior*, second edition. Noyes.

Waser, M. S., and Marler, P. 1977. Song learning in canaries. *Journal of Comparative and Physiological Psychology* 91: 1–7.

Watson, J. B. 1913. Psychology as the behaviorist views it. *Psychological Review* 20: 158–177.

Watson, J. B. 1919. *Psychology from the Standpoint of a Behaviorist*. Lippincott.

Watson, J. B. 1930. *Behaviorism*, third edition. Norton.

Wearden, J. H., and Burgess, I. S. 1982. Matching since Baum (1979). *Journal of the Experimental Analysis of Behavior* 38: 339–348.

Weisbord, M. R. 1992. *Discovering Common Ground*. Berrett-Koehler.

West, M. J., and King, A. P. 1996. Eco-gen-actics: A systems approach to the ontogeny of avian communication. In *Ecology and Evolution of Acoustic Communication in Birds*, ed. D. Kroodsma and E. Miller. Cornell University Press.

White, G. K. 1985. Characteristics of forgetting functions in delayed matching to sample. *Journal of the Experimental Analysis of Behavior* 44: 15–34.

White, M. J. 1985. On the status of cognitive psychology. *American Psychologist* 40: 117–119.

Whyte, W. F. 1972. Skinnerian theory in organizations. *Psychology Today*, April: 67–68, 96, 98, 100.

Wickens, T. D. 1998. On the form of the retention function: Comment on Rubin and Wenzel (1996): A quantitative description of retention. *Psychological Review* 105: 379–386.

Wiener, E. L., Kanki, B. G., and Helmreich, R. L., eds. 1993. *Cockpit Resource Management*. Academic Press.

Wilkinson, L. 1988. *SYSTAT: The System For Statistics*. SYSTAT.

Williams, B. A. 1988. Reinforcement, choice, and response strength. In *Stevens' Handbook of Experimental Psychology*, volume 2, second edition, ed. R. Atkinson, R. Herrnstein, G. Lindzey, and R. Luce. Wiley.

Williams, B. A. 1994. Reinforcement and choice. In *Animal Learning and Cognition. Handbook of Perception and Cognition Series*, second edition, ed. N. Mackintosh. Academic Press.

Williams, B. A. 1999. Value transmission in discrimination learning involving stimulus chains. *Journal of the Experimental Analysis of Behavior* 72: 177–185.

Williams, B. A., Ploog, B. O., and Bell, M. C. 1995. Stimulus devaluation and extinction of chain schedule performance. *Animal Learning and Behavior* 23: 104–114.

Wilson, M. P., and Keller, F. S. 1953. On the selective reinforcement of spaced responses. *Journal of Comparative Psychology* 46: 190–193.

Wixted, J. T. 1990. Analyzing the empirical course of forgetting. *Journal of Experimental Psychology: Learning, Memory, and Cognition* 16: 927–935.

Wixted, J. T., and Ebbesen, E. B. 1991. On the form of forgetting. Psychological Science 2: 409–415.

Wright, A. A., and Watkins, M. J. 1987. Animal learning and memory and their relation to human learning and memory. *Learning and Motivation* 18: 131–146.

Wynne, C. D. L., and Staddon, J. E. R. 1988. Typical delay determines waiting time on periodic-food schedules: Static and dynamic tests. Journal of the Experimental Analysis of Behavior 50: 197–210.

Wynne, C. D. L., and Staddon, J. E. R. 1992. Waiting in pigeons: The effects of daily intercalation on temporal discrimination. *Journal of the Experimental Analysis of Behavior* 58: 47–66.

Wynne, C. D. L., and Staddon, J. E. R. 1998. *Models For Action: Mechanisms For Adaptive Behavior.* Erlbaum.

Yoerg, S. I., and Kamil, A. C. 1982. Response strategies in the radial arm maze: Running around in circles. *Animal Learning and Behavior* 10: 530–534.

Zeiler, M. D. 1986. Behavioral units: A historical introduction. In *Analysis and Integration of Behavioral Units,* ed. T. Thompson and M. Zeiler. Erlbaum.

Zeiler, M. D. 1999. Time without clocks. *Journal of the Experimental Analysis of Behavior* 71: 288–291.

Zeiler, M. D., and Powell, D. G. 1994. Temporal control in fixed-interval schedules. *Journal of the Experimental Analysis of Behavior* 61: 1–9.

Zoladek, L., and Roberts, W. A. 1979. The sensory basis of spatial memory in the rat. *Animal Learning and Behavior* 6: 77–81.

Contributors

Giulio Bolacchi
Associazione per l'Istituzione della Libera Università Nuorese

Daniel T. Cerutti
Department of Psychological and Brain Sciences
Duke University

Mircea Ioan Chelaru
London Health Sciences Center.
University of Western Ontario

J. Mark Cleaveland
Department of Psychology
Vassar College

Robert H. I. Dale
Department of Psychology
Butler University

Rebecca A. Dixon
Department of Psychology
Eastern Oregon University

Valentin Dragoi
Department of Neurobiology and Anatomy
University of Texas-Houston Medical School

Stephen Gray
Department of Psychology
Wofford College

Jennifer J. Higa
Department of Psychology
Texas Christian University

John M. Horner
Department of Psychology
The Colorado College

Nancy K. Innis
Department of Psychology
University of Western Ontario

Mandar S. Jog
London Health Sciences Center.
University of Western Ontario

Richard Keen
Department of Psychology
Brown University

John E. Kello
Department of Psychology
Davidson College

Eric Macaux
Department of Psychology
Indiana University

Armando Machado
Departamento de Psicologia
Universidade do Minho—Campus de Gualtar

John C. Malone, Jr.
Department of Psychology
University of Tennessee

Kazuchika Manabe
Graduate School of Social and Cultural Studies
Nihon University

Susan R. Perry
Department of Psychology
University of Tennessee

Alliston K. Reid
Department of Psychology
Wofford College

Epilogue: Nancy Karen Innis, 1941–2004

This volume would not have come to pass without Nancy Innis. She organized a conference in my honor in the spring of 2003 at Duke. Students and postdocs, presumably with time on their hands, attended, some from as far away as Japan. Duke contributed generously to a truly moving occasion. Many speeches were made, some quite laudatory, and some accurate. At the high point of this affair, Nancy presented me with a fine wooden box. About the right size for 100 Cohibas but, alas (I thought), too heavy for cigars, it contained drafts of the contributed papers that were eventually to make up this book, and a promise from The MIT Press that they would publish it. I cannot imagine a more wonderful gift. (A bittersweet memory is of my distinguished colleague Irving Diamond, now deceased, when long gone in Alzheimer's, fingering each day a similar volume presented to him by his students. These things matter to old academics!)

Tragically, Nancy was not to see this project to fruition. In the summer of 2004 she attended an international conference in China that included a trip to Tibet, a place she had always wanted to visit (she was a great traveler). She died there suddenly and unexpectedly of a brain hemorrhage while visiting the 2,000-year-old temple of Yumbulakhang near Tse Dang.

The loss of Nancy put a serious crimp in this project. But others shouldered the burden (I must thank particularly John Horner, John Malone, Clive Wynne, and Richard Dale), and with Tom Stone's help it now finally sees the light of day.

Nancy Innis was my first student. She began as an undergraduate and a master's student in 1965, when we were both at the University of Toronto. We had already published four papers together when she finished her Ph.D. at Duke in 1970. Nancy went on to work briefly at the Ontario Addiction Research Foundation, followed by a postdoctoral fellowship and assistant professorship at Dalhousie University, from which she joined the faculty of the University of Western Ontario, where she moved through the ranks to full professor.

Nancy was always notable for her idealism and her devotion to experimental psychology. From her first experimental paper, which offered a simple timing account for "frustrative nonreward," she went on to do beautiful work on timing, including a Ph.D. dissertation at Duke on pigeons' unsuspected ability to track a changing sequence of intervals.

In the mid 1980s, Nancy's interest in the history of psychology led her to spend more of her time on historical topics, such as the evolution of comparative psychology, animal psychology in America, and early studies in behavior genetics. Her paper on the Berkeley animal psychologist Edward Chace Tolman was stimulated by his pivotal role in the 1950s California loyalty oath controversy. Soon, Tolman became her main historical interest.

Given Nancy's behaviorist background, her interest in Tolman and in a "purposive" behaviorism hardly distinguishable from what was later termed "cognitive" psychology is something of a puzzle. She was perhaps attracted as much by Tolman's open and decent personality and his political life as by his purely scientific work.

Nancy loved historical research and traveled far in search of records and people to interview for the book. She left behind voluminous notes and copies of letters and old papers that should be invaluable to future historians. Unfortunately, she was not able to finish the Tolman book before her death. Efforts are being made to see if it can be completed by another.

Nancy Innis was a true scientist, interested in finding the truth; not a careerist, interested in becoming famous. Apparently she died in a rather special place linked to the origin of Buddhism in Tibet. The locals felt that Nancy was "honored" by having her soul depart from that place. We are all honored to have known her.

John Staddon
Durham, North Carolina

Index